# YOGA MADNESS OR MEDITATION?

ZAHIR AKRAM

# Contents

# Acknowledgment

I would like to thank all those who helped me with various parts of this book, be it to check my grammar or to tell me what I didn't want to hear. To my friends, fellow teachers and students, Sara al Rikabi, Maria Longman and Mika Janhunen.

I would also like to thank the wonderful teachers at my studio (past and present) for putting up with me over the years. My issues with yoga teachers as you will read about throughout this book are in no way references to you all. I would like to thank Jessica Stretch for teaching me my first arm balance and Claire Berghorst for not only introducing me to yoga teachers, but also as she was next to me when I did my first ever hot yoga class (alongside Kim). Thank you again for your all help and contributions and my sincere apologies that I do not tell you all enough how much I appreciate you.

There are so many students of mine, I truly wouldn't know where to start. Tomomi, Cecilia, Ryoko, Lyn, Lopez, George, Adeline, Warren, Oliver, Yvon, Rowley, Julie, Tracey, Bethan, 'Heather', Boulet, Becky, Parm and little Jo. There are of course so many others. My apologies for anyone I have missed. They are literally too many to name. Teaching you over the years has been one of my greatest pleasures and I cannot thank you all enough for your continued loyalty to the studio. I have learnt more from conversing with you all than I have done from all the books I have on my book shelf.

Not forgetting The Flynn & Mr. Trimm.

Above all, I want to thank my beautiful wife, Laura. The energy source of my life. I absolutely love you and can't express my love and gratitude to you enough. I always joke and say how lucky you are to be married to me, despite everyone constantly correcting me it is in fact, I who is the lucky one. I disagree with them all the time, but in my heart, I could not agree more.

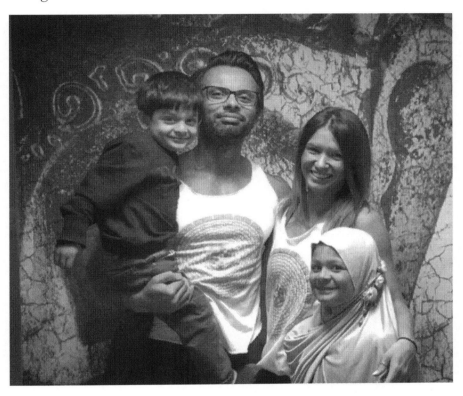

And how can I forget my niece and nephew? 'Kalegi ka Tukra' and 'Tingu'. I would not have known of my capacity to love so deeply if it wasn't for them.

"O Sathi re – there bina be kya jeena"

I want to thank my wife Laura again for the single defining moment in my ongoing examination of yoga and life itself. Whilst discussing with her the complicated and often contradictory subject of yoga, Laura eloquently quoted her favourite philosopher, Friedrich Nietzsche, "There are no facts, only interpretations."[1] This was my moment of enlightenment. Not in the sense that I was now a Buddha. Far from it. Although, since I married, I am starting to look like one.

This single moment changed the course of my investigation and study. I encourage you to remember that quote as you read this book and try to immerse your brain in understanding the subject of yoga so you can decide for yourself whether the yoga you do, will lead to madness or meditation.

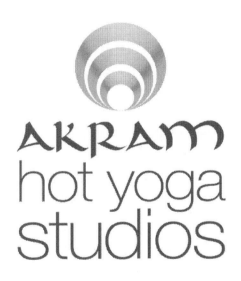

My name is Zahir Akram. I experienced my enlightenment (the goal of a yogi) whilst squatting under an apple tree on the banks of the Basingstoke Canal. In Surrey. Since this third eye opening experience, I have offered to anyone who wishes to listen, my enlightened punditry on life. And, especially on the subject of yoga.

Okay, I'm not being serious. That is a joke. Let's start again. My name is Zahir and I am not a yogi. This may sound a little odd as this is a book on the subject of yoga. But, bear with me. By the end of the book you will hopefully understand why I choose not to refer to myself as a yogi. I am just an ordinary person with an extraordinary love for yoga. I am a yoga teacher, but I prefer to refer to myself as a yoga 'tour guide'. I am on the same journey as you, but with a little more information at my disposal which will allow me to point you in a particular direction so you can explore the world of yoga for yourself. It's easy for us mere mortals to start thinking we are high and mighty yoga teachers. We are not. Sometime after referring to myself as a tour guide, I read a quote from George Bernard Shaw: "I'm not a teacher; only a fellow traveler of whom you asked the way"[2]. I realise how much better that sounds than my rubbish tour guide analogy. But I hope you get the picture.

I'm not a typical yogi. Far from it. I don't pray to the Hindu God, Krishna. I don't call myself a Hindu, wear mala beads and bust out an impromptu chant when there is a new moon. I don't wear OM t-shirts and I don't recite the Gita (a religious text) when I teach. I don't meditate and I certainly don't think my peacock is better than yours. But I reckon it is. I am blissfully in love with my wife. We are not vegans. We don't hug trees, and we don't claim to cleanse chakras. We do asana (yoga poses), we teach asana, we breathe asana, and we love Korean zombie movies. I'd like to think we are just a normal couple.

What is my intention with this book? It is to give the average yoga student not necessarily a complete understanding of yoga (which would be near impossible), but to provide them with a cultural interpretation of yoga. Or rather, my cultural interpretation of yoga. There is every chance, however, that you may finish this book feeling more perplexed than you were before. But this is what will open the door for further enquiry. I want you to understand the fundamentals (which themselves are open to interpretation) so you can strive to discover for yourself what yoga actually is, as opposed to what it can look like. This understanding that I share with you is based on my own odyssey which, at times, contradicts academia and much of what you may have read in the past. At times, it may even contradict itself.

Welcome to the wonderfully baffling world of yoga. This is not to say that I know best, that's far from true. I just want to give you an alternative view that does not involve the same old lifeless explanations and commentaries. I have intentionally tried to omit some academic dates as well as academic references as much as I can because this will not be another mundane, humdrum look at yoga. Not to say that academic books on yoga are boring or stuffy for everyone, they just are to me. I find most yoga books lifeless or lacking in soul, so I wanted to offer you something different. An alternative history of yoga inspired by the flair of Hindu mythology and my own reasoning, as well as a bias based on my own upbringing.

When a new student in my studio asked me questions about yoga, I found myself at a loss to recommend anything for her to read to help her with her inquiry. Most of the books I could think of would have left her confused and bewildered. I went over, in my head, the hundreds of yoga books that I own and have read over the years and was left just scratching my head. I recommended *Light on Life*, by the late, great B.K.S Iyengar, but that was not enough to cross the T's and dot the I's. When I myself was learning about this very convoluted subject, I felt like the authors of the books I was reading were always talking to their fellow authors or fellow academics. To me, an academic book on yoga is one academic's love song to another. And the books that did not fall into the academic category were for the more religious type of yogi. Very few books speak to the average Western yoga student who comes to yoga to "stretch" and would simply like to know a little more. This book is written for people like you and me who just want a little illumination and not academic exposure. So, this book will not be an academic book on yoga. I remember reading many years ago of how academia is a study for what is measurable, rather than what is meaningful. Don't overly observe life, you soon miss the whole point of living. Academic books on yoga explain yoga from a place of scholarship and "fact". This book will attempt to explain yoga from a place that exists somewhere between culture and my own logic and perspective.

I will try to explain the meaning of yoga as best I can, and then I will share some of my so-called wisdom on the subject of meditation, asana (poses), as well as the myths underlying yoga. These sections are likely to offend delicate yogis and yoga teachers who teach 'yogic meditation' and anyone who teaches that the knee should never travel over the toe. Anytime someone speaks their truth somebody is going to be offended. But my intention is not to offend anyone, but to explain as best I can my viewpoints and theories, this may inadvertently touch a few nerves. Or maybe not. Some will agree. Some will argue. Most, I hope, will just finish this book with a better understanding of yoga than when they started.

At an early stage of my own enquiry on yoga I would ask wise yoga teachers, "What exactly is yoga?" I would get answers like "Yoga is surrender", "Yoga is acceptance", "Yoga is life", blah blah blah. These answers were far too vague and airy fairy for me. I was looking for an actual definition. I realise now, after a long time, that often it's easier to give someone your viewpoint on yoga that it is to answer the actual question. To answer fully is not a straightforward process.

When students ask me that same question, I try not to give them a direct answer. I will often tell those students just to do yoga. Do the poses with all your heart. Once you have delved deep into the poses, those poses you thought were once impossible, you come back to me and then you tell me what yoga is. The answer is there inside of us, it just takes some examination and effort on our part to discover it. And what you discover is that yoga can be either madness or meditation. It all depends on the state of mind.

This book is for all the students over the years who have said to me that they would like to learn about or do yoga without feeling they have to be a vegan, or to chant, or to join a yoga community. No change in who you are is required before you do yoga or when you immerse yourself in trying to understand yoga. You are required just to be yourself, as you are. Your beauty is your individuality and you cannot compromise this for the sake of anyone or anything. Yoga only asks that you be daring enough to try and that you create a discipline. Nothing more is required. It's not yoga that expects anything from you, it's the yoga community. Or more specifically, it's what you think the yoga community expects from you. I want you, the casual yoga student, to understand that nothing is expected of you. You do not have to change. You don't need to chant to be accepted. You don't have to sit up straight like a perfect yogi and adopt certain mudras or hand gestures. You are not expected to be a yogi or to be yogic. You are not expected to have read the Bhagavad Gita. You are perfect as you are. All that is required is willingness to embrace this perfection.

Our inability to recognise our own unique and beautiful individuality is deep rooted from our childhood. How many times have parents said, or continue to say, "What is wrong with you?" How many school teachers have said that we need to change our behaviour? Or, that we should behave more like this kid or that kid? How many religious teachers make us feel that we are doomed for hell unless we change? It is part of our psychology that we think that there is something wrong with us and that whenever we step into something new, that something needs to change.

But, in yoga and especially in my studio, no change is needed. You will be further and further away from happiness if you feel you have to fit in with the yoga ideal. In the modern world, you are not allowed to be happy or content. If you are happy and content, you are considered arrogant by those who only wish they could love themselves. But yoga says you are perfect. You can be happy, and you should love yourself. What is there not to love? We believe that we need to add something to our looks or personality to be perfect, but what is required is just to remove the whispers that reside in the mind that tell us that we are not allowed to love ourselves. The mind is a theatre as you will learn throughout this book.

I once read a quote that has remained with me for what feels like my entire adult life. "Your whole idea of who you think you should be is taken from people who have no idea who they really are themselves." It's your individuality that makes you so beautiful. Embrace that and don't try to fit in. You never will. You were never supposed to. You were always designed to be free.

So this book is for anyone who is just interested in the enquiry that is yoga. Nothing is expected of you. There are no entry requirements. There are no dietary requirements. You don't have to learn Sanskrit. You don't have to go to India. It's okay if sleeping is your favourite yoga pose. You don't have to start juicing. There are no yoga police and there is no hell for bad yogis. Or, maybe there is. If there is a hell for bad yogis, then there are so many modern yoga gurus already residing in the Saraswati wing of hell[3], being adjusted inappropriately by Shaitan, that there is no room for us anyway.

You do, however, need to embrace your authentic nature and just be yourself. Yoga is for anyone and for everyone. Yoga is for the average Joe. If you have pulled a muscle reaching for a chocolate biscuit, then yoga is for you. If you only want to learn to stretch so you can fix your man bun, then yoga is for you. If you drink full fat milk, love a T-bone steak, hate avocados, think Lululemon is a girl band, then yoga is for you. If like the Henry vacuum cleaner you have lots of attachments, then yoga is, guess what, for you. Yoga is for everyone. All you have to do is to be willing to try.

On a final note, before I introduce you to the source of yoga, I would like to ask your forgiveness for any errors in this book, be they scientific or cultural. I am not a scientist or an academic. The inspiring Hellen Keller in The Story of My Life said, "Trying to write is very much like trying to put a Chinese puzzle together. We have a pattern in mind which we wish to work out in words; but the words will not fit the spaces, or, if they do, they rarely match the design." [4]

What follows is just the interpretation of an uneducated seeker. Many times while writing this book, I wondered if I was the right person to be sharing my thoughts with you. I am not a mystical yogi or an enlightened intellectual. Should I let this dishearten or intimidate me? Should I have stopped writing and just gone back to reading? How many people have a voice that they would like someone to hear? If we all stay silent, we remain prisoners our whole lives. Again, Helen Keller once said; "One can never consent to creep when one feels an impulse to soar." [5] If you have something to say, you should have the confidence to stand up and be heard. Even if this invites criticism. I want to encourage you to drop fear. We must not be afraid of our fears. They are not there to scare us. They exist to let you know that what you are doing has value. It is worth something. I do not think I am anyone special. I am just someone trying to make sense of how to fit my western body and mind, into this eastern tradition. Will it even fit? Does it have to? I hope that by the end of this book, I can at least help some of you understand that trying to fit your body and mind into this eastern tradition is what will lead you to madness.

Accepting that you are a western student with a western body (and mind) and making peace with who you are, and with what you are, is more likely to lead you to that place we all seek, a place of happiness. This is what I call meditation. It is not a practice but a destination or a way of being.

What follows is a not a book. It is a dialogue between me, as the guru (the "unenlightened one") and my alter-ego who is also my faithful, loyal and slightly confused disciple. The disciple asks and the guru waxes lyrical in response. Through some of the "wisdom" unearthed via the dialogues, you can decide if yoga will lead you to a place of madness or meditation. When I use the word "meditation", I am not referring to a practice whereby you sit with your eyes closed and try to de-stress. I am referring to "meditation" as a destination whereby one discovers a feeling of bliss and harmony.

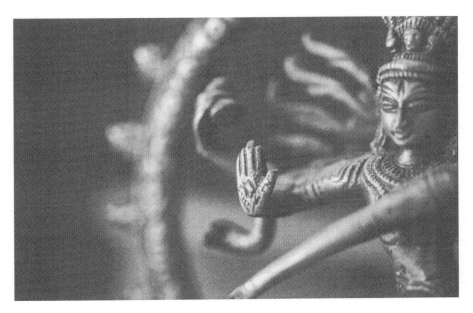

*Disciple - My master, what on earth is yoga?*

This is a complex question that has an extremely complicated answer. Yoga is India's greatest gift or contribution to mankind. That is, apart from Amitabh Bachchan (the actor). But what exactly is yoga?

In some ways it is easier to tell you what yoga is not. Yoga is not a religion. Yoga is not stretching. But yoga can form part of someone's religion and yoga can and does involve stretching. Yoga is not being on your head in headstand. But you have to overcome your fear of headstand to know yoga. Yoga exists in a paradox.

To fully understand yoga, or *joga* as my mum pronounces it (apparently a north Indian subcontinent pronunciation) and to answer the main question, I am required to introduce you to two central characters. The first of these men is the very first yogi, Adiyogi, or Shiva as he is more commonly known today. The second is a man called Patanjali. Although they 'existed' on this earth thousands of years apart, understanding a little about these two is central to the answer to the big question of what is yoga?

In a very humorous video you will find online, an interviewer travels around India asking the common folk "Who is the source of yoga?" The answers are comical. My favourite answer is the man who says,

"Shilpa Shetty?" Some of the other answers range from the Mongols to Mohdi (the prime minister). But it was none of them. Shilpa Shetty was a fun actress to watch when I was younger but no, she isn't the source of yoga. The credit for this, culturally speaking, goes to Shiva, or the Adiyogi. The following story and the various other tales within this book are all retellings of various stories I have heard and read over many years of casual reading and research. I have taken artistic liberties where I feel that this is appropriate because otherwise the stories lose much of their charm and grace. Unless accompanied by a footnote all dialogues are imagined by me. My intention with this story is to present Shiva to you in a way that is relatable, and in a way we can all understand. For this reason, I have chosen here to present him not as the Hindu God, but rather as the Adiyogi, the first yogi, whose system of realising the true self remains available and accessible to all, regardless of gender, belief and religion.

It happened.

*Disciple - Really?*

It's true. I saw it on Zee TV many full moons ago.

It was a very long time ago, thousands of years ago, before anyone had heard of chakras or healing crystals. A unique looking man was seen wandering around the Himalayas. No one knew his name. No one knew who he was. No one knew where he had come from. He looked beautifully wild. A mysterious stranger. He was enchanting, and he was the most alluring tortured looking soul anyone had ever seen. As time passed, his legend grew as well as his stature. He was seen very rarely but when he was, he was in cremation grounds dancing wildly, or he would be sitting completely still, his legs crossed, and his eyes closed. He would sit motionless for many months at a time. He was full of illusion, magic, madness and paradox.

At this time, only a few million people lived on earth, so the region of the Indian subcontinent was not as populated as it is now. All the people of that part of the world soon began to speak of this wandering loner. Some believed he was a myth created by the elders to frighten children. Others believed he was possessed by spirits. Those abandoned by society were hypnotised. Those who ruled were frightened. He was described as seven feet tall with long dreadlocks. His body was smeared in ash and sometimes even in blood. On occasions, he appeared to have no clothes on. At other times, he had the skin of a dead animal draped over his shoulders. He carried a trident in one hand and a skull in the other, and wherever he wandered he was followed by the few who believed he was of divine origin. "The gods have power to assume such beauty" they said. When he danced wildly, he seemed to be completely inebriated. His expressions were unique; his dance had energy and vitality. He was unlike anything that man had seen before. He was referred by many simply as 'the yogi'. Yogi at this time meant 'ascetic'. One who is a hermit and/or a recluse.

Another person who was enchanted by him was the beautiful Princess Parvati. She was the daughter of Himavat, the King of the Himalayas. It seemed that nature had lavished all the beauty of the heavens on Parvati. Virtue and modesty enlightened her charms and her lustre was brighter than the stars of the heavens. It was rumoured that, in her presence, even the heavenly damsels would blush with shame. When the glorious princess heard descriptions of this man wandering around the cremation grounds, she became spellbound. The descriptions she was given, the whispers she had heard, all matched that of the man she had been seeing in her dreams since childhood. When Parvati travelled to find him, she could feel her body, and even her soul, drawing itself towards him. She didn't need a map or directions; she just followed her heart. Her heart drew itself towards him as if they had been separated since the dawn of time. Although they had never met, Parvati longed to be with him. When, after many months of travelling, Parvati found him, he was sitting silently and motionless. Parvati just sat and watched him. She sat for many months just watching him as if she were under a spell, her mind, body and soul completely fixated on him.

After many months with his eyes closed, one day he finally opened his eyes. This was only for a split second, but it was enough for him to notice the angelic Parvati. They both sat hypnotised and just stared into each other's longing eyes. Shiva did not want to close his eyes as the reality in-front of him was more perfect than anything he had experienced before.

Finally, the ascetic spoke, "O thou who art beautiful beyond argument, who illuminates the sky with her lustre, thy scattered hair, thy fragrant breath, There are many beauties in this world, By the sight of you oh divine one, my internal darkness is dispelled." Parvati felt as if she had waited a life time to hear these words. Any fear she had about meeting him left her. They gazed lovingly into each other's eyes as the world seemed to stand still. The yogi could taste her fragrance in his breath and Parvati longed for him with each and every beat of her heart. Their souls had met, and their love was all-consuming. They were hypnotised by love.

Parvati had been with the yogi before, but only in her dreams. Parvati longed for him to fill her loneliness with music and dance. She desired him in the same way a dying person desires life. After some time, Parvati, respectful of the traditions she was born into, slowly walked away. She was uncertain and didn't want to leave but she knew that proper custom should follow if she wished to be with the wandering yogi. Parvati, returning home, instructed her dearest friend to inform the yogi that if he too wished marriage, he would have to ask Parvati's father for her hand. When the yogi was asked if he would speak to Parvati's father, the yogi agreed. Parvati heard the news and was euphoric. Her family, unsure at first of her wishes to marry someone they had only heard whispers of, soon joined in her celebration. Such was Parvati's joy her family couldn't not help but share her jubilance. Rumours have it that even Cupid breathed a sigh of relief.

After marriage, the ascetic would spend much time absorbed in meditation. His eyes remained closed and his mind peaceful. His body was free from illness and disease and his intelligence was far superior to that of anybody else. When he spoke, he spoke in a way that had never been heard. When he sat still, he sat in way that had never been seen. Parvati knew that her husband was experiencing another dimension of life. He was too far removed from the misery of the common man not to be experiencing a higher reality of life. The yogi was immersed in what seemed to be a completely separate reality.

One day the princess Parvati would make a loving enquiry that would form the basis of everything we know of today (in regard to Indian culture). She would ask; "O Shiva, what is your reality? What is your wonder filled universe?"[1]

With the above question, Parvati is more or less asking, "Oh Shiva, what is meditation? What is *Samadhi*? What is yoga? What is *Nirvana*?" - In this instant, Parvati used the words "your reality".

The ascetic, now referred to as Shiva (meaning the auspicious one), would explain to Parvati that man, if willing, can elevate himself and experience true awareness and realisation of life. This is man's true reality. Man must experience this reality to become free and peaceful. In many respects, the reality itself is freedom and peace. This freedom, Shiva would declare, is within the grasp of every human being.

(Note - The only prerequisite Shiva has for us to embark on our journey is to have willingness. He says, "man, if willing can elevate…..." This is the only requirement).

Shiva would briefly explain to his beloved that this highest reality that Parvati is enquiring about cannot be perceived by sound or any of our senses. "Nor can it be seen even in the obstructed half-moon, nor in the piercing of successive chakras, nor does universal energy constitute its essence. Ultimately the highest reality cannot be measured in terms of time, space or direction, nor can it be indicated by any attribute. The highest state a human being can reach cannot be characterised or described in any human language." Parvati would continue her inquiry. Parvati's loving nature wished to save mankind from its constant suffering. She felt that life itself was suffering. This is the great inevitability of life. To live is to find a purpose, and to seek solace is perhaps the meaning of life. She would ask, "By what practice or technique can one reach this higher reality? How may we enter this reality that is beyond space and time? remove my own doubts entirely" (This question of Parvati's reminded me a quote from Nietzsche, "The voice of beauty speaks softly; it creeps only into the most fully awakened souls"[2]).

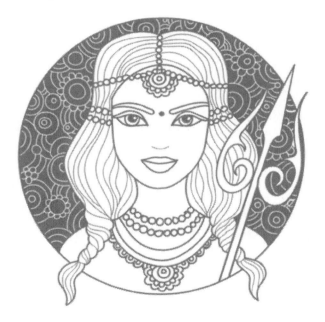

In response, Shiva would go on to explain 112 techniques that man could use to enter into this higher state of consciousness. This higher reality. The reality Shiva himself was immersed in. These are techniques (tantras) or more specifically, concentration techniques or exercises in concentration (dharanas). One is required to fix their focus and attention on something until they become absorbed into that point of concentration. These include several variants of breath awareness, concentration on various centres in the body, imagination, visualization and contemplation through each of the senses.

The 112 techniques or concentration exercises will be presented at the end of this book.

An example of one of these techniques is to visualise the emptiness of space. Upon mastery of this exercise in concentration, one's mind can become absorbed into space itself. The individual practicing this technique no longer feels he or she is concentrating on space but feels that he or she has actually become one with space. There is no longer a distinction. This is total absorption. If this occurs, the aspirant or seeker experiences the true reality of life. They have gone beyond the current state of their consciousness.

Take Gautama Buddha as an example. The Buddha is in a constant meditative state. Buddha is a man who is immersed in our reality on a physical level, but his mind sees life for what it really is. This is *Nirvana* to the followers of Buddha. Once our eyes open, we awaken. This is what it means to be a Buddha. To be awake. Once the veil has been removed, we remain eternally awakened. To some tantric yogis, this is referred to as a state of *Bhairava*. Others will call this *Samadhi*. A more contemporary description was given by the late B.K.S. Iyengar (author of the classic "Light on Yoga'), this reality he says, is "Ultimate Freedom"[3].

Sadhguru from India has said of this conversation between Siva and his wife, "It was on this day that the seed of liberation was planted in the human consciousness. It was on this day that it was declared for the first time in human history that biology is not destiny, that it is possible for a human being to evolve consciously. The finite can turn infinite. The particular can turn universal. Compulsion can turn into consciousness. It is possible for a piece of creation to become one with the source of creation. The human creature can become a divine entity"[4].

Shiva was referred to as the Adiyogi, the first yogi, because this science of realising our true reality was referred to by some as the system of yoga. In essence, yoga means to bring two things together. So, this system of yoga that Shiva revealed to his wife Parvati was a system that would bring you together with your true identity. Or, your true reality. These two seeming opposites join and come together until there is no longer a distinction between the two. You are now in yoga. Here you encounter the reality as it is.

*Disciple – 'Oh Son of Akram', Is this conversation between Shiva and Parvati universally understood as being the birth of yoga?*

The answer is no because nothing in yoga history is that straight forward. The conversation between Shiva and Parvati in the context of a text or scripture is called the *Vijnana Bhairava Tantra*. Tantra means technique, *Bhairava* is the name for Shiva given by the earliest writers and also means consciousness and *vijnana* (pronounced vigyun) means to go beyond or transcend. So, the text itself means techniques that go beyond consciousness.

The conversation took place many thousands of years ago. Anything from 5,000 to 15,000 years ago according to tradition. It depends on who you ask of course. Who knows when the original text itself would have been composed. The text itself was only discovered in early 1900. The first full English translation of the text was provided in a 1957 publication by the American author and poet Paul Reps. The first full commentary was printed in 1979 by Jaideva Singh (which is still the best translation available by far). This provided us with a basic understanding of the conversation which appears to be chanted in a language we have yet to fully understand. So, discovery of the text is fairly new compared to other more 'famous' yoga texts even though tradition says the basis of this text pre-dates everything else available – perhaps even the holy Vedas (more on that later).

It's possible that, before 1957, the understanding of this tantra or conversation was limited to the direct lineage of gurus and students who had been sharing this text as an oral tradition.

Tradition says the source of yoga is a loving enquiry by a woman asking her husband to clarify her doubts many thousands of years ago. There are also many different interpretations within the tradition. The understanding from this particular Tantra is that Shiva has given no philosophy.

So, to answer the question, is this conversation understood between two lovers (or god and goddess to many) to be the birth of yoga? Yes and no. It just depends who you ask. What they have been raised to understand or what academia has told them. From a cultural perspective, I have not met anyone who denies that Shiva developed the system of yoga. Whether they believe this conversation, in the context of the text, the *Vijnana Bhairava Tantra* to be the source of yoga is a constant source of discussion the answer to which we will never really know. It's an ongoing debate which in some cases can end up in full blown arguments. I have known it be a sensitive subject especially for some who say it is the Lord Vishnu (not Shiva) who 'invented' yoga. That is when the conversation tends to heat up.

Essentially, it's a case of saying that my dad can beat up yours. The ironic thing is that in the deepest part of the tradition, Vishnu and Shiva are the same entity. So the argument itself is ludicrous. But this is where things get complicated so we will stop there and perhaps expand on that in a future edition.

Is there any evidence to support the existence of Shiva all those thousands of years ago? The answer would be "no". In the same way, there is no evidence remaining today of the existence of many people we have read about throughout history. Our earliest evidence of The Auspicious One comes from a seal found at the Mohenjo-Daro archaeological site of the Indus Valley Civilisation (present day Pakistan). The seal, discovered around 1930, is believed to be dated from $2000_{BC}$. It shows a naked man sitting in a yogic position on a throne. Some scholars believe this to be the earliest form of Shiva. Others are not convinced. I prefer to let them debate amongst themselves.

There was also a bit of an archaeological revelation around 1960. A heavy chest containing an idol was discovered by Tibetan Monks. The contents of the chest (that was handed to the CIA for seemingly unknown reasons) included a small brass idol that depicted Shiva. The idol was referred to as *Kalpa Vigraha* and is said to be dated around $26540_{BC}$[5]. If this idol indeed represents Shiva, this takes our timeline back even further than the imagined 10,000–15,000 years ago. That is, only if the archaeological world would universally agree this to be a depiction of Shiva. Because they don't agree, we still have no real idea. And even if they did agree that it was Shiva, this does nothing to clarify whether he actually existed or not. All it tells us is that Shiva worship has been going on for longer than we first realised.

Back in time, the person we now call Shiva was referred to as *Bhairav*, and around $1000_{BC}$ he was referred to as *Rudra*. The word Shiva, which means auspicious, was understood to be a quality of *Rudra*. Some say they are not even the same person, and history has amalgamated them all into the one supreme form of Shiva we know today.

Most yogis and most yoga scholars and academics will confirm that yoga is credited as being manifested by Shiva based on the various salutations at the start of the texts they try to translate and understand. I doubt that the Shiva I speak about looks anything like the Shiva you see online, or the Shiva I dressed up as a few years ago at my fancy dress party. Blue skin, serpent around his neck and a six pack. The truth is that we know very little, if anything, factual about him. Everything is based on assumptions, legends, mythology, tradition and interpretation. How should we view these mythologies? Maybe there are truths in there somewhere? I remember reading that every religion and tradition is true in one way or another. It is true when understood metaphorically. But, when metaphors are interpreted as facts, then we get into trouble.

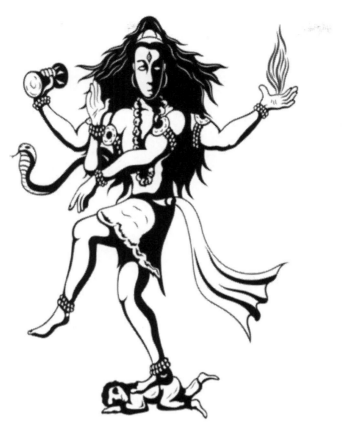

*Shiva as 'Nataraja', Lord of Dance. Here, Shiva is shown with his foot on the 'demon' Apasmara. The demon represents man's ignorance.*

There is a 112-foot statue of the Adiyogi, or Shiva, in Tamil Nadu, India. It was financed and designed by the Isha Foundation. This gives us our closest cultural depiction of what Shiva may have looked like. It is not for me to say if any artistic liberties were taken in portraying Shiva. The fact is that Sadhguru of the Isha Foundation claimed he experienced his enlightenment many years ago. This enlightenment allows him to view the world without the veil that the rest of us are apparently wearing. His realisation of the true reality allows him to see beyond academia and scholarship. So, when Sadhguru unveiled this image of the Adiyogi, and said that this statue represents Shiva, most people would trust that this is the closest we will ever get to knowing what Shiva actually looked like. That is, of course, if you trust Sadhguru. That is something you would have to decide for yourself. Or maybe, once you experience Shiva, you realise there is no way of depicting him in artistic form, So, it becomes easier to create something we already imagined ourselves. That may be the easiest approach. As I said, this won't be an academic understanding of Shiva. There are other people who would do a far better job of that. We are looking at Shiva as he exists in a paradox. Somewhere between culture and fantasy.

Sadhguru on Shiva has said; "In the yogic culture, Shiva is not seen as a God. He was a being who walked this land and lived in the Himalayan region. As the very source of the yogic traditions, his contribution in the making of human consciousness is too phenomenal to be ignored".

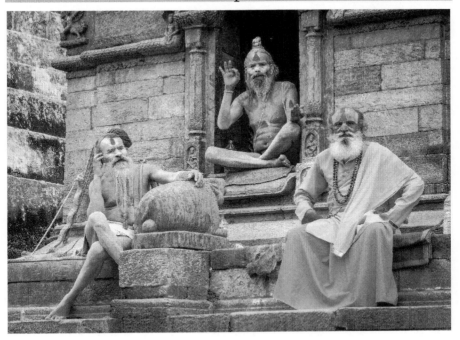

*Disciple – You have said that this text, this book of 112 techniques is called the Vijnana Bhairav Tantra. I know you said Tantra meant technique, but I thought Tantra was its own tradition? I have heard people in the past say that yoga and tantra are both different. What exactly is Tantra?'*

Remember this is book is not an academic study. The subject of Tantra can be very perplexing, and my aim is to make it as accessible as possible. To achieve this, I am intentionally omitting some words and concepts not only in his chapter but throughout this book to give you a less confused understanding of the subject. When I mention Tantra, I am not referring to Tantra as a whole, but I am using the word Tantra in context to this text alone – the discussion between Shiva and Parvati.

Tantra singular means technique. A tantra can mean a single method or technique, or it could imply a collective. So a tantra can also be a book or a collection of techniques. Tantra can also be looked at as a tradition for those who follow this book of teachings. In the context of this book and for the purpose of understanding, when we refer to Tantra, we are referring to Tantra as a tradition. Tantra is referred to the tradition of those who follow Shiva's teaching of the *'Vijnana Bhairav Tantra'*. The followers of this path can also be called 'yogis'.

Those who seek 'union' with the highest reality. They are one and the same.

*Disciple – Ok. Understood.*
*1 - So an individual technique is a tantra.*
*2 - A collection of these techniques (essentially the book) is also tantra.*
*3 - The culture or tradition of those who follow this book is called Tantra and that is how you will refer to Tantra from this point onwards. Got it.*
*      Is there any difference between Tantra and Yoga? If you follow Shiva's method's, you follow the path of tantra. I thought if you followed the path of Shiva, you followed the path of yoga. Which is correct?*

They are both correct. But for the sake of understanding, let's look at them both individually.

The Tantra Path –

Tantra and yoga can be looked at as slightly varying paths but with the same goal. Again, this just depends on the perspective you have come to understand. It can be said that if you fully understand the methods passed down by Shiva and immerse yourselves in them immediately and directly, you are a tantric. Essentially, you are a direct follower of the path of Shiva. This could be devotional in the sense that you believe he is god so nothing more is needed to attain a higher reality but submission to his direct words alone. So, if you fully understand a technique from the text or it has been transmitted or taught to you by a guru and you wholeheartedly dedicate yourself to that method, then the method you follow is Tantra and you are a tantric.

It is not easy to follow Shiva's path directly however as many of the verses in the *Vijnana Bhairava Tantra* are poetic and even cryptic. Earlier commentaries said that the language used was often secret, used on purpose to hide the real meaning from the uninitiated. Also, some of the words used in the text have no direct English translation, and, in some cases, the language used was not even understood by earliest Kashmiri commentators. Some have said that this text is written in the language of love. Love is the basic device to understand this tantra. Western seekers will attempt to understand ancient wisdom with a mind that is too logical. These earliest tantras were never written for the logical mind. When Parvati sits on Shiva's lap and enquires about reality, there is no logic between the two. Just pure love. So this tantra is written in the language of love that most commentators will not understand. The tantra of Shiva and Parvati is not meant for intellectual dissection. Very much like *The Yoga Sutras of Patanjali*. If you pick a flower, it immediately begins to die. When we pick and dissect the conversation between Shiva and Parvati, the essence can never be found. If a flower has no scent, is the flower the problem or is it our senses? A theory is that the highest form of intelligence is our ability to observe without analysing, without evaluating the content. We analyse and dissect because we want the content to fit into our limited maturity (or intelligence). If we cannot understand the tantra (and the yoga sutras), it means our intellectual senses have yet to mature. We are just not ready. It should all make sense to us in our own time (if it meant for us). Only then will the tantra have any meaning.

The Yoga path –

If the Tantra does not reach out to you or have meaning, perhaps you need a pre-requisite of sorts? You need to do something for your mind and body so you can better understand the wisdom of Shiva. If you partake in breathing exercises and bodily postures as a way of preparing mind and body for one of the 112 Tantra techniques, you are essentially a "yogi". So, yoga could be looked at as an indirect method towards the highest reality. In yoga, you breathe and "meditate" as a means to make you, your body, and your mind stronger or more durable. In Tantra, you just do this directly with no means of preparation. So, it could be argued that yoga is a pre-requisite for Tantra.

If we just think of modern-day Western yoga purely as an example, if I was to teach a handstand, the tantric approach would be to just do the pose with wholehearted faith in what you wish to achieve. There are no pauses or doubts. You just do it with pure conviction and heart. The yogic approach is methodical in that the pose is first analysed and then a pre-requisite is structured. You may well feel like you have to do many movements and exercises to prepare yourself (physically and emotionally) for your handstand. The tantric would say that the yogis are too full of doubt and the yogis would say that the tantrics are all too vain. Neither are right. Both paths lead to the same destination. The paths just differ in their own perceived wisdom.

Or you can easily say that Tantra and yoga are the same thing; just labels passed down by man to create division. At the time of the conversation (between Shiva and Parvati), I doubt there were squabbles over who was what because the words 'tantra' and 'yoga' didn't exist. Even today, if you ask many devotees whether they are yogis or tantric, they will just laugh at you. They say that they are "bakths", which means devotees. I read once in a book that Shakespeare said a rose by any other name would smell just as sweet. So, what is in a name?

Try to think of modern-day Western yoga as an example again. You could say there are Hatha yogis and Ashtanga yogis. Hatha yogis approach their poses more statically, with a greater emphasis on alignment. Ashtanga practitioners have a faster pace and focus on Vinyasa, which is moving with the breath. Both have different labels but aim to achieve the same goal of making you move and feel better. In many cases, it is not even those who participate that are called Hatha yogis or Ashtangis. It is labels given by people from the outside, because in our heads, we need order and organisation. We need definition and systems. But the individual who practices Ashtanga may just call themselves a yogi and not an Ashtangi. Definitions belong to the definers, not the defined. Of course, in some cases, Ashtangis want the world to know that their system is superior, so they call themselves Ashtangis. Labels are stuck on one's forehead by others seeking division and often by ourselves to satisfy our vanity. Just like Hatha and Ashtanga, Tantra and yoga can be looked upon as the same thing as the goal is ultimately the same. The methodology, however, can differ.

*Disciple — Understood my astute guru. But I always thought Tantra was like sex n' shit !?!*

There has always been a misconception over Tantra. Tantra is thought of, in the West, as representing mysticism and sexuality. Some people find tantrics culturally horrifying and associate them with the occult. Both do not represent Tantra as I have come to understand it.

To reiterate, the text itself and Tantra as a tradition may be dated academically to around the 1st millennium, but I am referring to the time the discourse was traditionally meant to have taken place. Not when the first texts on Tantra were discovered by European scholarship. This perspective I am presenting to you is more of a traditional way of thinking.

Many of the devotees who began following Shiva's path (of attaining the highest reality) years after he left the earth continued to follow his methods directly. These aspirants can be referred to as tantrics; followers or devotees of Shiva's original system (of which there are many additional branches of today, as you can imagine). These followers or aspirants can be considered to be Shiva's original disciples. Nevertheless, it could also be understood that the original path is not orthodox Tantra but is, in fact, yoga — the union of man and the highest reality. Thus, Shiva's original system is also called yoga by some. Tantra can also mean "expansion of the mind", and yoga is trying to achieve a stillness of mind. Both essentially the same thing again, just different methodologies.

It can be argued that yoga is a tradition developed from Tantra (it can also be the other way around). Those who followed Shiva's methods directly were seen as primitive and rebellious, and they would follow Shiva's example and smear themselves with ash and sing and dance at cremation grounds. They were adorned with a topknot and the three transversal stripes across their heads. This would become the typical dress of an ascetic. Just like Shiva, they were wild, untamed and free from the rules and rituals of society. The more "priestly" amongst society at the time found this behaviour to be embarrassing. Rather than rebellious, untamed yogis, these followers were seen more as barbaric and uncultured animals. Without a guru or guide around in the form of a Shiva, many sub-sects soon developed as a way for people to distance themselves from those they considered "low caste". The priests and the more orthodox devotees of Shiva began discussing and theorising on this higher reality. They sat on their high perches and had many debates and discussions, all feeling like they could add something new to Shiva's teaching. They spoke of morals, ethics and principles. They created sub-sections and caste systems as a way of establishing control and power.

The tantrics didn't care for such codes or the caste system. Shiva's only pre-requisite was to be "willing". So, the ash-covered tantrics saw no use in discussion with the priests. They understood the methods of Shiva that had been passed down. They understood that a union with "Shiva" or the highest reality/consciousness would not be possible through discussion and analysis. They just continued to practice and to dance away in the burial grounds, ignoring those who preferred analysis and investigation. They celebrated themselves and their bodies. These "tantrics" remained hidden in the gratifying wildness of nature, bound by no boundaries and tamed by no ruler or king. Thus, Tantra become understood as a rebellious path towards the highest reality and yoga was considered more cultured and orthodox. This is why Tantra is so unique. Or, more to the point, why the *Vijnana Bhairava Tantra* is so unique. It is only concerned with a "how". Not a "why" or a "when". This is why Shiva's method is a science, because it is all about experimenting with the methods. You don't sit and ponder "what" the highest reality is. You simply "do", and you will become aware of the answers.

Over the years, many, many more sub divisions were created, as you can imagine. But at the time of Shiva, there was no differentiation between what is Tantra and what is yoga. Both were one and the same.

*Disciple – Ok I heard that. I follow. Yoga may have developed from the Tantra tradition. Tantra is direct, yoga is indirect. Clear as mud. Another question on Tantra, like I said in the previous question, why do I associate Tantra with sex?*

Sexuality is a theme in some of Shiva's techniques but not in the way we view sexuality in the West. The techniques go beyond sexuality and become eternal bliss. In some of these "sexual" techniques, one loses all sense of the physical self and becomes dissolved in a divine energy. Jaideva Singh in his commentary of the wonderful dialogue between Shiva and Parvati says "It is a fool who takes this illustration as an injunction for carnal pleasure"[1].

Tantric sex or more appropriately, tantric union, goes beyond the physical realm. It is a deeply spiritual practice. When we view artwork of Shiva and Parvati in union, we in the West look at their physical bodies and attempt to replicate the various physical positions. What we miss are the two principals in this union, Shiva and Parvati, and the emotional connection that creates this union. Although Shiva referred to Parvati as a goddess on account of her divine beauty, and Shiva himself is referred to as *Sundereshvara* (beautiful lord), their union went beyond the physical. When Parvati sat on Shiva's lap, their souls were one. They are soulmates, which means all of their energy centres meet naturally. When Shiva and Parvati embrace, they are completely dissolved in the feeling of oneness. All feeling, external and internal is lost and all that is experienced is a divine state.

Shiva and Parvati are thus perfectly balanced. The male and female energies are in perfect equilibrium. It is the balance of energy, and the union of their souls that makes their union beyond sexuality.

*"I listened mesmerized, visualizing the goddess with her divine mate, wondering if it was possible for humans to replicate this perfect relationship. Would I be blessed with such a love in my life?"[2] –*
*Chitra Banerjee Divakaruni, The Forest of Enchantments*

Once in a while, there is a Shiva and a Parvati. A Laila and Majnu. A Heer and a Ranjha. A Kajol and a Shah Rukh. The universe created these couples as one. Even if they are born in different lifetimes, they will still find one another. This is pre-destined love. This is real love. It is rare like lightning or a real guru. You cannot create this. This is not something you can experience or feel on a tantric weekend in Brighton. You cannot create this by reading one of the many nonsensical tantric sex books you can buy online. When Shiva and Parvati make love, this is the union of tantra and they both are lost. There is no "I". There is no sun and moon. Both have merged and become lost in one another.

In tantra, the word "love" is misleading. This word implies that there is also the possibility of hate. But tantra is beyond the dualities. When we love someone, it is also a possibility to hate them. When we cry, we then laugh. Our compassion and cruelty, our peace and violence, our madness and meditation, mind and no-mind, silence and sound are all intertwined with one another. We live and then, we die. Our life is a play between the opposites of nature. We are never one, we are always a mixture or a dance between the two. In physics, this is referred to as antimatter. Nothing in the universe can exist without its opposite. However, tantra transcends this. "Love" is inadequate as a word to express the love of Shiva and Parvati. In tantra, "god" or the highest reality does not love. "It" is not capable of love as this is a human quality. God IS Love. So Shiva and Parvati who leave our reality and enter the highest realms of reality are no longer lovers or loving each other. They are simply love itself. They breathe love. It is within their cells. It is their blood and veins. They can never fall out of love. There is no opposite to love in tantra. However, such a concept will feel absurd to Westerners. If it does feel absurd, then we have had our first glimpse into and our first real understanding of tantra. The same is true for the word "sex" in Tantra. This is not sex as it is known in the West. Both "love" and "sex" are not enough to describe the union of Shiva and Parvati yet there are no other words. This is because words are secondary as the experience comes first. The shame is that most, if not all, books on tantra are not written by yogis or tantrics but by people who just want to sell books.

The only comparable love that we experience that is close to the love of tantra is the unconditional love between a mother and her child. This, in many respects, is divine love. This love is god according to tantra. There is no opposite in this love (most of the time anyway). But can this type of love ever be experienced outside of the mother and child relationship? If it can, like it was for Shiva and Parvati, then the tantra can be fully understood by anyone who wishes to learn. Until then, it is like reading a foreign language. The tantra thus remains a mystery and source of constant enquiry.

The tantrics would say that we (in the West) confuse love and sex. This is why there is so much misunderstanding about tantra. Tantra is not all about sex – far from it. Sex is biological whereas love is emotional. Sex can exist with love, but without love, sex (as a means for the yogi) only fulfils immediate needs.

The yogis say that we can only comprehend tantra when we understand and experience "true" love. The original text, the *Vijnana Bhairav Tantra* is written in the language of pure love – the divine meeting of two hearts, two souls, two beings or two bodies becoming one. This is why I have a statue of "*Ardhanarishvara*" inside my studio. This image is not a religious symbol. I can see why it looks like I have a Hindu deity in the studio because let's face it, it can make the studio look more traditional.

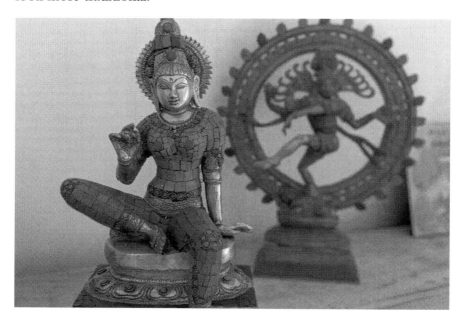

*above - Statues of Parvati and Shiva at my Teacher Training studio that Laura and I have collected on our travels. Both statues have a unique stone and colour design. Parvati is from Nepal and the Shiva statue is from Goa.*

But this is a tantric statue that symbolises the union of Shiva and Parvati as if they are one. This is union or yoga if you will. You could say that union or yoga means "love". When there is a merging of two and there is no longer a distinction between the two, they are blessed. So this murti in the studio, that is half Shiva and half Parvati, is a tantric symbol of pure love – the type of rare love that has no opposite.

Love is the basic tool that one needs to understand tantric wisdom. Without this love, we are blindly reading and guessing. We attempt to understand ancient wisdom with our logical minds and misinterpret it. The tantras however were never written for the logical. When Parvati sits on Shiva's lap and enquires about reality, there is no logic between the two, just pure love. Thus, tantra is written in the language of love and not sex. If we continue to read about tantra with lustful minds, we will never make sense of it. We will interpret it as our minds perceive "love" at that time in our lives.

In tantric union, there is total bliss and harmony. Because of this harmony, peace arises. There is no conflict, drama or emotion. There is a total transformation from animal to divine, and the finite becomes infinite – this is tantra.

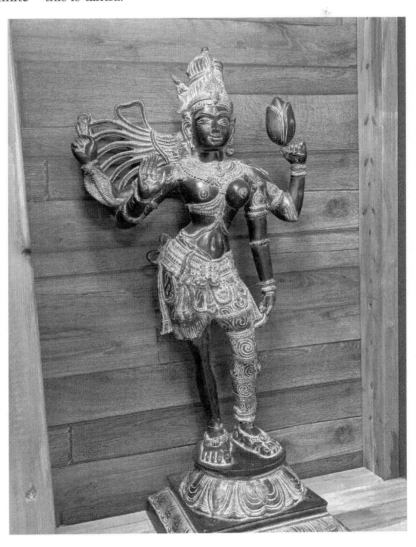

*above - The 'murti' of "Ardhanarishvara" inside my main studio. The right side of the murti is Shiva. The masculine 'Sun'. The left side is Parvati. The feminine 'Moon'. We look at this murti as Shiva and Parvati to help us understand but in reality, there are no two sides. Ardhanarishvara is one being. Once they unite, there is no longer a distinction between the two.*

*Footnotes for the curious* - There is of course, different 'types' of Tantra in the same way there are different types of yoga. All similar themes yet contrasting and often contradictory views and practices. Some elements of Tantra are not as poetic as I have described above. According to some Tantric scriptures the inner energy is concentrated in the sexual fluids of women who embodied the creative power of the great goddess (Parvati). There was often ritualised sex as well as alcohol and meat consumption. So, just like most of us then! There is also an even more misunderstood branch of Tantra and they are the '*Aghoras*'. It does kind of mean 'white people' for those who have heard me reference that in the past. It actually means 'filled with light'. Sex again is very central to the *Aghora* tradition. They say however it is cosmic sexual union of universal dualities. The aim of the *Aghoras* is termed '*Laya*'. This means the union or return of the seeker to the undifferentiated existence. *Aghoras* are considered the 'left hand path' by the orthodox yogis down to misunderstanding the tradition. The misunderstanding is generally through fear and ignorance. So, Tantra as a whole is a large subject like yoga that has many sub-divisions and at times contradictory methods and opinions. Some tantric and *Aghora* traditions are simply oral traditions and have no real doctrine or dogma so it is very hard to understand their methods and practices.

In the context of this tantric text, the dialogue between Shiva and Parvati, Tantra is love and love is Tantra.

*Disciple: O prudent one. If Tantra is Love (as you say), why do so many modern-day yogi's (of the lived tradition in India) abandon love? I have heard many yogi's (in the subcontinent) say that love is attachment and should be discarded. They renounce love once they become wondering 'holy men' or monks. But you say that love can be a method in itself to reach the higher reality?*

In my opinion the yogi (in the subcontinent) has chosen to renounce love (and life to a degree) because in the core of his being, a lot of these cultural yogis do not really believe in a type of unconditional love. The yogi may believe it exists within their relationship with their mothers, but they do not believe it can exist otherwise. Outside of the sacred mother-child relationship they have no understanding of love. Or, with the ascetic who was once a family man, he becomes an ascetic because he does not understand love.

So, the answer as to why a holy man can renounce love and life in the sub-continent is a combination of not really believing in love and also not understanding love. My argument, as you read on, is if you know and understand real love, how can you renounce it?

I remember once speaking to an ascetic who was married at eight years old. This may come as a surprise to Westerners, but this remains a very common practice in the Indian subcontinent. Child marriages are tradition (in some parts) and have been for a very long time. When I was in Kashmir, I tried to trace my family tree to get an idea of how old my great aunt would have been when she got married (she isn't an actual aunt but a "desi" aunt – meaning she is just a neighbour). She got married in pre-partition India when I imagine she was no older than my niece is today: nine years old. What these child marriages do is build companionship and not love. They create a business arrangement where two people have to work together to survive. There is very little actual love that exists. In most cases, in their youth, responsibility is confused as love. The ethical and cultural bond of marriage, which is sacred, is called love, but it is not. It is just duty. It is *dharm* or *farz*. It is nothing more than a business transaction - honestly, it is even less than that. In a business arrangement, both parties can benefit, but more often than not, only the man benefits in an arranged marriage. It is one of the hardest places in the world to be born a woman. Parents often arrange children's marriage to maintain or improve their respectability within the community. It has nothing to do even with the parents' love for their children. It is *izzat*. It is all a show. No love exists at all. So how can we expect such children to one day become loving adults or be loving or understand love when their parents were perhaps married as part of a business transaction and so were they. If no love is ever present in their lives, then how is there any hope for them to find love or even understand love as adults? The ascetic I spoke with who was married at 8 years old also had no mother. He was raised by his grandfather. Can someone be loving when he was never raised with the impression of love?

This is why the holy man renounces love. Because he does not know what love really is. He renounces what he thinks is love. A mother would die for her child. This is love. When you are willing to die for your husband/wife. This is love. The ascetic who leaves his household, leaves his responsibilities, his wife, his children. How can such a man know love?

So the soon to be holy man approaches mid-life and realises deep in his heart that his heart is devoid of real love. This is why he abandons life and goes searching for "god" (to fill his void) and becomes an ascetic, sadhu, pundit, yogi or holy man. But, if he had known real love, I argue he would never have left. Because the ascetic does not understand the meaning of love or has not had an experience of real love, he believes his "love" for his family is an attachment. He believes love can create misery and suffering, so he leaves his wife and children and becomes a wandering monk (perhaps fulfilling his Hindu obligations). But he is not a monk as he believes he is. He is no more than a beggar – a literal and spiritual beggar. He is simply begging for love and begging for god. But if he truly loved, he would never have left as true love is not attachment. Real love is a freedom from attachment. Love is not draining and challenging. It does not keep you in a bondage. Love is nourishing and purifies the soul. Real love does not lose its splendour and meaning over time. It continues to grow and fulfil you for the rest of your life. However, it is clingy behaviour and attachment that destroys love.

When you really love someone, you are attached to nothing. We become attached to something due to the fear of losing it. But if the love is pure, it can never be taken so it cannot be an attachment. I love my wife, but I am not attached to her because I have faith in our love. There is nothing to fear. If I feared, I would pester her all day long. This is not love. This becomes possession. And if I am possessive and afraid, how can god (or reality) enter my heart? Without love, life remains something with potential and nothing more - a "what if". We end up simply drifting around and wasting life. For the holy man or the seeker, no love should equal no god.

Swami Vivekananda said, "But unattached love will not hurt you. Do anything - marry, have children, do anything you like - nothing will hurt you. Do nothing with the idea of 'mine'. Duty for duty's sake; work for work's sake. What is that to you? You stand aside."[3]

Thus, the answer to your question is that the culture these men have been raised in does not support the idea of true love or even help them understand what love is. They are always in a cultural agreement – first with their wives, and then with god. With their wives they say, "I will support you if I can. In return you be a good wife and take care of me". Then when they renounce life, they say, "I will worship you dear god daily. In return, take care of me and save me from returning in the next life as a lower form. Don't forget that I left my wife and kids for you". Again, this is not love. This is fear. The hidden desire of a reward from god for all his prayers and penance makes the ascetic's offerings unholy and unwholesome.

For the ascetic and the holy man, life is all about self-preservation - nothing more. Ascetics are just customers trying to buy love. In their minds, love is a business. Kahlil Gibran once said, "Love gives naught but itself and takes naught but from itself."[4]

I read somewhere that this is the bizarre economics of life. When you love, love returns to you. When you love, you simply give and do not desire anything in return as my mum has always taught me. The greatest success of a man would be to have lived and made themselves worthy of love as well as to have received and given their love wholeheartedly. There is no success in life without love as such a man just wanders through life headless and heartless looking for sympathy. Sympathy is a poor man's substitute for love. Life becomes a daze and a constant source of bewilderment. Men, rather than trying to conquer life and death, should attempt to find true love in a partner. This will be his most significant success. Through giving this love, his heart will almost certainly fill itself so there is no void that he feels only god and his begging bowl will one day fill. The conqueror is the man who may be poor, but rich in love.

My mum once said (referring to my future wife), "You know she will be the right one for you because she won't look into your pocket and say that you are poor, she will look into your heart and say that you are rich". And then Laura came into my life. I could have worked hard my whole life and not been receptive to love and been the richest man I could ever have dreamed of. But without love, without Laura, I would still have been poor. Then all the riches would have become a burden because deep down a void would always have existed. Now that I have my Laura, I may be broke, but I have never felt richer. I have never been more happy, or more alive. Love has been a rebirth. Without love, you are the poorest man alive. This is why an ascetic will remain a beggar his whole life. This is why the ascetic rarely experiences the bliss he desires.

*"One word frees us of all the weight and pain of life: That word is love."* [5] —
*Sophocles*

The subcontinent and Bollywood, in particular, has two significant words that help us understand love. The first word is *"pyaar"* or *"mohabbat"* - they both have the same meaning. *Pyaar* refers to love but a more romantic type of love such as teenage love or first love. It is something that can grow and be developed. *Pyaar* comes from the Sanskrit word *priya*. My Sanskrit dictionary defines *priya* as loosely translating to "beloved". *Pyaar* is a word used so commonly in India that the word itself has very little meaning. We see this in many Bollywood movies: A bustling young man notices his *raani* from across the school cafeteria for the first time and instantaneously falls in "love". He will then tell her, and a choreographed dance sequence will follow. This is *"pyaar"*. We have come to understand this word to mean "love", and in many ways, it does imply it, yet it is not a poetic enough word. The word itself is too flimsy and lacks the magic that encapsulates the feeling that is beyond a teenage crush. What word can be used to describe love that is beyond lust? If *pyaar* is love in the presence of lust, what word can be used to describe love beyond lust - a type of divine love? This word is *Ishq*. *Ishq* is an Urdu word that means almost obsessive love. This level of love is beyond *pyaar*. *Ishq* can develop from *pyaar*, but you cannot experience *ishq* and then fall back into *pyaar*. This would imply that the love you experienced was never *ishq* in the first place.

Various streams, random as they may seem, all lead to the sea. To paraphrase Vivekananda, love itself is a stream. The sea is existence, god, the highest reality or the purpose of life. Love leads you to this reality. Love is a device that leads you to the highest reality even if that reality is simply happiness itself. In disregarding love, these holy men are committing a crime towards themselves.

Nietzsche once said, "Be careful when you cast out your 'demons' that you don't throw away the best of yourself."[6] The ascetics in my opinion are all just too brain dead to realise that this is what they are actually doing.

Kahlil Gibran has said; "When you love you should not say, 'God is in my heart', but rather, 'I am in the heart of god'.

'God', bliss, happiness, Zen, *nirvana* or 'ultimate freedom' (whatever you wish to call it) cannot enter an empty, joyless and bewildered heart.

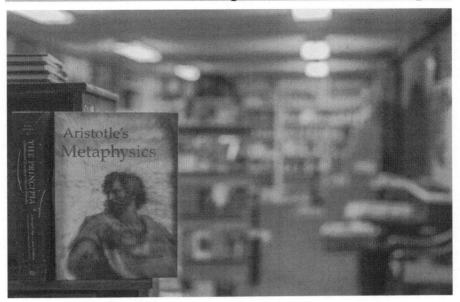

*Disciple — Getting back to those 112 methods of reaching a higher dimension of life for a moment, just so I've got this straight, man, over time has labelled this revelation as either yoga or tantra. If we were to separate them for the sake of argument, Yoga is an indirect method. Tantra is direct. Is that right?*

Correct. Although the argument continues to this day whether Shiva's revelation is Tantra or Yoga. For the sake of continuity, we will call it Yoga.

*Disciple — And thus Yoga philosophy can also be looked at as a philosophical interpretation of the Tantra created by man?*

Shiva did not reveal a philosophy and did not give an actual definition of yoga (just techniques), so the priests and the holy men decided to make up their own philosophy. And they did so. In huge numbers. The higher caste decided they would create a philosophy to suit their needs and requirements. Thus, yoga philosophy was born. This way of thinking was a more 'cultured' approach at reaching the highest reality. Some claimed this new philosophy was just an expansion of Shiva's methods, other said it was a more refined and cultured way of reaching or realising this highest reality.

*Disciple - What happened to Shiva and Parvati after their famous conversation?*

After Parvati was satisfied with the content of her discussion with Shiva, Parvati asked that this information (the 112 techniques) be passed all around the world. She longed for man to be free from endless suffering and idol worship. This awareness, insight and knowledge of yoga would then be passed to the holy men of that time who travelled to the far reaches of the world sharing this science of self-realisation with whoever wanted to learn.

But, after many years of mis-use, blindness and ignorance, these masters and holy men hid themselves away in order to avoid all people during what they referred to as an age of ignorance.

Shiva, however, also wished to enlighten the world, so he once again shared his knowledge. Seeing as Shiva himself was too wild to be a scholar, he decided to teach the theory of the *Vijnana Bhairava Tantra* to the sage Durvasa. It is said, in a legend, that, once Shiva taught the tantras to the sage Durvasa, "he disappeared into the ether". Shiva was never seen again.

*Disciple – The methods that Shiva declared are techniques whereby man can attain or experience - 'ultimate freedom'. Understood. But when you say ultimate freedom, or the highest reality, what does this mean? Once you experience true realisation of life, how can it be described?*

It is the same realisation of the Buddha. For the followers of Buddha, this reality was *Nirvana*. This is where you come to experience your true being. The word *nirvana* actually means cessation of the self, arising from a no-self, emptiness. This emptiness is not empty, as the word suggests, but it means empty in a way we cannot yet grasp. This emptiness is said to be tremendously beautiful. Even the word beautiful is too lame a word. It is an opening of space, a space that has no limits and no boundaries. A non-existence, an emptiness, a void that pulsates with life, that has a feeling, a vibration to which words cannot do justice, a reality that is beyond the bounds of artistry, fantasy and imagination. An exquisite expanse of life awaits us. This is liberation from the self. The ego's ultimate failure. Here we are isolated but never alone. We are eternally connected to the cosmos. It is here we come to the realisation that, far from being a bystander, we are vibrating along with the vibration of the cosmos. We are one and the same. There is no longer a drop and an ocean. The drop merges and becomes the ocean. This is our infinite nature and always has been.

Abhinavagupta who was a mystic from Kashmir ($950_{AD}$) has said; "A viewer with emotional capacity loses sense of time, place and self.

Thus, transcending the limitations of ego-bound perception, the sensitive viewer has a foretaste of enlightened detachment, which takes the form of melting expansion and radiance".

Interestingly, Shiva, the man who brought to light the science of yoga, gave us no philosophy. He simply gave us methods. He didn't explain the essence of this reality nor did he define it. This is why, yoga is not a philosophy. Yoga is a practice. A practice for the daring. You can sit and have intellectual or academic conversations about yoga. You may leave this discussion with your intellect satisfied. But you cannot really know yoga. Yoga is something you must do. Doing is knowing. Shiva indirectly says to Parvati, "Here are the methods, try them, then you will know". All these questions asked by Parvati are very philosophical questions. But they do not get a philosophical answer as a response. Parvati gets a scientific response. She is given methods or techniques. In our modern understanding, it is like asking "what is meditation?" The question cannot be explained using philosophy. You have to follow methods and work the answer out for yourself. Because, unless you do this for yourself, you are only temporarily intellectually satisfied. But there remains a doubt because, deep down in your core, you know that you do not really know.

Because no philosophy was declared by Shiva, anyone of any background or any culture is welcome to try the original form of yoga. There is no pre-requisite of faith. If you have discipline and you are daring, then the exploration of yoga is for you. Discipline means that, if your life is an ordeal, you will take the necessary steps to find happiness. It is not a quick fix. That would not be discipline and it would not be yoga. Discipline means to have self-control and self-respect. These elements are the roots of discipline. Shiva says, "if you are willing". That is all that is required.

For around 12,000 years after Shiva, man theorised on the goal of a yogi. Man also theorised on what yoga was. Man created further systems, beliefs, pre-requisites and even elevated Shiva to the status of God. You see, he was the first one to share with us that the universe was ours, that, if we wished, we could attain this higher state of consciousness. We could also be a Shiva. We could go beyond our limitations and we could experience this true realisation of life. Because he imparted this science, the people of that time said that Shiva himself must be the highest reality. If there is no difference between us and the universal reality, once we ascend to it, then we ourselves must be this reality. Since Shiva was the only one who had experienced this, he must be divine. Maybe he is this reality in human form on earth trying to save us, his children, from making a hell out of earth. The people of the earth at that time said he must be God. The history of man has taught is that we will worship many, and any, natural phenomena we do not fully understand. Shiva was logically speaking, just a man. Just like the Buddha.

So again, for around 12,000 years since Shiva, man has theorised. There are so many theories now on yoga, so many philosophies that it is indeed almost impossible to understand the meaning of yoga. Who should we listen to? The reason that there are so many philosophies is because man had become restless. Man found this self-realisation an arduous task. As you can image, man didn't want to work so hard. Ironically, these seekers and so-called holy men didn't have the patience of a saint.

These holy men didn't have the patience or the willingness (Shiva's only prerequisite) to take a leap of faith. These holy men first needed a clear-cut map that shows the destination before they would embark on this journey. So, these holy men, the sadhus and the pundits, created doctrines and wrote many texts and created many philosophies. They held many debates to find the answers. They discussed the methods of Shiva. They broke them down, analysed and created further systems. Here yoga philosophy was born. From the starving brains of celibate holy men who one after the other, refer to themselves as an avatar of Shiva. And what is yoga philosophy? A route of many streams all leading from somewhere mysterious and all arriving at precisely nowhere. From the undeveloped, restless, anxious and disturbed human minds (in the sub-continent) grew the doctrines of modern-day religions and the tree of yoga itself. All this was created by the minds of men because they had not experienced the 'experience' themselves. Shiva gave no philosophy because once you know the reality, you realise this is beyond intellect. And, if you have not experienced but continue to desire this experience, you over-analyse until you have tackled the problem. The problem with that is you will never really know. Nor did these sadhus and holy men. So many of these ancient texts and doctrines and theories are just blind men trying to lead more blind men. What you are left with is a continent full of blindness and ignorance with so-called men of God all bickering about something none of them have experienced for themselves and they are asking you to follow them. "We will show you the way" they say. These holy men or so-called God men couldn't show you water if you were sitting in a boat.

*"Man is so intelligent that he feels impelled to invent theories to account for what happens in the world. Unfortunately, he is not quite intelligent enough, in most cases, to find correct explanations. So that when he acts on his theories, he behaves very often like a lunatic." - Aldous Huxley[1]*

In my opinion, if women had first spread the teaching of Shiva, we would perhaps have a less conflicted idea of what yoga is. Women would not have been so petty and obnoxious. Women would not have been so hungry for power; they would not have been so anxious to be taken seriously as gurus and they wouldn't have wanted the world to stare at them as they preach and shout in their orange robes, seeking attention and notoriety. Maybe there were plenty of female devotees and real yoginis. Maybe they just preferred to remain in the background while the men, the sadhus and the sages and the pundits all squabbled between themselves. Or, knowing the nature of men through history, maybe women were ousted in this very male dominated movement of self-realisation. Most of these so-called men of God believe in Parvati as a great goddess, the energy source 'adi-shakti' of the cosmos, yet ironically there is no room for women in their system of yoga.

*"The world which worships Mother Mary and goddess Durga also has experienced such heinous crimes against her daughters."[2] - Debajani Mohanty, The Curse of Damini.*

Man has dominated the Indian subcontinent since the dawn of time. Man dominates today and has done so throughout history. Most of the problems that have arisen in that part of the world are because of the imbalance between men and women. A woman cannot possibly lead or revolt or seek, because if women did and were successful, compassion and love would prevail in our lives. When there is compassion and love there is no space for man's instinct to conquer. A woman wants to enquire about love and the nature of being loving. And the nature of God. As was the case with Parvati. Man, on the other hand wants to know God or become God. There is a huge difference.

A woman wants to understand the secrets of life, but a man simply wants to conquer life. Because of this, man has written theory upon theory and doctrine after doctrine. Because, as we know, there is no stronger force on this planet than the collective ego of men.

*Disciple - So just to re-cap, yoga is the journey and yoga is the destination. The journey is to raise awareness of our true reality. The destination is union with this reality. Correct?*

Yes, that is correct. The word yoga is used both in the sense of the communion with the highest state of consciousness and the means for that communion. Yoga is transformation from the human consciousness into the divine consciousness. Our human consciousness is blurred. Our divine consciousness is free from illusion. This is our true reality. This is ultimate freedom.

*Disciple - Got it.*

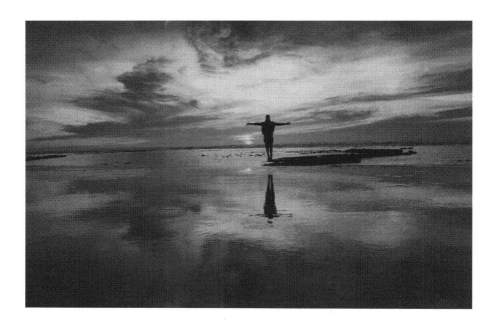

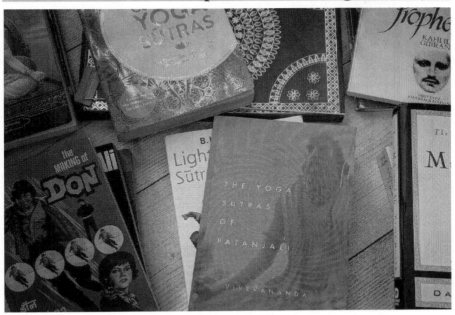

A few hundred years before Christ, a distinguished man decides it is time to define yoga once and for all. His definition will be total. He will study and research his whole life until he has in his hands a masterpiece. A masterpiece on yoga. The author of this masterpiece is the sage Patanjali, the second character I promised to introduce you to.

Was Patanjali a myth? Was he an incarnation of Ananta, the loyal serpent of the Hindu deity Vishnu? Mythologically speaking, yes. But, logically speaking, perhaps not. It's more likely that, if he existed at all, he was simply a brilliant man way before his time. It is also said that Patanjali may have "defined" (as we will see in a moment) yoga under the instruction of his guru, Mahirishi Nandinatha. It is said that his guru Nandinatha sent his eight disciples around the world to spread the teachings of "*Shaiva Siddhanta*". This is how man can become an "enlightened" soul through the grace of Shiva. Interestingly, some people believe that Nandinatha is the "real" adiyogi. At the very least, the first yogi and that Shiva is just a "god" and not the man who manifested the existence of yoga. In truth, we will never know for sure.

On the subject of Adiyogi, Sadhguru from India has said the following: "Everybody on the planet should know that He is the one who offered this science to the world. In the last five to six years, four major books were published in Europe contesting that yoga did not come from India but, is the evolution of European exercise systems. If they write another ten to fifteen books like this, that will become the truth. Whatever you read in your textbook as history, you believe is the truth. It is not, I am telling you, it is just written by some vested interest largely. So, if they write twenty-five to fifty books like this in the next ten to fifteen years, after some time everyone will say yoga came from United States or from California, or that Madonna invented yoga. It is not a laughing matter; it can easily be done. There are people who are willing to write anything. Some very famous books are saying this. Dan Brown, in his book Angels and Demons, says yoga is an ancient Buddhist art. Gautama is only twenty-five hundred years, Adiyogi is fifteen thousand years. Now you say Gautama, tomorrow you will say Madonna. If you write a few books that will become the truth. So, I want to make sure, before I am dead, that everybody should know yoga came from Him, nobody else but Him"[1]

I am not asking anybody to believe Sadhguru. That is a decision you should arrive all by yourself. I just wanted to provide you with the cultural reasons as to why Shiva is regarded as the first yogi. Patanjali is someone who may have simply spread his teachings. Back to Patanjali......

Patanjali was an academic and having compiled so much knowledge from reading man's numerous interpretations, decided that man needed a more complete philosophy. Since Shiva manifested the existence of yoga in conversation with his wife some 12,000 years ago, man has been crying out for complete philosophy. Yoga is crying out for a 'universal' definition.

Patanjali gave us this much needed definition. In his brilliant work The Yoga Sutras, Patanjali clearly and logically defines yoga as…"stillness of mind".

This is not the universal definition for yoga as there is no such thing. Man will always debate and squabble. But this is our definition and one that has been understood by many in the yoga tradition for some time. Yoga is the cessation of the fluctuating mind. This allows us to awaken to our true reality. A state of no-mind allows us to experience and to be in tune with this reality.

*Disciple – 'O Killer of Ego's'….What does stillness of mind mean?*

The mind is the element, part, substance, or process (that is the part of the brain) that reasons, thinks, feels, wills, perceives, and judges. The mind enables man to be aware of the world and of experiences, to think, and to feel. It is the faculty of consciousness and thought. The mind is the process of thought. A stillness of mind, or a cessation of the fluctuating mind, allows us to drop the negative aspects of the mind (fear, judgement, anxiety etc.) and to only retain the positive aspects. There are no negative thoughts, no feelings, no judgements, no anxiety, no fear, no emotions. Just a constant state of bliss and harmony. This is the goal of traditional yoga. To create stillness of mind. So, although stillness of mind or a state of no-mind (both meaning the same thing, just different translated versions) implies that the human mind must be dropped, upon further reading Patanjali's sutras we understand that they refer to the negative aspects of the mind. So, a fuller modern definition would be, "yoga is the cessation of the negative aspects of one's mind", or, "yoga is the stilling of the unfavourable parts of the mind." "Stillness of mind" is used because Patanjali does not give us long drawn out statements. He gives us a thread of his knowledge so we can come to know the real meaning over time. He does not elaborate or offer detailed explanations. Very much like Shiva's 112 techniques, the sutras or threads of Patanjali are short, concise and poetic. It could take a lifetime to explore the hidden depths of these sutras. Perhaps that is the point. Yoga is a life-long immersion not a weekend study.

*Disciple – 'Hang on a minute'...you said, that Shiva said, that yoga is our journey to our ultimate reality. Now you say that yoga is stillness of mind?*

Shiva did not say yoga was anything. Shiva just gave methods. If you remember, Shiva said that man can attain a higher realisation of life but what is this realisation? Or how does one attain this higher reality? When one can control the fluctuating thoughts of the mind, when the mind can be controlled, you can then experience the highest reality for what it is. So, in many ways, Patanjali logically defined the doorway to the highest reality. One must first control the fluctuating mind, or create stillness of mind, or create a state of no-mind for there to be an entry into the highest state of consciousness.

An academic, a scholar, a genius by the name of Patanjali decides there is too much talk of the universe. People are getting too caught up with defining the universe before they have even tried any scientific techniques to realise the universe for themselves. Too much talk and not enough action. If you remember, this is the opposite to what Shiva wanted.

In Shiva's methods, doing is knowing. So, Patanjali says that the universe can be defined as a state of no-mind. He gives the definition in the hope that now that we have a total definition, maybe we can get back to work. We can get back to doing rather than trying to know through debate and literature.

There is an old Zen saying, "In matters of religion, most persons prefer chewing the menu to actually eating the food!"

You can also say that Patanjali has given a method in itself. A state of no-mind can be a technique in itself. Or, it defines what each of Shiva's techniques are. They are concentration techniques that can create a state of no-mind. Once 'no-mind' is reached, reality is presented to you.

*Disciple – Okay, I think I follow.*
*1 - Shiva's 112 methods are just techniques or tantras, or Dharana's (all meaning the same thing).*
*2 - Patanjali defines these techniques as saying that they will help you achieve a state of no-mind. Or cessation of mind. Or stillness of the fluctuating mind (all mean the same thing).*
*3 - Once this state has been reached, the seeker is enlightened. They become like a Buddha. They experience Nirvana. The great homecoming. They experience the true reality.*

Exactly. Patanjali's stillness or state of no-mind is just a definition. Yoga has been given many definitions. Before and after Patanjali. This does not mean that some are right, and some are wrong. Most of them are saying the same thing, if you look beneath the surface.

The Bhagavad Gita (meaning God's song - a text on the various types of yoga), says that yoga is deliverance from pain and sorrow[3] (I am not the Gita's biggest fan, but I do love this definition).

In the sixth chapter, the Gita says, "When the restlessness of mind, intellect and self is stilled through the practice of yoga, the yogi by the grace of the spirit within himself finds fulfilment. Then he knows the joys eternal which is beyond the pale of the senses which his reason cannot grasp. He abides in this higher reality and moves not therefrom. He has found the treasure above all others. There is nothing higher than this. He who has achieved it, shall not be moved by the greatest sorrow. This is the real meaning of yoga - a deliverance from pain and sorrow."[4]

*Disciple — 'Lovely haired one', Can I ask, not that it matters as I appreciate the message is more important that the man, but did Patanjali actually exist?*

Most great talkers on yoga have always found a way to avoid answering that question fully, so it is hard for us to know. Some grow up believing that characters like Shiva, Krishna, Dattatreya, Patanjali and others are all real people. So, to them and their conditioned upbringing, there is no real argument. They will adamantly state, "Yes", they existed on this earth many years ago. The basis of their opinion is their faith. Historians and scholars have always been sceptical (it is kind of their job to be). This open mind is what ignites their passion to always seek their truth.

The Patanjali we speak of, the author of the Yoga Sutras and the man behind our definition of yoga supposedly lived two hundred years before Christ. He apparently wrote more than just the yoga sutras. He has also been credited with having written books on Sanskrit grammar as well as Indian medicine (*Ayurveda*). I have also read in the works of academics that they place Patanjali to have written the book on the sutras around the third century CE[5]. And it is said that the Sanskrit grammar and Indian medicine texts attributed to Patanjali are in fact "other" Patanjali's and not the author of the book on the sutras. This is something of a yoga trend that many old yoga texts never appear to be composed by just one author.

What is the traditional view on Patanjali?

B. K. S Iyengar (1918 – 2014) the great yoga teacher from Pune, India said, "Patanjali, of whom you will hear much in this book (Light on Life), is considered the father of yoga. In reality, as far as we know, he was a yogi and a polymath (a person of wide knowledge or learning) living around fifth century BC India, who collated and elaborated existing knowledge of the yogis' life and practices. He wrote the Yoga Sutras, literally a thread of aphorisms about yoga, consciousness, and the human condition. . . . What Patanjali said applies to me and will apply to you. He wrote, 'With this truth bearing light will begin a new life. Old unwanted impressions are discarded, and we are protected from the damaging effects of new experiences' (Yoga Sutras, Chapter I, Verse 50)"[6].

Sadhguru Jagi Vasudev has said "Today's scholars argue that this is not one man's work, that many people must have worked to make this happen because it is so big, it cannot fit into one man's intellect. It is one man's work. He is probably one of the greatest intellects ever on this planet"[7].

The above offers a fairly biased view on Patanjali. As per tradition, he existed and walked the earth. Scholars may however say otherwise, but I remember a Sufi saint telling me that often scholars become scholars because they lack imagination and soul – it is a bit harsh but that is his view point. The Sufis say, "Understand with your hearts what the most learned scholars cannot understand with their minds".

Thus, tradition and academia will always be in conflict. A friend of mine who is a scholar says he means no disrespect to the tradition at all. He only goes by the evidence that is available and exists. Tradition would say that academics are always looking for a way to disprove yoga and specifically Indian tradition as a means of asserting authority. The viewpoint (from my Hindu friend) has been that Western scholarship continues to belittle Indian tradition because it is in their DNA to do so. I assume that is a reference to the British Raj.

I am not sure I totally agree, but I am just playing the devil's advocate for a moment. I believe that the Eastern tradition and Western academia will always be in conflict. I have met many scholars and academics on yoga, and I believe their intentions to be good. They are just academics and mean no disrespect when their research or findings contradict the traditional way of thinking. Some scholars are arrogant for sure, but that is true in every field. I assume it is these men that Nietzsche was referring to when he said, "They're so cold, these scholars! May lightning strike their food so that their mouths learn how to eat fire!"

David Gordon White who authored the "Yoga Sutras of Patanjali: A Biography" tells us that the sutras fell into relative obscurity for nearly 700 years from the 12th to 19th century. He says, "It (the sutras) had become a moribund tradition (terminal decline), an object of universal indifference. The yoga sutras had for all intents and purposes been lost until Colebrooke found it"[8].

Henry Thomas Colebrooke has been described as the first great Sanskrit scholar from Europe. He "discovered" the yoga sutras of Patanjali around 1800 during British occupation. It is said that several decades later and due to the efforts of the great Vivekananda, the sutras made a comeback. Vivekananda introduced yoga to the world in and around 1900 and aimed to popularise it once again having nearly lost the sacred science to those in the tradition who simply wanted to keep this secret to themselves. So, there was a huge period of time in which the sutras had little relevance to the lives of those who were traditional until it was 'discovered' by European academics. I imagine the Bhagavad Gita was a more fashionable read, at the time, and also served the Hindu establishment better but that is a rant for another book.

When I look at the material available for me to work or quote from regarding Patanjali, it is vast. Western academics have found this text fascinating since its ascension by Vivekananda and its increased popularity in recent times, which owes much to B. K. S Iyengar. But to simplify the answer to your question, "did he exist on this earth"?

Like 99.9% of the contents in this book, it just depends on who you ask. This goes back to the start of the book where my wife eloquently quoted her favourite philosopher: "No, facts is precisely what there is not, only interpretations".

*Disciple — 'Strong armed one', What is your opinion on scholarship vs the traditional way of thinking?*

We are raised with certain romantic notions handed down through generations and, sometimes, drilled into our brains by our parents and "gurus" or religious teachers. These notions may not be factual but are lapped up by us in the name of tradition and culture. Basically, it means that at times, empty words have been passed on from one generation to the next. When these ideas and traditions are labelled as 'mythological' by some or when they say that no evidence exists of such traditions, our primary instinct is to feel offended. That, however, is no fault of scholarship. We are offended simply because we want to protect our parents "way of thinking" and traditions, even though me may actually agree with logic of scholarship. We then 'lash out' at academics, when in fact, it should be our parents and gurus/teachers whom we should be angry with for feeding us such nonsensical romantic notions in the first place. We must be more open to accepting the "truths" as life continues to school us, and scholarship continues to create and assimilate more material.

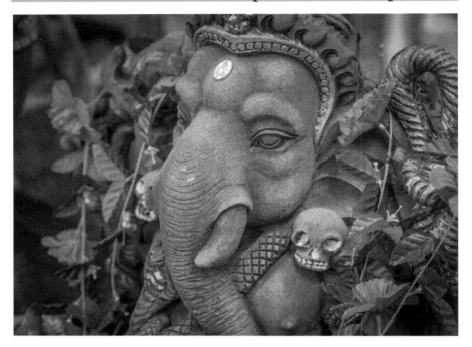

Yoga has always been a relentless journey of self-exploration. We often feel that true happiness is external and that it is something to achieve or gain. The mind wants more, and, the more we gather, the more we accumulate and collect, the more the mind wants. The mind will never be satisfied. If we believe that happiness is something to gain, we can never be happy. It will always be a chase. We will always be running after it. The yoga path calls for an inward search. Not an external search. It asks that man look inside for answers. Through a period of hardship and reflection, one is able to realise that all that we seek (happiness, contentment, bliss etc) is not outside of us. It has always been within. This is our true nature. This state of no-mind is not an achievement, it is our reality. In this reality, we will know what it is to be known. Or simply, what is worth knowing.

## Ganesh & Kartikeya

It happened (there are many variations of this story).

The half man half elephant deity Ganesha (don't ask) had a younger brother called Karthikeya. They got along well but, just like all other siblings, they would have moments of arguments and fights. On one such day, the brothers were summoned by their parents. The parents just happened to be Shiva and Parvati.

Shiva, wishing to challenge his children, made a proposition. He asked Ganesha and Karthikeya to circle their world three times. Whoever did so first and returned to Mount Kailash (their home) should explain to their parents the meaning of true happiness. Could they find and/or experience such happiness on their travels?

Karthikeya immediately hopped onto his pet peacock and flew speedily across the Earth. Ganesha was a little more 'big boned' compared to the chiselled Karthikeya. Ganesh's pet was a mouse who couldn't fly. So Ganesha was stymied. Having listened to Shiva's proposal attentively, Ganesha sat silently and meditated on the proposal. He wanted to ensure that he used his intellect or else he would not win the challenge. A few hours later, Ganesha got up from his contemplation exercise and started walking around Shiva and Parvati and then sat back down sitting cross legged in the manner of a very serious yogi. A few days later, Karthikeya returned. He looked glum and despondent. Shiva asked his son if he was okay. "Yes father" replied Karthikeya. "But I have failed. I travelled afar. I went around the world on three occasions and I saw no happiness. All I saw were problems and suffering."

Shiva then asked Ganesha what he could have learned not having left Kailash at all since accepting the challenge. Ganesha replied that Shiva had asked them to circle their world three times. And he did just that. For Ganesha, his parents were more than the world. They were the entire universe. So, all Ganesha had to do was circle them three times. He explained to his brother and parents that you can travel far and even cross the boundaries of the universe, but you will always be searching.

True happiness, bliss and freedom, Ganesh said, are all closer to home than one realises.

B.K.S. Iyengar has said, "You do not need to seek freedom in some distant land, for it exists within your own body, heart, mind, and soul. Illuminated emancipation, freedom, unalloyed and untainted bliss await you, but you must choose to embark on the Inward Journey to discover it."[1]

It is said that all hope, wisdom, clarity, knowledge is inherent in man. No knowledge comes from the outside. Man should not seek something new but discover or unveil what is already inside. The great Swami Vivekananda once gave the example of Isaac Newton. Vivekananda says that Newton discovered the law of gravitation. He asks if the law of gravitation was sitting in some corner waiting to be found? Or, was the knowledge already in his own mind? The falling of an apple gave the suggestion to Newton, and he studied his own mind. The secrets say Vivekananda, are already ours. The infinite library of the universe is in our own minds.

The Sufi are a mystical branch of Islam. I grew up fascinated with the Sufi path and my family, although not directly Sufi, are hugely influenced by its teachings. The Sufis, like yogis, have an inward approach to life. In one of my favourite books on the Sufi's, Recognising Sufism, the author Arthur Buehler starts with one of the most well-known stories involving Mullah Nasreddin, a wise-fool character used to convey a particular message.

Once, the great Mullah Nasreddin was searching for something on the ground outside his house. His neighbour asked the Mulla what he was looking for. The Mulla replied that he was looking for his keys. His neighbour asked him, "Where did you leave them?" The Mulla replied, "Inside the house".
        "Then why are you looking outside?" asked the confused neighbour. "It's dark inside" replied the Mullah.

This has been the issue for man. Even when we know the keys are inside, it is almost our nature to look outside. Outside is safer for the Mullah. There is strength in numbers. Outside there is light, everything is open. Inside is dark and claustrophobic. Man searches and searches outside and what is found never fills the void. Man is going to the moon. Man is trying to reach further, from earth into space, and man has not yet learned the nearest part of his life. The answers related to the cosmos exist closer to home. They exist within. The problem for man is that the distant drum is so appealing. Even hypnotic. We are drawn by distant dreams. Ashtavakra (you will learn about him later) says, "You are what you are seeking." Man is perfect, and according to the wise men of yesteryear, we have always been free. Our projections have always been our barrier. This is why we need yoga. The wise man does not need yoga to recognise his true nature. One day he just wakes up! It dawns on him that we have always been free from these negative emotions. We have just created an attachment to them. The everyday person like you and me cannot just wake up and be like a Buddha or a Sufi saint. We need to stumble on our true nature in stages.

*"You are the one observer of all, and in reality, have always been free."*[2] *- The Gita of Ashtavakra*

In an interview for the documentary "Who owns yoga?" The legendary Dharma Mitra was asked if he ever studied in India. Dharma Mitra replied, "I have never been to India in my life. What's the point? I would love one day to see all these holy places. But there is a point in yoga when you find something inside, you find that India is inside of you."[3]

This is the path of yoga. The goal may be deliverance from pain and sorrow (when a state of no-mind is reached, you can no longer feel pain) but the journey is inwards.

One must remember that we will always be running if we think that no-mind means that there is something to gain. Let's not call it no-mind for now, let's just call it happiness. Every human wants to be happy. There is no question of this. If we learn to look inside, through reflection, silence, breathing, visualisation etc. (all of which combined are sometimes referred to as meditation), one can achieve this life-long quest of discovering happiness. I use that word very carefully. You do not find happiness. You discover it. It has always been there.

A Zen master was visiting London. He went up to a hot dog vendor and said, "Make me one with everything." The vendor fixed up a hot dog with fried onions, gherkins, and mustard and handed it to the Zen master, who paid with a £20 note. The vendor put the note in his register and snapped it shut. "Excuse me, but where's my change?" asked the Zen master.

"O my brother" said the vendor, "change comes from within."

*Disciple - 'O judicious one'. So, one can arrive to this state of no-mind by turning inwards? By this you mean meditation, concentration exercises etc?*

Yes. The 112 techniques declared by Shiva are just that. Techniques whereby the yogi stops looking outside for answers to explain the mysteries of life but turns inwards. You can call this soul searching. The proper term is introspection, meaning to look from within yourself to find the answers. The actual definition of introspection is – "the examination or observation of one's own mental and emotional processes". When you direct your awareness internally, all of the deceptions and delusions of the outside world begin to fade away. As your inward eye reflects upon its own nature, you find that there is nothing but a pure presence of empty awareness, one that's free from all thoughts, feelings, memories and opinions. You realise that inside, you are vast. There is no beginning and no end. You are limitless and your potential knows no boundaries. You are infinite.

You could say that looking inward is the process of looking at and becoming aware of your thoughts and feelings. It could be listening to your body and observing your mind. Also, watching your breathing or observing the colours behind your closed eyes. This can be done with your poses as well as in meditation. This is why, in a classical physical yoga class there is no music. How can you turn your attention inwards if you are creating such a commotion on the outside? This is why when I teach, I try to get students to just listen to their breathing while in postures (and close their eyes). I want them to feel the breath inside their bodies, to feel and internalise the very subtle influence the breath has on their body. You can only achieve this if there is no music, no distractions and your eyes are closed. Here the outside world disappears. There is a reason there is no music in an Iyengar or an Ashtanga class. In many respects, what makes the pose *'yogic'*, or consistent with yoga principles, is not the pose itself, but what we do when we are in the pose. This is why 'yoga poses' continue to evolve and develop. Because the essence of the pose is not the posture, it's what we do whilst creating the shape of the pose. You could do one of the earliest and most traditional yoga poses, say *Padmasana* (Lotus). If there is no internalisation, it is just a form of contortionism. You can do a pose that has just been 'made up' in the past year by Tara Styles and if you internalise, it is the most *'yogic'* pose you have ever done. So, the art is not what you do, it is how.

I have heard that if you want to stop all your senses, all one has to do is hold their breath. Once this happens you become lost to the outside world. And Shiva says so in the conversation with Parvati.

One of the techniques to experience the highest reality is to focus on the pause between breaths. We can do this in a yoga pose. We are in such a hurry to Inhale-Exhale, we forget there is point between breaths where there is no breath. This, according to Shiva is the most important part of our breathing. And it only needs to be for a split second or as long as you are comfortable. If we want our yoga practice to ascend to celestial heights, then we must observe the pause between breaths. Shiva says at this point we are beyond the world. The Tantra says that this exercise in awareness of 'non-breathing' can be done in any activity, not just sat silently with legs crossed.

Our yoga poses seem to lose their soul and their substance more and more with each passing day. The only way to preserve the integrity of what you do is to remember to internalise. You will find a whole new zest for doing so. So, although many of us are doing yoga poses for external gain (flexibility, aesthetics etc), we can create a sense of internal calm by 'turning our intention inwards'. I say that this is the very essence of a yoga pose. If there is no internal awareness, then the pose is just stretching, or gymnastics. You want to create a deep intimacy between the intelligent part of your mind and the inner workings of your body. The most obvious of these inner workings is your breath.

There is a story I remember reading, maybe from the teaching of Sadhguru. Although, there is also a similar story told by the Sufi's.

A man had been begging under a particular tree for his entire life. He just sat under a tree and begged. One day this poor man died, and his lifeless body just remained lying under the tree. He had no friends, relatives or family. He had no one to carry his body and no one to bury him or arrange his funeral. Out of compassion, the locals who would see this man begging everyday decided that they would bury him. And they decided to bury him right there, at his hermitage, right under the same tree he sat under for his entire life. As the locals began digging, they came upon a huge treasure. Just a few feet beneath where this man had sat and begged, there was richness beyond belief. A giant pot full of gold existed directly under the very spot that this beggar sat for his whole life. "If only he had dug down" the locals said. "He was sat under a treasure this whole time and he had no idea. He was a vagabond his whole life not knowing his could have been richer than in his wildest dreams".

Often, the inward search has been described as the discovery of treasure. It has been described as life's real riches. A beggar is really an emperor. An emperor is really a beggar. The beggar believes that wealth will make him happy. His condition cannot allow him to see past this. He is convinced that the emperor is fulfilled and happy. The emperor has all the wealth. But, deep down, the emperor is just like the beggar. He is lost. As was Alexander the Great. In fact, I will just call him Alexander. He was just a beggar. He conquered and conquered and what was left for him? I remember reading of how fascinated he was with Indian holy men who appeared to have nothing, but who had had everything. No wealth, no luxury, no army. And for some, not even clothes. When Alexander killed them in the search for his immortality, some died smiling because they had conquered the purpose of their lives. They had no fear of death because they were fulfilled. They had arrived at a state of no-mind where there is no fear of death. They literally died smiling.

These men are the real Alexanders. The real conquerors. In one of my favourite Bollywood songs as a child, Amitabh Bachchan's character Sikander travels on his bike in the crowded street of Bombay and sings, "Everyone arrives (in this world) crying, but the one who exits laughing is the conqueror of his destiny. Life is unfaithful, one day it will leave you. Death is a lover; it will take you with it. The one who will teach the world how to live after dying, will be called '*muqaddar kaa sikandar*' (the conqueror of his destiny)."

The holy man, a beggar in the eyes of Alexander, was the real conqueror, the real emperor. Alexander was not a conqueror. He died unhappy. He died a beggar.

*Disciple - I get it. Shiva's 112 techniques are concentration exercises designed to help the 'aspirant' turn their awareness and attention inwards?*

Correct.

*Disciple - The methods of internalisation is called yoga?*

Correct.

What did the sign in the monastery searching for new monks say? Inquire within.

*Disciple - Oh God! Laura warned me about your bad jokes. So, the goal is reached when one is no longer trying to look in, but ends up falling into this state of no-mind? The finite becomes infinite. The drop has merged with the ocean?*

Correct. I couldn't have said it better if I was having a conversation with myself.

*Disciple - Just one more question, I thought yoga was like, stretching n' shit !?!*

The yoga poses help us discover this state of no-mind as explained earlier. We can strive for this by turning our awareness inwards when we practice. We cannot have a pure mind if our physical body is suffering in any way. Whatever happens in the body affects the mind, and whatever happens in the mind affects the body. They run parallel. That is why there is so much emphasis on the body in modern times.

If the body is not blissful, your mind cannot be. Many traditions of thought claimed that there was a distinction between mind and body. The reality is that this just an illusion. The mind is born of the body and the body drives the mind. Let me repeat, just to emphasise, whatever happens in the body affects the mind, and whatever happens in the mind affects the body. Alcohol is ingested by the body, but overconsumption can affect the mind. A hypnotherapist talks to your mind and affects your body. He talks to your mind and says you are a chicken, which transfers to your body and makes you dance like one. Mind and body are two sides of the same coin.

The earliest Hatha yogis had a theory. The mind affects the body. This we know. When you are sad, it shows in the way you stand or the way you slouch. If you are happy, you act and create a very different type of posture. Your mind and what it is experiencing are displayed in your body. You can tell that someone is sorrowful by the way they carry their bodies and their body language. The earliest yogis, who first gave yoga poses the attention they deserve, thought, "If the mind can influence the body, can the body influence the mind?" Can we reverse this pattern? Can we stand and sit a certain way? Can we change our posture? Will this change our minds? Can we create purity in our bodies? Will this then create purity of mind? That essentially is the science of physical yoga poses. We are using our body to influence our minds. This is why there is such a modern day need for meditation (more on this later). People are not gaining anything from meditation; they are not even meditating. They are gaining something from sitting still and from breathing. They just call it meditation. But the real reason this mediation works is because you sit still for 10 minutes. Here, you bring about what is referred to as the relaxation response (more on this in the meditation chapter). When you are sitting still, the monkey mind will slowly stop the mayhem that is brought about by jumping around from one thought to another. Eventually the monkey stops jumping. So, the mind is not racing and jumping as much as it was. This, in itself, creates a sense of calm. The body is affecting the monkey mind. The monkey wants to jump but you are sat still so it has nowhere to go. Then the breathing can function optimally. Now there is calmness and a sense of bliss and it all started with the body. Yoga, in its purest sense, is purely psychological and deals with the workings of the mind. Instead of exploring the outer world as other sciences do, Patanjali's science is concerned with exploring the inner world.

*Disciple - But Shiva didn't mention the asanas (yoga poses) in any of his 112 techniques?*

Strictly speaking, no. The asanas were added to yogic lore much later on. Maybe 15,000 years ago humans were not as physically pathetic as we are today. If that was not the case, then maybe Shiva would have mentioned poses as part of his 112 methods. Shiva set out some techniques that, in theory, you can try while in a yoga pose, but he did not specifically prescribe yoga poses in that particular conversation with his wife. Not to confuse you, but Shiva may have mentioned asanas, or yoga poses in conversation with his wife, he just didn't mention them as part of the original dialogue or conversation. He may have mentioned them much later on in time, after the knowledge of the 112 methods had already spread. We will get to that in the Asana Chapter.

# Chapter 6 – Mind

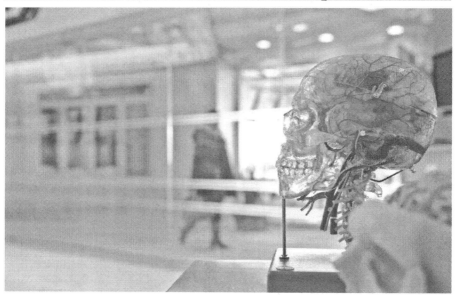

Fifteen thousand years ago, Shiva gave us methods enabling man (if willing) to attain a reality that is, for us now, totally beyond our comprehension. Twelve thousand years later, Patanjali defines this reality as a state of 'no-mind'. Or, more accurately, a state where the mind is under conscious control. Man is no longer a slave to the wondering mind. This is Yoga.

You could say that the mind itself is not the problem. The problem lies with the default setting of the mind, which is to wonder. The wondering mind is the problem. I get annoyed when I see Instagram posts of the same old things. Over and over again. That is why I do not post a lot as I find posting almost as lugubrious as seeing. I find Instagram a reflection of my wondering mind. We get annoyed and irritated as to why our minds cannot just be still for a moment. Why is the mind always wondering? Instagram shows me the same default yoga poses over and over again. How many more posts do I have to see with a yogi pointing his or her toes? I become so bored I just switch off. I look for an escape (which, to be fair, should just mean logging off). I find the same with my mind. The minds recollection system brings up the past over and over again and it also thinks about the future. I just see the same old images. This whole process (which again is just the default mode of the brain) just gets so boring. I want to switch off and stop the monkey mind from swinging from one branch to another. I do this via the poses of yoga. They give the monkey something to do rather than just throw the same old thoughts into my head over and over again.

In the opening of the Dhammapada, (a collection of sayings from the Buddha), the enlightened one said, "What we are today comes from our thoughts of yesterday, and our present thoughts build our life of tomorrow - our life is the creation of our mind. If a man speaks or acts with an impure mind, suffering follows him as the wheel of the cart follows the beast that draws the cart. If a man speaks or acts with a pure mind, joy follows him surely as his own shadow."[1]

There is a Sufi story that I remember from when I was younger.

It happened. It did.

A horse suddenly came galloping quickly down the road. It seemed as though the man riding the horse, the Sufi seeker Mullah Nasreddin, had somewhere important to go. Another man, who was standing alongside the road, shouted, "Mulla, where are you going?", the Mullah replied; "I don't know! Ask the horse!"

In this story, the horse symbolises one's mind. The story tells us how we live. We are literally slaves of our mind. Our mind will drag us here and drag us there and we are ultimately left lost and exhausted.

Yoga is controlling one's mind. Yoga means to create a union between you and this state of 'no-mind'. Here, the mind exists, but it is no longer pulling you here and there. The mind is your slave. This is our true reality.

*Disciple - Stepping aside from yoga slightly, Where is the mind? Is it located in your head?*

The scientific answer to that is the brain. It is common knowledge from what I have read and understood, that all the fascinating features of our mind, are born from the grey matter inside our heads. Our brain. The brain is the organ of our behaviour.

The brain's 100 billion neurons and its some 100 trillion connections contain the physical embodiment of our personalities, knowledge, our character, memories, thoughts and emotions. Science would say that technically there is no such thing as the mind. The mind is only an expression of the various neural circuits that are part of our brains. If, for some reason, the coordinated electromechanical activity within the brain was to cease, our mind would disappear from the face of the earth. Our minds would be no more. Our mind is made up of these 100 billion neurons, all sending electrical signals among themselves. This network of neurons is the human mind. Saying that, very recently a bunch of neuro scientists and other clever people got together and, after much discussion, decided to redefine our understanding of the mind as, "The emergent self-organising process, both embodied and relational, that regulates energy and information flow within and among us."[2]

The surprising aspect of this definition is that, supposedly, our mind now extends beyond what we once thought. Our mind is not simply our perception of experiences, but it is those experiences themselves. Dan Siegel (a really clever guy) argues that it's impossible to completely disentangle our subjective view of the world from our interactions[3]. This more recent understanding of the mind brings us closer to the yogic understanding of the same subject.

The science of yoga has a view that is in conflict with those who say the mind is an exclusive product of the brain. In yogic science, there are five layers of the body. These layers are called koshas. These koshas are like energetic sheaths, similar to a set of Russian dolls. Each layer unearths something distinctive, something rare and unique. In the words of Shrek, "Ogres are like onions. Onions have layers." Just like our favourite ogre, we have layers too. Five, to be precise. Yoga seeks to create a harmonious union between all these layers. This creates the wholeness that we all crave. B.K.S. Iyengar says, "True health requires only the effective functioning of the physical exterior of our being, but also the vitality, strength, and sensitivity of the subtle levels within."[4]

I won't go through all these layers, just the first three.

1 - The first is known as the *annamaya kosha*. This is the physical sheath. The physical/anatomical body. The food body, the earth body, which is made of earth and is constantly to be nourished by food. Food comes from the earth. The right amount of food and the correct type of food are needed for the body to remain alive and to preserve vitality.

In the yogic system, there is no such thing as the brain in isolation from the body. The brain is part of the physical body. The heart, the muscles, the liver, the lungs and the brain are all part of the physical body. The external body.

2 - The second of these layers (behind the physical body), is what the sage Patanjali (from the Yoga Sutras) calls the *pranamaya kosha*. This is the energy body, the electric body (or even the *chi* body). This sheath is influenced by your breathing. This is why such importance is placed on the purity of breath. Your harmonious breathing pattern adds vitality and life to this kosha. This layer is more subtle than the first.

3 - The third layer is what Patanjali calls the *manomaya kosha*, or the mental body. Essentially this sheath is your mind. Unlike neuroscience that says the mind is just an expression of the brain, yogic science says that mind is not just in one particular part of the body. Every cell in the body has its own memory and intelligence, its own mind. The physical body is the hardware – the mental body is the software.

On the subject of *manomaya kosha*, Sadhguru says, "The second layer is the *manomayakosha*, or the mental body (he calls it the second layer not the third). Today, doctors are talking a great deal about psychosomatic ailments. This means that what happens in the mind affects what happens in the body. This is because what you call the mind is not just the brain. It is not located in any single part of the human anatomy. Instead, every cell has its own intelligence, so there is an entire mental body, an entire anatomy of the mind."[4]

*Disciple - Last science question O educated one. Because I know this is not an academic book on yoga. What about consciousness? Is the state of no-mind or a higher state of consciousness the same thing? What is the difference between mind and consciousness?*

For the sake of simplicity, a state of 'no-mind' and a higher state of consciousness are the same. One invites the other. You could argue that your thoughts (the clouds) block out the clear sky (your consciousness). We are not as conscious as we should be as we are always entertaining our thoughts. We are entertaining our imagination and memory. We are entertaining our monkey minds. When we can stop doing this, stop the entertaining, stop the juggling acts, and the other circus tricks we do to stay in tune with our monkey minds, we start to see the possibility of connecting more with our consciousness. And what is our consciousness? Because the prefix 'con' means 'with' and the root 'sci' means 'knowledge', the word 'conscious' simply means 'with knowledge' or 'with awareness'.

Human consciousness is the functional expression of the brain. It is what creates our basic awareness of being alive. Our intelligence is consciousness. The only reason you are alive, and you are reading this book is because of your consciousness. Consciousness allows us to experience our reality. Consciousness is the brain's response to its surrounding stimuli. Consciousness is essentially a complex dance of the circuits within our brains. For over six million years the human brain has reorganised itself, increased in size and in complexity to the point where, today, man is supposedly at the peak of consciousness.

The brain is the organ of creation and it is the most complex organised structure in the whole universe.

Our consciousness is our undisturbed nature. Our authentic nature. This is the real part of us. Each time you pay attention to something, you listen, you think and perceive, is your consciousness. Our everyday consciousness is like the tip of an iceberg. Underneath the water, there is an uncharted mysterious realm of consciousness to be explored. It's this additional state of consciousness that we aim to experience. This additional state is much more complex, vast and advanced than our everyday consciousness.

The mind is not the real part of you and me. It is different in everybody because it is manufactured. Our mind is created by us, and we feed the mind and we make the clouds darker, and we multiply them by adding fuel. The mind doesn't make just one cloud, it creates many. We don't have one mind. We have many minds. Hundreds and thousands of minds. Each circumstance calls for a different mind. Our minds are a reflection of how we feel about society and our place in that society. We are anxious, afraid, alone, lost. With all these emotions we water the seeds in our minds. They may not flower right away, but, over time, they will. Then our consciousness, our real nature, becomes even more blurred as it gets even more lost behind the clouds of our mind. Our mind is now, our consciousness is eternal. Our mind is not our own. It is a collection of mini-minds that has influenced us over many years. It has been shaped by our parents, our teachers, our bosses and our philosophers. Buddhists say that we even store seeds from our previous lives, and our parents pass their seeds onto us too. When we identify ourselves with our minds, we soon realise that this is not the real us. This is 'Maya' in yogic speak. Maya is not an illusion as is commonly understood. The world is real. We just can't perceive it through our mind. Our mind is a store of thoughts, fears, threats, quotes, words, teachings, dogmas and doctrines, all passed down and ingrained in us, some before we even had a chance to blink.

This state of no-mind, or this state of full awareness or highest state of consciousness is our truth, our true reality.

*"How can you prove whether at this moment we are sleeping, and all our thoughts are a dream; or whether we are awake, and talking to one another in the waking state"* - Plato

Once there is a state of 'no-mind', no thought patterns, once we stop entertaining the mind, we become consciously aware of our reality. Our perception of reality is altered because we have nothing distracting us. We remove our thoughts; we remove the clouds. We see the clear sky. We experience *Nirvana*.

This is why I prefer to use the phrase 'no-mind' rather than 'stilling of the mind' (although they do mean the same thing). 'Stilling of the mind' implies that for now you are in control. But the mind is just still for now. So, the clouds have cleared the sky, but they will be back. In a state of 'no-mind', the clouds have not just gone, they have disappeared completely. It's only a matter of small words but they have big consequences. 'Stilling of mind' is also a little contradictory for me. The mind can't be still. In the East this is referred to as the monkey mind. The monkey cannot sit still. That said, in Nepal they do stop and pose for photos but, in general, monkeys cannot be still - this is in their nature. There is no point getting cross with Bubbles the monkey when he won't sit still. This is his nature. The monkey mind is jumping here and jumping there. So, 'stillness of mind' as a concept doesn't quite work for me. It's a bit like the word's tolerance and acceptance.

Some people say we should tolerate immigration. It's only a word, but what harm is there in the word tolerance? The thing is it just doesn't fit. Once, my friend Sangeeta said in conversation that she hated the word tolerance.

It made it sound as if people were grudgingly agreeing with immigration, but the truth is that, deep down, they were against it and that society has shaped their opinion. Sangeeta preferred the word acceptance. We don't tolerate other religions and beliefs and people. We accept them. A small word is the difference between love and hate. A small word is the difference between understanding yoga and not understanding yoga. So, for me, in my opinion, a state of 'no-mind' is purer than 'stillness of mind'. But, that said, I don't mean 'no-mind' in that mind does not exist. That is impossible. The mind is a functional expression of the brain. The mind is, in essence, what the brain does. So, for the mind not to exist would require the brain not to be working. So, you would have to be dead for there to be no-mind. 'No-mind' should be short for 'No longer a slave to the negative emotions of the mind'. No-mind for me means freedom from these negative emotions. The mind is beautiful and much more fascinating and captivating than we realise. It would be very easy for us to feel in awe of its grandeur, such is its sophistication. So, I can see why the idea of 'no-mind' could imply that yoga is against the mind. This is not the case.

*Disciple - What happens once you are able to experience this state of no-mind?*

Well I can't talk from experience. My mind is not under my command. It is fair to say that my mind is most definitely my sidekick. I remember a scene where Homer Simpson speaks to his brain and says, "All right brain. You don't like me, and I don't like you. Let's work together and get through this so I can continue to kill you with beer." This is a perfect summary of my relationship with my mind. We don't get on and we don't agree on anything. But there are times when we must work together.

If you allow the mind to become your master, then madness will surely follow. But the man who can tame his mind and become master of his mind has mastered meditation. This is the ultimate freedom.

In one of my favourite quotes, the Sufi Idris Shah once said, "Man (and woman) has an infinite capacity for self-development. Equally, he has an infinite capacity for self-destruction. A human being may be clinically alive and yet, despite all appearances, spiritually dead."[5] This is a consequence of the mind. By allowing your mind to be your master, you are creating spiritual suicide.

*Disciple - How can one defeat the mind?*

One way is to show heart. Have heart. Have courage. Whenever you are down in the dumps or feeling low, an instinctive response by someone is to tell you to take heart, to show courage. Courage resides in your heart. This is why (again instinctively) no one says you must learn to be courageous. This would imply that courage is something external to be gained. But it is not. Most people will say "show courage". Or "be courageous". This is our nature. So, one must take heart.

Interestingly the word courage comes from the Latin root cor, meaning heart. The original meaning of the word courage was to speak one's mind by telling all one's heart.

*Disciple - Does courage really reside in the heart?*

Yes. And, no. When we talk about 'heart', 'taking heart' etc. We are not talking about the biological heart. We are actually talking more about the romantic notions of the heart. Courage does reside in your heart but not in the biological heart that serves to pump blood around your body. I don't think in the whole of human history that the biological heart has ever shown any emotion. Or, any thought.

Courage resides in the metaphorical heart. This metaphorical heart is the part of the mind that is not your nemesis.

You can say that this metaphorical heart that we speak about is part of the intelligent side of your mind. The positive aspect of the human mind. This heart that I am asking you to use in your duel with your mind exists, like everything else, in the brain and is itself a part of the mind. But, we like to keep the metaphorical heart and the mind separate for the sake of explanation. The various emotions that we speak about, taking heart, courage etc. all arise from the neural activity of the limbic system - right above the brain stem. So, when a thought or emotion arises, which we associate with our heart, it is simply our brain talking to us in a foreign language. It's the foreign language which makes us think that this voice has come from a different geographical location. But, it has not. Like everything else, this comes from the activity of our brains. Our brains are our organs of behaviour.

It can get complicated to say that our struggles are all in our heads. And they are. The very mind that is the source of our madness can be the source of our salvation. The mind is a paradox. The very circuits in our brains that create meditation can also create madmen. So, courage does exist in us, the geographical location changes depending on how logical you want to be. For the sake of logic, the heart we speak of is metaphorical. For the sake of romance, our biological heart does have emotions and stores the courageous side of our personalities that wishes to make its grand entrance into our lives (it's just not scientifically correct). We only need to open the door to let this courage out so it can fight our demons. Our demons also reside in our minds (doesn't everything?). Essentially our lifelong fight is between the positive aspects of the human mind (courage, heart etc) against the negative parts (fear, ego etc).

## Durga & the Demon Mahisha

In Indian mythology, the *Asuras* are demons that represent the unfavourable parts of the human psyche. They are always up to no good and most, if not all, mythological tales end with Shiva (representing courage – the positive aspects of the mind) defeating these demons and putting them back in their place. If it is not Shiva, then it is Durga (a badass version of his wife Parvati. Just as Bruce Banner becomes The Hulk when he gets mad, Parvati becomes Durga). She slays the demons and she represents our innate qualities. So, your mind is made up of thousands of tiny pesky demons. Your heart has more than enough courage to defeat the 'bad guys'.

It happened. In Mysore, in India, a long time ago.

The demon king Mahisha used to go to war to expand his kingdom. Empowered by a gift from God that meant that no man could kill him (don't ask why he got the gift - that's a different story altogether), Mahisha's power and might was unparalleled. He ruled all over the earth for many years. However, Mahisha did not just conquer kingdoms, he destroyed them. People feared him but they did not know what to do or how to escape his rule. The wounds he inflicted would take centuries to heal. Anyone who stood up against the mighty Mahisha was mercilessly killed. The ruthless Mahisha was not satisfied with conquering the earth. He set his sight on the heavens. He invaded the heavens and defeated Indra, the king of the heavens. Indra's army was defeated, and everyone was driven out.

The people prayed fervently to Parvati (the great goddess of Indian mythology) to come and protect them. They knew that, because of the divine gift that Mahisha had received, only the goddess could overthrow him and restore harmony. One day, the unforgiving Mahisha sat proudly on his throne on earth. Like all great kings throughout history, he portrayed himself as mighty and noble. Yet, the world he ruled over was drowning in bloodshed and oppression. On this particular day, Mahisha heard the sound of footsteps which made the earth quake. Anxiously, he looked around to see who was behind this commotion. He was shocked that someone would make such a racket in his palace. The barbaric Mahisha heard a roar that filled the sky. Then he saw her. At first Mahisha was blinded by light. He covered his eyes in fear but slowly the brightness dimmed, and Mahisha saw the goddess Durga. Her divine form was majestic.

She was the perfect balance of divinity and danger. She was enchanting yet threatening, flawless in her majesty, immaculate yet slightly ruffled, impeccable yet vicious. She was utterly beautiful and enticing. Her glamour seemed forbidden and her presence mesmerising. Mahisha didn't know if he should bow in affection or fight with humility. She aroused his passion, but she also evoked his deepest fears. For a moment there was silence as Mahisha just fixed his eyes on Durga's ravishing form. He remained open mouthed as his body was consumed with lust. Lust soon turned to despair as Durga sat on a lion and let out a chilling roar. The roar was so loud that the earth began to rumble and quake. Durga personified the earth as it shook and broke apart under the violence of her roar. The earth and the mountains began to break up. The powerful vibrations of the roar destroyed everything in their path. This sounds a bit like my Laura after I have eaten the last of our Haribo.

During the upheaval, Mahisha's heart nearly stopped and his army feared for their lives. Durga spoke, "Roar with delight while you still can, O illiterate demon, because when I will kill you, the gods themselves will roar with delight." Then a great battle began between Durga and Mahisha and it raged for nine days. Land was destroyed, armies were killed, the earth was ablaze, and it looked like it has just experienced Armageddon. The stars had fallen from the sky, the moon was no more, and the sun would not set. On the tenth day, Mahisha knew that he could not keep this up any more. Finally, Durga let out a huge roar and jumped from her lion. She leapt on Mahisha and pinned him down. She used so much force that Mahisha was unable to move. Durga then looked at him and with a flash, she brought out her trident. Before Mahisha could even understand what was happening, it was over. Mahisha was no more. Game over. The demon was defeated by the goddess.

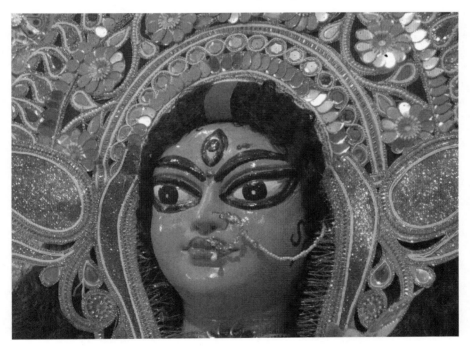

*above — Durga*

*Disciple - Mahisha is short for Mahishasura correct? The anglicised version of that is Mysore (a city in India). So Mahisha was the demon from Mysore? That sounds like...*[3]

Woooooow don't go there. Ashtangi's are very delicate people. Anyway, moving on.

The metaphor behind the story is that over time, Durga has become a symbol of hope for many women from the sub-continent. When Durga slayed the demon Mahisha using her trident, she told every one of her devotees that she had given them all that they require to slay their own demons. Durga used her trident to slay Mahisha. The three spikes of Durga's trident symbolise will, strength and courage. Durga has blessed her devotees with the same three qualities within their hearts (their metaphorical hearts - remember?). She won't appear and destroy your demons, but you have to trust these three qualities to slay the demons that already exist within you. When you call for the goddess Durga, you will find her within yourself.

I read somewhere, or maybe I imagined it, (I don't remember), if one is courageous, if one uses heart, then one is like a house where lamps are lit – the demon Mahisha is afraid to enter. When there are no lamps and the house is dark, Mahisha can enter easily. The person who learns how to show heart, to listen to their heart, is like the house where there is a guard at the door, fully awake. It is difficult for the demon Mahisha to enter. He cannot gather courage because this is not his quality. This is a quality that comes from the heart. The mind wants to enslave your consciousness. The heart can defeat it. The weak part of the mind does not want you to have a heart. Supposedly Nietzsche once said, "One ought to hold on to one's heart; for if one lets it go, one soon loses control of the head too". This is a constant battle between 'heart' and mind until the state of no-mind is reached.

The weakness of the mind will make you feel weak, hopeless and guilty. In the trailer for the new X-Men movies, Professor X says, "The mind is a fragile thing. It takes only the slightest tap to tip it in the wrong direction."

A story. It happened.

A warrior and the son of Shiva, the young Kartikeya came to the holy sage Narada, and asked, "Is there really a paradise and a hell?" "Who are you?" inquired Narada (He knows who he is. He is just doing what wise men do.). "I am a warrior" the young Kartikeya replied. "You, a soldier!" exclaimed Narada. "What kind of ruler would have you as his guard? Your face looks like that of a peacock." Kartikeya became so angry that he began to draw his sword, but Narada continued, "So you have a sword! Your weapon is probably much too dull to cut off my head." As Kartikeya drew his sword Narada remarked, "Here open the gates of hell!" At these words the young warrior, perceiving the master's discipline, sheathed his sword and bowed. "Here open the gates of paradise!" said Narada.

Hell and heaven and not geographical locations, they are products of the human mind.

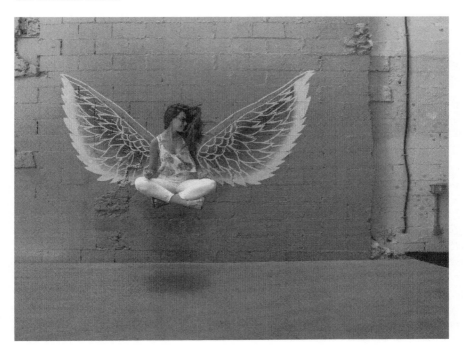

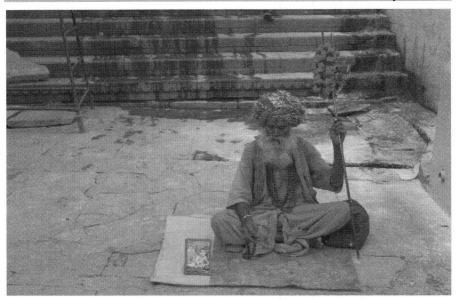

*Disciple - There have been many so-called yogis and holy men who have made claims of enlightenment. Claims of 'seeing' Shiva or 'meeting' Krishna (another God). They have attempted to articulate their experiences and I for one do not believe most of what they say. The few who I believe had experienced the highest reality would not make such cheap claims. So why do these holy men and yogis make such claims?*

The first reason is ego. How can we ever escape from this rascal? He is a shadow that will forever follow us around. Maybe the key to life is to ignore his existence?

Many holy men and yogis from the Indian subcontinent (as well as many other so-called religious men) are blind lost men as I mentioned earlier. They are driven by their egos and their desires. Their egos are fed because they are on display. They wear robes and beads and they place themselves in shop windows. They are deep into how they will be perceived. One holy man wants to be holier that the other.

In the subcontinent, we have the word '*izzat*'. This can be translated to mean reputation. How one wants to be perceived by others. There is nothing in sub-continent culture that is more important than *izzat* (be it for a Muslim, a Hindu or a yogi). For many of these holy men, the pursuit of God is second only to *izzat*. *Izzat* is the greatest display of man's ego. It is the most powerful force in the world. The ego is the part of us that hankers after anything that attracts us. This is our sense of identity. The ego is not a real aspect of ourselves, but it is self-born out of fear and self-denial and then it is watered through years of insecurity. The ego is the most negative aspect of our minds, but ironically, we are always trying to feed our egos. This is particularly true for these 'great' yogis and holy men.

These gurus and yogis play tricks on their students and westerners and all this does is feed their inflated egos, their desires and their bellies. They thrive on the attention they get from vulnerable westerners by being yogis. In an amusing scene in a Bollywood movie I watched recently, the so-called holy men stopped having face-to-face meetings with westerners. They preferred to do their consultations on WhatsApp and get their money through Western Union. They claim to be modern gurus. The scene finishes as these orange-robed men of God high five each other and compare gold watches. It was a scene that was amusing but disturbing. The director is making fun of a situation, which he knows is common in India. This is why I say you should avoid so-called yogis. They are con artists of the highest degree. Don't let the garments fool you. They are as clever as the devil. Ironically the biggest trick or con these men are playing is on themselves. They will never reach meditation they are simply on the verge of madness and it is in this madness (when they get there) that they will probably find their freedom.

One day an illiterate man came to Mullah Nasreddin with a letter he had received. "Mullah Nasruddin, please read this letter to me." Mullah Nasreddin looked at the letter but could not make out a single word. So, he said to the man. "I am sorry, but I cannot read this." The man cried, "For shame, Mullah Nasreddin! You must be ashamed before the turban you wear (i.e., the sign of education)."

Mullah Nasreddin removed the turban from his own head and placed it on the head of the illiterate man, saying, "There, now you wear the turban. If it gives some knowledge, read the letter yourself."

Don't be fooled by the sadhus or holy men or the yogis wearing all their yoga uniforms. Under the robes are naked bodies and under the headwear there is nothing but broken brains.

It happened.

A young doctor named Sam went off to India to find himself. He had suffered a terrible break-up and he wanted to fill the void left in his broken heart. Many months went by and his mother had not heard a word. She was so concerned that she booked a flight to India. She needed to find her son and to bring him back home. Many more months passed, and her search brought her to the wisest guru in India. She was directed to his ashram and told she had to wait another two months before she could have an audience with his holiness. The waiting list was huge. The mother was told that, so important was silence to the great guru, that she was only allowed to utter three words in his presence. Before entering she must bathe in the Ganga and cover her body in orange robes. Once the rituals were done, she waited patiently to see the master. When she was finally ushered in to the private chambers of the wise guru, she said to his holiness, "Sam, come home!"

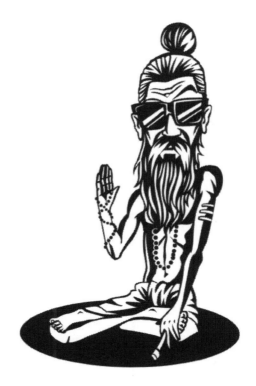

For as long as stupidity remains a human trait, gurus will always exist. The reason this guru needed silence was perhaps, at times, foolishness can sleep very soundly. Any man with a beard and a man bun can become a guru. And the only people more idiotic than this guru will be his followers.

The other reason for such wild claims of God realisation by some of these holy men is simply down to malfunctioning brain circuits (from a science perspective). If a man makes a claim that he sees God or that God sent him a message, there is every chance that he suffered temporal lobe epilepsy. Individuals with this condition often report vivid hallucinatory experiences of a mystical nature, such as an encounter with God. Or, Krishna. Or, Shiva. Or, whatever Godhead the patient has come to associate with his God. So, these encounters with God are actually epileptic seizures. The patient has created a supreme being, a God, in his own mind. The resulting seizure is just his unconscious desire speaking to him.

Hippocrates once said; "People think that epilepsy is divine simply because they don't have any idea what causes epilepsy. But I believe that someday we will understand what causes epilepsy, and at that moment, we will cease to believe that it's divine. And so it is with everything in the universe".

Continuing on the science path for a while, at times, the temporal lobe can trigger a frenzy in the amygdala (the part of the brain that deals with emotions). So, when someone suffers from temporal lobe epilepsy and has a seizure, the amygdala is triggered, which can lead to a feeling of bliss and the absolute meaningfulness of the universe. This encounter with God completely overrides the logical circuits of the brain and convinces the person of an experience with the divine being. Not that I plan on telling someone who says they saw God that they probably had a seizure. That would not be one of my smartest moves. As a quick scientific summary will show, temporal lobe epilepsy is at the root of many kinds of spiritual experiences. Science has an answer to those who make bold claims about God, Shiva or religious realisation.

The neuroscientist V.S Ramachandran has said the richness of our mental life never ceases to amaze him. All our feelings, our emotions, our thoughts, ambitions and importantly, our religious sentiments are all activities of the "little specks of jelly" inside our brains. "There is nothing else", he concludes.

To summarise, people with brains do not know God. And those who claim to know God have no brains.

*"In the event of this kind (seeing god) the door between the subconscious minds opens. What follows is like a dream. People believe it is coming from outside them, but it is actually coming from their subconscious. The voice they hear is real. It speaks to them. But it is their own voice, coming from inside their own mind"[1] —*
*Richard Holloway, A Little History of Religion*

*Disciple - So any guru or yogi who makes claims of reaching samadhi or enlightenment should be ignored? You believe they are all fake? And science would say even those who think they have seen God simply have a brain dysfunction?*

Not all of them of course not. Just most unfortunately.

Once a holy man who was the new holy man in the holiest of towns told Mullah Nasreddin, "I have come out here to make an honest living." "Well," said the Mulla, "There is not much competition."

*Disciple - But many books on yoga talk about the need for a guru. Including Patanjali's Yoga Sutras.*

True. One of the go-to texts for western yogis the Bhagavad Gita also says, "Learn the Truth by approaching a spiritual master. Such an enlightened Saint can impart knowledge unto you because he has seen the Truth. Inquire from him with reverence and render service unto him, bow unto him, be thou unto them a servant."[2]
 We are told that our egos can only be slain by our guru. The way to achieve this is to offer our obedience, humility, devotion and complete openness to whatever our chosen guru gives us or wants for us. There is an absolute need for a guru to show us the way. This is written by a guru, remember? No, thank you, Mr Guru. I would much rather be ego driven and have lost my way than give you any more power. A guru today ties our hands in chains and ties an anvil around our ankles and asks us to swim in his ocean of knowledge. They want us westerners to simply massage their egos and their bank balances. They want the student to be a prisoner their whole life. They will tell them when to eat and what to wear. We are infinite beings with infinite potential, but this infinite nature is imprisoned. The student asks the guru, "What is yoga? What is spirituality?" The real questions should be "What is life? Is this life? Is this my purpose?" We need to lift our heads and look to the sky. Look away from the ground where we are expected to crawl. There is an open sky where we can fly.
 In many respects no guru can teach yoga. Yoga is something to be understood with time. You cannot teach yoga. You can teach the poses of yoga for sure. But not the system of yoga itself. When the poses are taught, it generates an inquiry in the student. And this is all we as teachers can do. We open the door or switch on the lights. When the students develop a hunger, a thirst for yoga, the teacher has done their part. But the modern-day guru (or even the modern-day teacher) does not want you to be enquiring. They want you as an eternal student. The guru has no wish to let his students off his leash.

Aravind Adiga in his book The White Tiger has said, on the subject of how being a faithful servant is considered honourable in India; "Do you know about Hanuman, sir? He was the faithful servant of the god Rama, and we worship Hanuman in our temples because he is a shining example of how to serve your masters with absolute fidelity, love, and devotion. These are the kinds of gods they have foisted on us sir. Understand, now, how hard it is for a man to win his freedom in India."[3]

These men are no longer the gurus of old. Times have changed. The guru no longer exists in my eyes. To use an expression from Nietzsche, the guru is dead. A true guru would never tell you what to do. But he would give you the knowledge with which you could decide what would be best for you to do. But today all gurus just want you to do as they say. It is not about shining a light, it is about being your light, so you are blind without them. The blind are leading the blind into more blindness. These gurus, swamis and religious teachers fear our real identity and our innate nature, and this is why they want to re-dress and even re-name their students. The whole time their student lives under a new name, that student is like a child who is dependent on their parents for survival. Renaming or rebranding a student has nothing to do with yoga. It is one of the oldest psychological tricks in the book. All it does is keep the student subservient to the one who has re-named them. But why change your name under your guru's direction? What is it about you that needs to be changed? There is that word again - *change*. You change your name meaning you take a new identity to make something new or different. But what was wrong with the old you? The old you is the one who got you to the present. It was the old you who survived all the trials and tribulations of life and carried your carcass to this stage of your life. And, your guru sees that. He can see your fortitude and it is this that makes him nervous. He fears your inherent nature. He feels that this innate nature of yours is what will one day no longer need him or will reach the conclusion that he is not what he says he is.

The real you just reminds him of his own forgery and deception. It is all the cunning work of a devil. Or, maybe all that psychoanalysis is mumbo jumbo. The guru probably just thinks you have a silly name. It's one or the other. And what is so wrong with your name anyway? It was probably your mother who gave you that name and out of respect to your mother, the woman who gave birth to you, a guru should never ask you to change your name. The guru or swami is just another clown in this circus we call life.

*"If his Mama named him Clay, I'm gonna call him Clay!" - (referring to Muhammed Ali) - Eddie Murphy's character in the movie Coming to America.*

In the West we have learned and gained knowledge through the Socratic tradition. This means that our education and learning system was influenced by Socrates himself. This western tradition is based on consistently questioning the wisdom that is taught and learned. We do not accept any conclusion until we question and theorise everything until we arrive at our own truth. It is a forum for open-ended inquiry. This method of learning is perhaps Socrates' most important contribution to western thought.

The Eastern or Indian spiritual system is the Guru-Student (or disciple) tradition in which the student gives his body and soul up to his guru in exchange for wisdom, knowledge and/or the absolute truth. The actual word for this is *'parampara'. Parampara* translates as something along the lines of 'succession from guru to disciple'. Ironically, Guru means a dispeller of darkness. The Guru in question is not an ordinary spiritual teacher (or a yoga teacher), but one who has attained union with God and is therefore qualified to lead others to that same goal. The word, disciple, has roots in the Latin word, discipulus, which means learner.

The eastern *parampara* tradition perhaps started as far back as Shiva and Parvati. It could be argued that Shiva was the guru and Parvati was the first disciple or student of yoga. Shiva gave Parvati techniques whereby she could find for herself the answers to the questions she sought. Shiva did not feed her mind with nonsense as is done today.

Shiva did not ask Parvati to wash his feet or to bathe him. He gave her a gentle prod. And that is all. As a result, Parvati was able to leap towards the sky. Shiva was just the conductor of an orchestra, and, as a result, Parvati was able to hear the music that existed already within her own heart. Was Shiva not creating the Socratic tradition himself by simply giving her the methods to educate herself? Shiva did not give any answers or conclusions, just scientific enquiry. Shiva educated by enquiry rather than by giving answers. The modern-day guru does not encourage enquiry, but he wants to give you his answers. He wants to sow nothing but seeds of weakness and inferiority in the minds of his vulnerable devotees. The guru says that God can only be experienced and known through devotion to the guru. Gurus only create slaves, who, over time, are nothing but weak creatures with no sense of identity or self. They say they are killing your ego but all they do is take your self-esteem to feed their own self esteem at a significant price. The student finds that the choices offered are the guru's choices and that their freedom also belongs to their guru. The student becomes a nobody. This man-made system of guru/religious teacher worship must change for man to ever be free. How can we realise our own authentic selves when we are tied in bondage by our so-called gurus?

*"Gurus are no more than the teachers we had at school. You may find them when you need to learn, but you have to outgrow them in order to grow."* [4] *- Indu Muralidharan, The Reengineers*

Why do we westerners go to India and assume each man in his yellow turban (signifying knowledge) is a potential guru? Why are we so sold on his supposed God-realisation? Does our need for a guru-student relationship go back to our childhood? Are we always looking for a father figure throughout our lives? A father figure should mean a biological father, but we seek a more psychological one. Are we just trying to fill a deep void? Does life not have more meaning than just to be a psychological slave?

As get older, we create surrogate fathers to show us our way. Some turn to God as their spiritual father, their guide. Others turn to a guru. Some find a legitimate guru. Others meet Gopal, the delivery driver, and make him their guru. Why do we still feel we are so lost in our adult lives without a surrogate father? Why do we give everything up for these gurus? We are grown men and women. We are adults with responsibilities and well-respected jobs. So why do we make the first Indian with a moustache that we meet our guru? Freud had a theory. He theorised that most people do not really want freedom, because freedom involves responsibility, and most people are frightened of responsibility. We will happily allow a blind man to lead us than walk for ourselves. Are we really that pathetic?

Our psychological need to re-create child-like devotion towards someone is the biggest problem of them all. This state of helplessness we crave, this place of no responsibility and wholehearted faith in someone else is creating a guru worship culture that is doing the exact opposite of its original intention. A guru was needed to support the aspirant as he ascends towards his destination. Now guru worship is nothing more than a foot on the neck of the seeker.

B.K.S. Iyengar was affectionately called Guruji his whole adult life. But he was not a guru. I personally love the man and his teachings. But, I cannot delude myself and call him a guru or even my guru. He was not a realised soul. He was not a Buddha. He was an amazing man with an amazing gift for teaching and inspiring, and he said so himself. I have never heard him refer to himself as a guru. It is us westerners who put him on such a lofty perch. Pattabhi Jois was of the Ashtanga tradition and he was not a guru either. However, Ashtangis all refer to him as 'Guruji'. I appreciate that this is done out of respect but after so many years of being called 'Guruji, Guruji', Mr Jois probably felt he was a legitimate guru. And he was not. He was just a yoga teacher like Wendy from the church hall. He just happened to be Indian and a student of the great Krishnamacharya, who was probably also just a yoga teacher. Pattabhi probably convinced himself that he was a guru and that he could do whatever he wanted. This is exactly what he did.

If you have been raised in the Asian culture, as I have, you witness and hear so much about how these so-called gurus laugh at the naive westerner who goes to India in search of their guru. It's an ongoing joke. The Indian's themselves laugh at their country's so-called yoga gurus. Yet, we westerners think the Asian subcontinent is the spiritual centre of the universe. It may have been at some point in history. But no longer. I remember reading an article in the Guardian by Anuradha Roy. Roy said; "The India I grew up in has gone".

The true God in the Indian Subcontinent is not Shiva or Shakti, it is money. What won't man do for money? Who won't he deceive? These men genuinely believe that money is everything. So, they will do anything and everything for money. These men sell their underage daughters for money and you think they won't rip off the vulnerable westerner as they jet off to find themselves? Swami Vivekananda has said; "Whenever any religion succeeds, it must have economic value". Bill Gates, a few years back, wished to eradicate polio from India. It was a magnanimous gesture. I wonder if anyone will ever rid the subcontinent of this other disease. This disease is dragging the continent backwards.

The Indian subcontinent is not what it used to be. Yoga gurus and spiritual guides are no longer what they used to be. Find a sadhu or a guru, or the hundreds of so-called religious teachers (of all faiths) open his skull and look into his brain and all you will see is the colour of money. The author Aravind Adiga once said, "In a socialistic economy, the small businessman has to be a thief to prosper."

*"You can go to the Indian subcontinent and you are sure to find lots of yoga. But there are very few real yogis" – Guru Zee*

What we have to do today, in 2019, is to walk our own path, with guidance. With someone pointing us in the right direction (a yoga teacher perhaps) and that is all. We need a teacher just to open the door for us and show us our path and nothing more.

In the Prophet, Kahlil Gibran says, "For the vision of one man lends not its wings to another man…No man can reveal to you aught but that which already lies half asleep in the dawning of your knowledge."[5] We no longer need gurus to hold our hands and to lead us down the wrong path. This is what they have been doing for so long. We have to create our own path by simply walking. There is no ready-made path that is just there lying waiting for us. It is just like the sky. The birds fly, but they don't leave any footprints behind or any trail. They just soar. We cannot follow them. We must have the heart to fly all by ourselves.

On the heights near Shiva's abode on Mount Kailash, an old guru stood next to his much younger and naive disciple while they both contemplated the great void of misty space. Referring to the great void, the guru declared, "Ah, my son, one day all of this will be yours."

*Disciple – These godmen, holy men and sadhus are not all bad, are they?*

Absolutely not. I have met some very honourable holy men on my travels. Honest and sincere sadhus and yogis. In Nepal I met more good apples than bad ones. One in particular, to whom Laura and I became very attached. We met in Pokhara. He was a lovely man. You could see the honesty and gentleness in his face. All he wanted was oneness with his Lord. He didn't want anything from us, and it was a struggle to get him to join us for breakfast. He was a special person who we were fortunate to meet. He restored some of my faith in these holy men and in the system of sadhus. Unlike many sadhus who find it difficult to smile, our sadhu had a permanent smile. I would like to think he smiled because Shiva, to whom he had devoted a life of meditation, is not a sad bewildered and disillusioned being. Rather, he is a smiling, dancing and joyful one. His god is the Nataraja (the Lord of Dance). I think it was Nietzsche who said, "I would only believe in a god who could dance." Our sadhu friend was always smiling but he was rare. Most of the sadhus I have met cannot or do not smile. Why have so many sadhus lost their smiles? Maybe it's because deep down they know that their Shiva or their God is just a figment of their imaginations? They are waiting for God to arrive at their abode. There are 100 billion stars in the Milky Way and 170 billion galaxies in the known universe and these holy men think they are so significant that God will arrive and take them away on his divine chariot. The more they pray, the harder they try, the further from reality (ironically) they get. The more penance they perform, the more they come to the realisation that the god they have spent their entire lives worshipping and fearing is just man made. A hallucination or paranoia or fear created phenomenon that has been passed down through generations. For a sadhu, yoga is their religion. In a religion, your seriousness is your credibility. Hence, they do not smile. Or, maybe they are miserable because their robes are too tight. I will investigate more.

So, despite my attack on sadhus, gurus and holy men. I admit there are some very nice and genuine ones. In my experience, and again this is just me sharing my experiences with you, they are few and far between. Most gurus will give you such a strict and difficult sadhana (practice to follow) that your whole energy and effort is spent trying to break through the walls of this task and make progress with this exhausting assignment. While you are consumed with your task, you don't have the time, strength or the foresight to question the so-called wisdom and credibility of your guru. This is the gurus' most Machiavellian, cunning and calculating strategy.

For anyone who wishes to seek a guru one day, or already has one, the hardest thing for you is to make a judgement. How wise is your guru? Can he lead you? Has he seen the way for himself?

There was a yoga guru who fell into the river Ganga while washing away any last remnants of sin. The problem was that he couldn't swim. When a boat came by, the captain yelled, "Do you need help, swami?" The guru calmly said "No, Bhagwan (god) will save me." A little later, another boat came by and a fisherman asked, "Namaste babaji, do you need help?" The Guru, getting ruffled, replied again "No. Mahadev (god) will save me." Eventually the Guru drowned and went to the life after. The 'Guru' arrived at Shiva's abode and asked Shiva, "Why didn't you save me. I am your loyal devotee?" Shiva replied, "Fool, I sent you two boats!"

India is a beautiful country and it has some beautiful people. I feel great love and affinity towards the country of my ancestors. I see my own mother in the women of India, and I see my sisters in all the young ladies. One of my favourite human beings ever, Amitabh Bachchan, also just happens to be Indian. It is just that the fake gurus and swamis living in their glass houses that get on my goat. The way these so-called gurus act and display themselves is what troubles me so much (that and their treatment of women, but that rant may have to be for another day).

Even with Vivekananda and Sadhguru, I still echo the words of Gautama the Buddha, and I question everything they say. I do not doubt, I simply question. This may certainly be a reflection of me and my shortcomings as a person, or more likely, a reflection of society where being realistic is often judged as being pessimistic. Maybe I am a little too harsh. "How can we expect men to rise from poverty and somehow still smell sweet?" Perhaps this is what Kahlil Gibran meant when he said, "For what is evil but good tortured by its own hunger and thirst."[6]

I only ask that you approach the system of yoga gurus with caution and you never allow someone referring to themselves as a swami or a guru to take or assume your power.

*"Over the years the Indian leadership, and the educated Indian, have deliberately projected and embellished an image about Indians that they know to be untrue, and have willfully encouraged the well-meaning but credulous foreign observer to accept it. What is worse, they have fallen in love with this image, and can no longer accept that it is untrue."[7] - Pavan K. Varma (Being Indian: Inside the real India)*

*Disciple - Final question on sadhus. How is it that these men who dedicate their lives to yoga as a means of God-realisation can act so immorally? I have researched the actions of modern gurus over the past 10 years and I am horrified. Why do these so-called men of God, who clearly wholeheartedly believe in God, behave in a manner that is so opposite to their belief?*

Have you heard of Pascal's wager? This is an argument, or a wager, presented by the philosopher Pascal in the mid-1600s. The basic premise is that we should believe in God. Just in case. If we don't believe in him and it turns out the big guy does in fact exist, then we will all burn in hell. When you read some of the biblical descriptions of hell, it does not sound like a place you want to visit. Pascal says that it is logical therefore that we believe in Him, so if he is real, we can spend our afterlife moonwalking with Marilyn in heavenly bliss, as opposed to being molested by Mussolini in depths of a burning hell. If that were a choice, I think most of us would reach for our dancing shoes. So, the argument is that you should believe in God. Just in case.

*"Belief is a wise wager. Granted that faith cannot be proved, what harm will come to you if you gamble on its truth and it proves false? If you gain, you gain all; if you lose, you lose nothing. Wager, then, without hesitation, that He exists."[8] - Blaise Pascal, Pensées*

Many sadhus want to believe in God/Shiva because they have been conditioned to believe. They have been raised as children with a belief in Shiva (and/or Krishna) and they have never dreamed of questioning his existence. When they immerse themselves into their sadhu lifestyles as adults, the time they spend alone allows them to think and to contemplate for themselves for the first time in their lives. During this reflection, a question pops us. What if Shiva does not exist? What if all this penance and hardship turns out to be pointless? Then they slap themselves for daring to question the existence of the blue-skinned one. They ignore their thoughts, have a smoke (a sadhu custom) and forget about that moment of pondering as it never happened. The problem is, the seed of doubt has been planted in the sadhu's foggy brain. He continues through the rest of the career as a wondering holy man in service of God but doubt now remains whether he likes to admit or not. This doubt is the seed of immorality. The sadhu, although still in service of Shiva, believes in Shiva and believes that faith in Shiva will save him from an eternity of re-births (the suffering cycle of Hinduism). However, there is a part of him now that thinks - "What if Shiva or God does not exist?" So, he performs his first immoral act based on this thought. Then, when there is no obvious or immediate repercussion, the holy man continues to act more and more immorally as time goes on. He does so because his belief is now only half as strong as it was. He either believes in God, or, he acts like a degenerate in case there is no God. Or, he behaves with no scruples, and then he acts like a good man just in case God does exist. He is trapped in a paradox. In Pascal's wager.

*"What I wanted to express very clearly and intensely was that the reason these people had to invent or imagine heroes and gods is pure fear. Fear of life and fear of death."[9] - Frida Kahlo*

This is not just limited to the sadhus, the so-called Muslim men in Pakistan who abuse children. Much has been made of this in the press over the past few years. A case in point is the horrific rape and murder of the young girl, Zainab. Her attacker was a regular at the mosque and lived and breathed and dressed as a Muslim. To the casual observer, Islam was in his blood and bones. But, deep in his heart, he knew he didn't really believe in God. He was only going to the mosque as a precaution. He was going just in case God exists. The crazy thing about all of this is that since any god worth believing in, or the gods these men believe in, would prefer an honest disbeliever rather than a calculating degenerate who claims a belief. How do these men go through life so blindly? Who is it that they are deceiving?

These degenerates are the most vile and inhumane beings ever born. Blame it on the devil. Or, blame it on man. Sometimes there is no justification. There is no devil. There is no reason. There is just pure evil. I was once told that the reason human beings are bad is because they have no desire to be good. They are as they are.

You may feel like at this juncture we have got side tracked off the subject of yoga, but we are still very much on track. This chapter on gurus and godmen is the most specific chapter to this book.

Yoga: Madness of Meditation?

When someone goes to the subcontinent in search for themselves, what is it that you think they find? Madness or meditation? With the so-called godmen waiting to rip you off, amongst other things, what is it that you expect to discover? I have always been baffled by those who wish to find themselves. What is it that you think you will find in that faraway land? Go for the weather, go for the food, go to do yoga, yes, but don't go in search for yourself as all that we seek already exists within. To use that word again, all it takes is introspection.

I do not believe that 'meditation' can be discovered in modern times in the presence of a guru. In the presence of a "realised" guru, yes, but not the fancy self-made gurus that plough through the subcontinent like cows in the street. You are probably more likely to garner wisdom and sanity talking to the cows than you are the so-called enlightened men of god.

There is a myth that tells is that at the dawn of time, Shiva became angry at his loyal disciple Nandi and discarded him to earth. The faithful Nandi was told he must live at a specific place of worship in the Indian subcontinent. This sacred place of worship supposedly the centre of the spiritual world has a thousand steps. Each day, Nandi is allowed to climb the steps alongside a pilgrim. If a pilgrim is able to make it all the way to the top step, this will signify - 'enlightenment' for the seeker. Nandi cannot ascend alone. He can only climb alongside a pilgrim. If Nandi is able to reach the top twice, he will be returned to his former-self and only then will he be allowed back to the heavens.

The myth says to this day, Nandi has only been to the top once. That occasion was when he walked alongside the Buddha. To this day, the poor Nandi is still waiting to walk alongside a pilgrim who can make it to the top, to the peak of human consciousness. The outside world to Nandi is a disheartening enigma. Nandi waits heavyhearted and demoralised.

The myth is telling us of enlightenment and what a rare occurrence this is. This is not a 200-hour Alliance verified teacher training. This is the experience of the highest reality. The highest state of consciousness. In enlightenment man is in the presence of the cosmos. Blessed is he who has walked into the unknown.

It is said a thousand pilgrims walked those stairs every day and only one man in thousands of years was able to reach the top. This is the complexity of enlightenment. This is what you must experience for you to be a true 'Guru'. You must have seen or known the way for you to lead others. You must have sat in the very presence of 'god'. You must have died and been reborn. Spiritually speaking.

There must be no difference between you and a Shiva. Between you and a Buddha for you to be a guru.

Yet in every corner of the world you will find men who make claims of 'enlightenment' waiting for you to call them 'guruji'. The psychologist Steve Taylor (author of The Leap) has said that best thing a spiritual seeker can do is avoid yoga gurus.

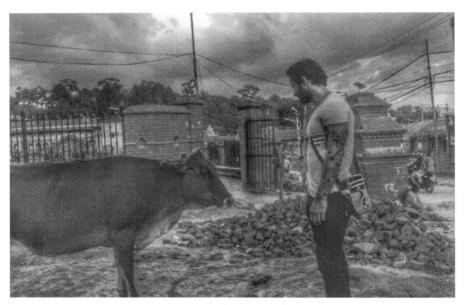

*Above - Conversing with a "yogi". Never has more sense been spoken.*

The reality is that man's desire, and the ego of man has made it near impossible for us to trust anyone who talks of enlightenment. Trust is the hardest thing to give but knowing who to trust has never been harder.

I was once told; "Nobody knows all the answers to the mysteries of the universe. For your own sake, be wary of anyone who claims they do".

# Chapter 8 - Understanding the Mind Via The Bhagavad Gita

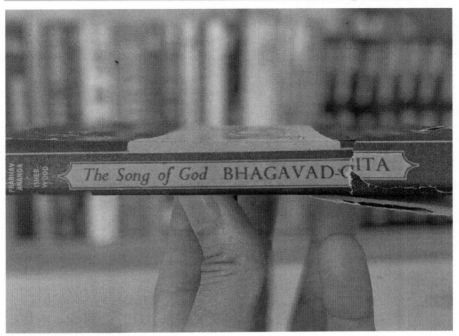

I have grown up surrounded by Hindu culture and have been seeing and reading about the various Hindu gods ever since I saw my first Bollywood movie as a child. In the 1973 classic, *Deewar*, Amitabh Bachchan's character Vijay visits a Shiva temple, and that is the first time I was exposed to Hindu iconography. And although I never believed them to be god in my own heart, I have been fascinated with the culture of these man-made gods ever since. If anyone wishes to learn more about the God culture in India, I would highly recommend the Bollywood movie PK. It was part of the Netflix schedule the last time I checked. It's a brilliant, astute, yet totally rational way of seeing the gods as they are viewed in India today. Just don't judge this movie on the songs. They are truly awful.

There is a great conflict within Indian ideals, and they revolve around the words of a 'god'. Or more specifically, the song of a "god". I am referring to a book that western yogis love to sit and discuss at their book clubs while they ponder and smile as the passages are all recited. The book in question is the 'Song of God' or the Bhagavad Gita. I do not get on with it completely, but I cannot ignore certain parts of its philosophy that aims to help us better understand the psychological battle we are all in with our minds. It is not the literal word of god as no such thing exists.

"God" in this book is simply used as a metaphor.

Tradition says that 5000 years ago, two branches of the same race were about to go to war over the right to rule the Indian empire. The war was between the *Pandavas* and the *Kauravas*. Just before he proceeded with what was referred to as a "holy war" (*dharma yudha*), the archer Arjun, who represents the *Pandavas*, was in great conflict. He did not know what to do. His heart had given way and he did not want to proceed with the war because the army on the other side was full of his old friends, family and even his old teachers. They all represented the same race, and for Arjun, this war was madness. Such is life that he had arrived at a time where he must fight them and even kill those who he once held dearly for so long. Arjun understood that there are conceivably many causes worth fighting and potentially dying for, but there appeared to be no causes for Arjun worth killing for. Such was the nobility of the man. Arjun dropped his famous bow and declared that he would rather be a slave of war than take the life of another man. He did not wish to fight, so he sought counsel from his cousin Krishna.

"Why go to war?" Krishna responded, "Arise, O Prince! Give up this faint-heartedness, this weakness! Stand up and fight!"[1]. For the remainder of the Gita, Krishna reminded Arjun of his duty and educated him on "Hindu dharma". You could call this the law of Hinduism. Within Hinduism, no man truly dies. Krishna says, "Though this body has its beginning and end, the dweller in the body is infinite and without end"[2]. His soul would be reborn, so there should be no fear in killing. All he would be doing is upholding his duty and responsibility. Krishna reminds Arjun that a warrior's "religion" is to fight. He warned Arjun that he was becoming weak. A warrior needed to show heart.

As Arjun continued to ponder war, Krishna, his charioteer, spoke to him and more or less said, "I know you well, Arjun. I have known you very personally and intimately as a great warrior. And I know you better than you know yourself; your innate nature is that of a warrior. And so, I am just reminding you of it. I tell you who you are. Know it rightly and then do what you choose to do".

Arjun explains (referring to war), "It is painful to kill my own people. I won't kill them even for the sake of a kingdom and a king's throne. I would rather go begging in the streets, rather commit suicide rather than kill my relatives, friends and teachers who are on the other side". For the next eighteen chapters of this book, or song, Krishna waxes lyrical on the merits of going to war and mentions devotion, karma, duty and more. And finally, when he cannot convince Arjun of his duty to fight, uses "divine intervention" to get his message across. He proclaims himself to be god incarnate and says, "It is God's will! You cannot get out of the war. What God has chosen has to happen". So, Arjun eventually agrees to war recognizing his dharma, which refers to his duty and or responsibility to his innate or essential nature.

The great Swami Vivekananda's commentary is as follows; "Let the whole world stand against us! Death means only a change of garment. What of it? Thus fight! You gain nothing by becoming cowards. Taking a step backward, you do not avoid any misfortune. You have cried to all the gods in the world. Has misery ceased? The masses in India cry to sixty million gods, and still die like dogs. Where are these gods? The gods come to help you when you have succeeded. So, what is the use? Die game. This bending the knee to superstitions, this selling yourself to your own mind does not befit you, my soul. You are infinite, deathless, birth- less. Because you are infinite spirit, it does not befit you to be a slave. Arise! Awake! Stand up and fight! Die if you must. There is none to help you. You are all the world. Who can help you?"[3]

So, the scene has been set. Both sides are about to go to war. Arjun is apprehensive and does not want to fight. Krishna explains to Arjun that it is his responsibility to fight and go ahead with this war as planned. It could be argued that the whole book is just a metaphor for a man trying to understand his own struggle through life. It is said that the battlefield represents the physical body itself. Arjun is the representation of the soul - the perfectly polished diamond that is lost in the chaos of the human body. The horses are symbolic of the senses and finally, Krishna is Arjun's consciousness and intelligence. This is the constant war that man is fighting from birth. From the womb to the tomb, man is in conflict and at war within himself until he is able to defeat himself and recognize his own divinity via listening to or recognizing his 'consciousness'. The soul, or the diamond that is Arjun, is unaware of his divine nature. Through the context of the dialogue, the intelligent voice inside his own head, which is his consciousness (Krishna), speaks to him and tries to help him understand through the concept of duty and righteousness that he is in fact, a perfectly luminous soul. He is a diamond and once he can work this out, the realisation will hit Arjun unexpectedly, and he will know that he is of divine nature as are we all. His soul belongs to the universal soul. Arjun has the spark of divinity within him.

Krishna is just a metaphor and not an actual being. To think Krishna has stated that you should all have a statue of him in your yoga studio simply for your salvation is slightly insane and profoundly missing the point of what could be a very clever metaphor. Krishna's message for Arjun are not universal but very specific for Arjun and for his own individual growth. This implies that that the revelation is not from god itself but the part of Arjun that is divine (his own consciousness). Essentially, this dialogue occurs in the fascinating conflict of Arjun's own brain. The verbal exchange may have seemed to last an eternity, but it actually took place in a few short moments as Arjun contemplated his obligations before going to war. In Arjun's brain, his pesky mind was fearful of war and tried to convince Arjun that he should walk away while there was still time. His mind tried to persuade Arjun that life as a slave to his enemy was better than that of a murderer. The other part of Arjun's brain, his consciousness, later explained to him that there is no death in the grander scheme of things - in Indian culture, no one ever really dies. The soul is infinite and will always be reborn. It is just the physical body that turns to dust. There is no sin in fighting this war as Arjun is not murdering to gratify his sick innate nature, rather he is simply fighting for honour and freedom. This is Arjun's "dharma". His consciousness explains that sometimes an act we consider bad can ultimately result in good.

*Disciple - So how does the dialogue between an archer and his charioteer, Arjun and Krishna, on the battlefield help us understand the human mind?*

It is said that if we want to be passive with our lives, we will end up like Arjun. You see Arjun is a simple and good man, a man with a good heart. He does not want to get involved in any conflict. At the point of going to war, he is filled with uncertainty as he does not want to go to war. He is caught in a conflict in his mind between responsibility (to fight) and his feelings on what is right and wrong. This is similar to our own conflicts. We are undecided about our own battle with our minds. Arjun is so caught up in this struggle: he feels that choosing war will forever chase and haunt him and choosing not to fight will completely delude him. He is in a desperate conflict that is echoed by the sadness on his face. The once luminous Arjun is now a shell of his own self. Arjun's doubts and fears about going to war could have enslaved him. They would also have enslaved everyone else around him too as he was the leader. Students and apprentices (or in this case, soldiers) are reflections of their teacher or leader. The central message is that man should strive to be more like Krishna. Krishna in this story acts as Arjun's consciousness and talks to him of why he should go to war.

Essentially, Krishna is the voice in Arjun's head that is the intelligent part of the mind - the part that is often clouded by the rest of the mind. Arjun is the visible part of one's consciousness, the body.

Krishna, on the other hand, is the invisible part of the body, the consciousness. When Arjun is in a vast space of anxiety and worry, he is trapped in his own paradox, somewhere between duty and death. If Arjun represents this anxiety and confusion, Krishna is a celebration of life. He is literally the other side of the coin. Krishna wants Arjun to remove his metaphorical veil and see life as it is.

Despite not being a warmonger, Krishna was determined to go ahead with the war. He reminds Arjun that "This is all play acting; killing or dying is only a drama". He also speaks to Arjun of his responsibility, his position in life and what he is ultimately worthy of. His dharma or duty unto himself is to be the very best version of himself. In doing so, he may have gone to war, but this way, he was never enslaved.

I feel like there is a parallel here with the battle we have with our own minds. Many students of yoga can be too passive with themselves and their bodies (I know I have been there). They don't quite appreciate how amazing or divine (as Krishna says) their bodies are designed to be. The way I see it, they enslave themselves and I have witnessed their insecurities also enslaving others. This is especially the case with yoga teachers who do not practice certain poses and in doing so, limit the advancement of their students. They literally enslave their students and keep them within the safe parameters of their minds.

Perhaps, going to war is the correct metaphor. You go to war with your mind and you push yourself, so you never become enslaved. Of course, you also don't want to become bloodthirsty as many did during the Mahabharata War; instead, you should seek to find the middle way. You simply need to find the courage to fight the war within yourself.

Imagine you are Arjun and in class, you are told that we are about to do a headstand or a "tricky" arm balance. Listen as your mind tries to talk you out of it. The yoga teacher is the voice of Krishna. He or she desperately believes in you and your self-worth. There is a conflict: Do you listen to your own mind and be enslaved in your insecurity or do you listen to your teacher who only wants to elevate your awareness of who you are and what you are worthy of? Staying within your own conflict and insecurities does not just affect you in that moment in time on your yoga mat. It has a much greater consequence. Not going to war does not mean the war will not happen. What this means is you are inviting others to also wage war on you. Being passive before a pose may psychologically affect you at a much later time after we have left our yoga mats. Does this clinging to insecurity invite others to wage war on us - at home or at work? When you achieve a certain pose for the first time, your body language reflects this. It is obvious. You dance like a young Krishna, singing and laughing. When you fail or don't even try, does this reflect on your body language or in the way others perceive you? It does because we observe this ourselves on others.

Very few teachers teach "advanced" poses because they want to show off what they can do themselves; most teachers who get to this stage just want to inspire you. My Laura or a Claire Berhorst (who teaches at my studio) say, "Look what I can do! All it took was faith (in myself) and practice!" We too can do all the things we see the "show off" yoga teachers do. Are we an Arjun or a Krishna? It's our journey. It's our war.

*"Your mind can be either your prison or your palace. What you make it is yours to decide" - Bernard Kelvin Clive, Your Dreams Will Not Die*

*Disciple: Can reading Bhagavad Gita help me, the modern-day yoga student, in other ways too?*

It's difficult to say. I don't think I can give you the answer until you yourself find a parallel between the Gita and your own life. I was at a loss for so long as to how reading the Gita could or would help me. Then I found my answer while reading Light on Life by B.K.S. Iyengar. Although not my own experience, I read for the first time how relative Krishna's Gita can be and the inspiration it can provide.

B.K.S Iyengar says; "Everyone sometimes finds themselves in the awful dilemma when every course of action or behaviour seems to be wrong. Arjuna, in chapter 2 of the Bhagavad Gita is on the horns of such a dilemma. To do nothing is an action too, with inevitable consequences, and so that is not a way to escape pain and suffering either. With Krishna's help, Arjuna follows the path of dharma, of the science of religious duty, and so reconciles what is on the human and material level, irreconcilable. In my own youth, it seemed impossible to be accepted by my students and by my family. But by persevering on the yogic path, I attained a level at which I am not only accepted but even now honoured by my students and my family. This would have been impossible without the evolution that yoga provided."[4]

So just because the Gita does not add up or make sense now, life experience tells me that at some stage you will find relevance whether it's an indirect experience or not.

*Disciple: Not to overly digress from the subject of the mind, can I ask some questions regarding the Bhagavad Gita itself, seeing as we are on this subject?*

*I have read the Gita in the past and struggle with some of the overly religious content (although I appreciate it not referring to god itself but being more of a metaphor). The Gita can itself be sometimes contradictory and confusing, correct?*

It is the same for me and many other people I know. I have found that you do not necessarily need to read the whole of the book to find some inspiration. I have often found myself more put off by Krishna than the entire Gita as a text, but that does not stop me from finding meaning within the text itself. Maybe the problem lies with my own understanding of the Krishna character.

Perhaps I have failed to understand him in the same way that I have struggled to understand myself over the years. Jung once said, "Everything that irritates us about others can lead us to an understanding of ourselves".

Since I first saw the image of Krishna as a child on Zee TV, I have been intrigued by him. I have been looking for faults in Krishna and, with time, I have come to understand that the faults I find are simply faults that man himself has given Krishna (through the various stories) and are no fault of the "man" himself. Maybe I have lacked the maturity to understand him. Just because I failed to understand Krishna does not mean that Krishna is at fault. This reflects on me. I remember trying to read and understand the complex mathematical system that is "Kashmir Shaivism". This is a Shiva-worshipping culture from Kashmir. Supposedly, it is the world's oldest religion. I was intrigued, as my family is from Kashmir and I felt obligated (for some strange reason) to simply understand it. I was desperate to, at minimum, comprehend the fundamentals of what looked like very complicated system. After a few attempts at reading and absorbing the works of Swami Lakshmanjoo, I became fed up and irritated and remember saying that this work is all nonsense. That it doesn't make any sense. My wife, the wise oracle that she is, very eloquently (as always) pointed out that my failure to understand the text is not a reflection on the text but more a reflection on me. Perhaps I am simply not ready in so many different ways to understand the intricacies of this system. Just because we fail to understand something does not mean that an explanation does not exist. And she was right. I believe that Krishna falls into that same category.

Maybe, over time, I will learn to separate the myth from the man and appreciate the character of Krishna for the way he is meant to be and not the way my limited maturity sees him.

I was reading A History of Western Philosophy by Bertrand Russell some time ago and came across a passage that perhaps sums up more than anything else my often-limited understanding of what others argue is a very profound scripture. Russell says, "A stupid man's report of what a clever man says can never be accurate, because he unconsciously translates what he hears into something he can understand"[5].

So yes, the Gita can be confusing for whatever reason. But a casual read of the Gita without overly seeking meaning will help you find meaning and inspiration, I believe. Like so many things in life, it is down to our over-eagerness for answers that we miss obvious truths. I know that to be the case with me. The Gita of Krishna, it has been said, requires a lifelong immersion for one to fully absorb and understand its secrets and often the wisdom that is very obviously on the surface. It's just hard to comprehend when so many of us read with our limited understanding of the subject. But as my friend and yoga academic Daniel Simpson has pointed out to me, perhaps the Gita is not meant to make sense as a whole – in that one aspect of it will appeal to some more than others.

Ultimately, the Gita and Krishna remain confusing to me at times because I was not raised with the Gita as my Bible and with Krishna as my god, therefore the text is not speaking to me. You see, I can appreciate a love song if it was written for someone else, but would the person who the song was written for hear the words in the same way as me? The words of a love song written for someone would penetrate their soul. It would enter their hearts and reach their core. I would simply hear the superficial words that only reach my ears. It can be argued that I will never fully understand a love song written for someone else in the same way that I will perhaps never fully understand Krishna and his words because it was never meant for me. The casual Western yoga student who reads the Bhagavad Gita needs to understand this too. The Gita is a love song that perhaps was never meant for you, either. So read the Gita if you wish, but don't go looking for answers, meaning and inspiration. If parts of the Gita are meant for you, it will find you at the right time.

Gandhi once said, "The Gita is not for those who have no faith".

*Disciple - How much of Krishna's words do you think are lost in translation?*

The Gita is hard and near impossible to fully understand because you and I can only read words. We can only read the words of man. These man-made words will always contain flaws within them, because man is not perfect. So, is there any surprise when grown pundits have Gita debates and it all ends in tears? Arjun understood the word of god because Krishna appeared before him. He experienced Krishna and was able to absorb his words and feel his presence (if the whole thing actually happened, of course). Arjun was captivated by the man more so than his words. This is how Arjun was able to fathom the wisdom of Krishna. Maybe that is where we go wrong? When Laura and I watch a Bollywood movie and Amitabh Bachchan gives his customary poignant and heart-breaking speech, I am always frustrated with the subtitles. Laura reads the subtitles and I hear Bachchan's voice. Bachchan's words are so powerful that I feel them in my bones. I can feel the pain in his voice and see the agony in his bloodshot eyes. I am mesmerised by his onscreen presence (I am referring to his speech on stage in Mukaddar Ka Sikander). Laura, on the other hand, is emotional in spite of reading only the subtitles that have not captured any of the heartbreak and poetic nature of the dialogue. The subtitles are very direct in English, and so much of the sincerity is lost. As an example, at one point, Bachchan's character Sikander says, "When I first became aware of life, I had neither a mother's lap to lay my head on nor a fathers security... The footpaths replaced a mother's warmth and I was accompanied through life by hunger and poverty". You know what the translation said? "I had no parents and I lived in poverty". Strictly speaking, that is not an incorrect translation, but at the same time the heart of the dialogue has been taken away. I was aching for Sikander, yet the casual observer would not see what the big deal is. The translation is so direct, it makes the characters devoid of life and charm. Even my English translation word for word fails to capture the emotion of the dialogue once it has been taken away from its original language.

There is another iconic scene from the 1983 movie Coolie where Bachchan's character, on the verge of being killed, says, "Tere haath mein maut ka samaan hai toh mere seene pe khuda ka naam hai... chala golee!" When I first heard that dialogue as a child I was mesmerised. On the brink of death, he utters the most exquisite dialogue I had ever heard. We were kids and I remember my English friend Mark Welsh asking me, "What does it mean? What does it mean?" And I was at a loss to explain. I didn't and still don't have the artistry or the poetic nature to translate it without compromising everything that is so sublime about the dialogue. For anyone who understands the dialogue, how can you seriously explain it without it sounding corny and dumb? In English, it roughly translates to, "If you have an item of death in your hands, then I have God's name on my chest... So fire your weapon!" You see what I mean? You are probably thinking, "Really? What is so sublime about that?" My response would be, "Exactly!".

Sometimes the original should be left untouched and unblemished by man's constant need to understand and add his own commentary. It's ok sometimes to leave things as they are. But such is the ego of man.

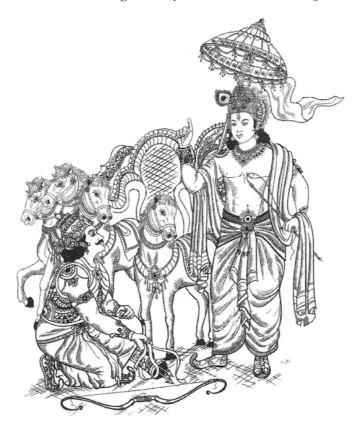

*above - Krishna standing talking to a kneeling Arjun during the 'Song of God'*

This, in a weird way, is the same as the Gita. We want to hear Krishna and we are all aimlessly reading the subtitles and what we are left with is a jumbled up and very direct translation that loses most of its magic, eloquence and beauty. Word has it, especially from The Hare Krishna Group, that one is required to be a sincere devotee of Krishna to fully understand his words. "You must have a feminine receptivity to Krishna's words. You have to allow Krishna words to impregnate you". Those are the literal words I have heard from a 'guru' of the 'International Society for Krishna Consciousness'. Unless you do so, his words are lost. It is like a blind man trying to read a map. All you have are blind interpretations.

Like I said, I don't think that the Gita was meant to be fully understood by us. Inspiration is definitely there; it can sometimes take time to rise to the surface. The point is, don't think you are expected to understand the whole thing.

*Disciple: Krishna asks Arjun to submit to Krishna. To submit to the "whole". Why must Arjun surrender to Krishna on the brink of war? Why submit to "god" or the understanding of a higher being/reality/consciousness as a means to prepare for the upcoming conflict? What wisdom is Krishna trying to instill in Arjun before Arjun goes to war?*

It is said that the true sign of a man's power is the measure of his surrender. Krishna wants Arjun to drop his attachment to the world and to all his actions and surrender to him because, through this submission, there is no ego. If there is no ego, there is a state of "no mind". In this state of illumination, Arjun can see the world for what it actually is. A drama. A play. A hallucination and nothing more. Once Arjun comes to the realisation that what awaits him (the war) is not "real", he will uphold his duty as a warrior and fight this war. All of Arjun's fears would have left him in an instant. Arjun would no longer fear killing his family and friends (and killing in general) because it dawns on him that no one will really die, anyway. All of life is a cosmic theatrical piece with Lord Krishna as the divine architect.

Krishna informs Arjun that he cannot be attached to a life that does not belong to him. How can you be attached to something and claim it as yours when it is so dependent on the universe for survival? Can a human survive without oxygen?

Can man survive without water? Can life itself survive without the sun? This is all nature. Man is dependent on external forces for survival, so how can we think that this body belongs to us? It belongs to that which it cannot survive without – nature. We cannot be attached to that which we have zero control over. If the sun never shines again, if the sun went cold tomorrow or if it was extinguished, how long can the human species or life itself survive?

On the subject of the Sun, Sadhguru has said, "This body is a piece of Earth powered by the sun. You are a solar powered life. If the sun does not come up tomorrow, the scientific data says in eighteen hours' time, all the water in the oceans, your blood, your brain – everything – will be frozen solid"[6].

The sun is nature's work. Water is nature. Oxygen is nature, and without nature man would not exist. Life could not sustain itself. Einstein has said, "A human being is a part of the whole, called by us universe, a part limited in time and space. He experiences himself, his thoughts and feeling as something separated from the rest, a kind of optical delusion of his consciousness".

So Krishna says don't be attached to this body that in many ways does not belong to you. It belongs to nature. Or, in the context of the Gita, it belongs to Krishna, as he is the embodiment of the universe. He is nature and the cause of nature. Each atom and each cell in the universe are a reflection of Krishna. So, give it to me, he says. Man did not create man. Something else "out there" created man. We may not believe in god, but we believe that something supernatural is the architect. We didn't design and make ourselves. There is a divine architect that is the source of creation. We have no say in our role in the cosmos. It could be taken from us as easily as it was given. According to the wisdom of Krishna, only a man who has removed his attachment to life can see the bigger picture and perform his duties as an instrument of nature.

*"Man is the most insane species. He worships an invisible God and destroys a visible Nature, unaware that this Nature he's destroying is this God he's worshiping." – Hubert Reeves*

According to Krishna, surrendering will transcend Arjun's struggles. Surrender is beyond the ego. I have heard before that surrender is synonymous with serenity. Serenity is the state of being calm, peaceful and untroubled.

We have spoken about Shiva's 112 techniques to attain a higher reality and go beyond the mind. Maybe this is Krishna's one and only method. For Krishna, nothing else is needed to attain the highest reality but "surrender". According to Krishna, Arjun can experience Nirvana, Samadhi, Bhairava, his true reality if he surrenders and submits his will wholeheartedly, whereby not a trace of Arjun is left behind.

This idea of surrender has helped one of my students recently. She has read the Bhagavad Gita since childhood, but she never really found meaning or inspiration. Lately she has been in a real war or battle with her troublesome son. Her husband and her are battling a raging war with their son for various reasons, and both parties are on the edge of madness as a result. After discussing the Gita with me, my student all of a sudden came to the realisation that the root of the problem is that she is overly attached to her son. Not only attached, but dangerously attached, according to her. She had to see her teenage son as not just something that belongs to her, but a child of nature just traveling through her. When she was able to see this bigger picture, her husband

and her were able to give their son the space he desperately needed. Remember, Krishna more or less says that only when man has removed his attachment to life, can he see the bigger picture and perform his duties as an instrument of nature.

In the Prophet, Kahlil Gibran has said; "Your children are not your children. They are the sons and daughters of Life's longing for itself"[7]

This is just a specific example of why one should read and just allow the wisdom to reach us when we are ready and not feel like meaning should always be there for us right away. I have been guilty of this more than anyone else. I constantly reject something when it does not talk to me right away. The reality, again, is that it will talk to you when it is relevant to your life.

*Disciple: The Gita can be a bamboozling read if you struggle (in general) with the word "god", etc. Is any pre-reading required before one sits down with a cup of Earl Grey and starts to read this book?*

Many people I have met and many commentaries I have read emphasised the need to fully understand the complexities of the Sanskrit language and the writing of the author, Vyasa, before they read the Gita. Part of the confusion (or even ignorance) lies in not understanding the writing style. "Realised" yogis or those who claim to have an insight on the Gita say that it also requires the wisdom of a god-realised guru to fill in the gaps. It is not as straightforward a text as implied by some.

I have met some scholars and yogis who say that the Gita sold without an accompanying commentary is part of the reason why there is so much delusion and ignorance regarding the text. There are many religious teachings within this text, but there is also much universal wisdom. Through your own engagement in yoga and your examination of the Gita, you will find explanations and interpretations for yourself. And you can then decide, after much soul searching, just how relevant the Bhagavad Gita is for you. Don't be distressed if reading the Gita leaves you feeling puzzled and perplexed. Getting lost along the way is part of the journey in trying to wrap your brain around the often bewildering "philosophy" of yoga. It is worth remembering that some beautiful paths can't be discovered without first getting lost.

I used to find the Gita baffling and, at times nonsensical. But writing my thoughts, hearing myself out loud and having discussions has helped me see things with more clarity. I used to be against Krishna and the Gita, and now I am not. I believe that time has brought me maturity, and that is what yoga students often dismiss: The time it can take for the knowledge to penetrate.

Over time, as life evolves and maturity develops, opinions will change as various thoughts and philosophies enter our minds. I don't have the same opinions on certain subjects today as I had a year ago. Life is constantly schooling me and proving me right or wrong. So not only do you have to give reading time to penetrate your mind, you also have to expect that, over time, opinions and views will change. This is growth.

Muhammad Ali has said, "The man who views the world at 50 the same as he did at 20 has wasted 30 years of his life". The yoga teacher who teaches the same way today as she did a year ago is wasting her talents. The thinker who has the same opinion today as he did a few years ago is exhausting his growth. Life evolves, and so should we.

*"The snake which cannot cast its skin has to die. As well the minds which are prevented from changing their opinions; they cease to be mind."*[8] *— Friedrich Nietzsche*

*Disciple: Some people do genuinely believe that Krishna from the Gita is real and is God itself. The supreme figure of godhead. He is not a metaphor for consciousness to these devotees, correct?*

Yes. There are many groups and cultures who believe that Krishna is very real, and this war actually took place. But don't let that put you off from reading the text and finding some value. Read the Gita and decide for yourself whether you see Krishna as an obvious metaphor or if you see him as God in human form. There are plenty of Western yoga teachers who also think that Krishna was a real "personality" and have statues of him in their 'studios'. I find it mind boggling that they think that, but then some Star Wars fans think the 'Jedi' are real too. I guess we all want to believe in something. In traditional yoga circles, the belief in Shiva or Krishna as God is prised. It is very much ingrained in everyday life as you can see and experience for yourself whilst in India.

The western yoga student/teacher who wants a sense of belonging feels it is in their best interest to believe in Krishna whether they truly do or not. It just helps the western student/teacher fit into what they think is the yogic ideal.

*Disciple: You obviously think Krishna is just a metaphor?*

Respectfully, yes.

When I imagine Krishna, I see a man with blue skin standing in the streets of India wearing a crown of peacock feathers encrusted with diamonds and gold. His body is covered in the finest yellow silk. He is playing his flute as his wives all dance around him, open-mouthed at his splendour.

Captain America in The Avengers says; "There's only one God... And he doesn't dress Like that."

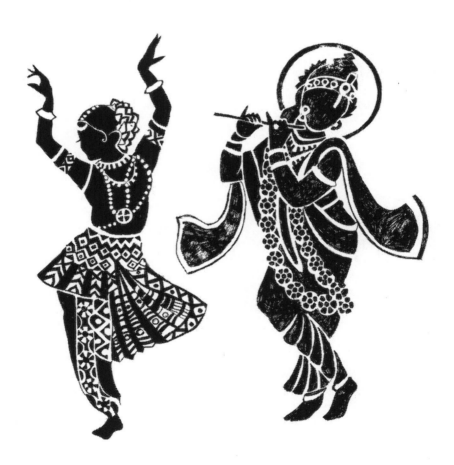

*Disciple: So, it's ok if I don't believe Krishna was real or if I find the Gita perplexing and not for me? Or will I go to yoga hell for not liking it?*

Yoga students need to have the courage and faith within themselves to disregard anything that does not agree with their way of thinking at that time. This is not being rude this is just being honest and staying true to who you are. So, if I came to a teacher training and you taught me the Gita and told me that Krishna is my salvation, am I to just sit there with a fake smile and nod along the whole time (even if parts of it do not agree with my upbringing/religion/way of thinking etc.)? Do I grin along in fake approval, or do I have a responsibility unto myself to speak up when something does not sound right? Many students out of respect for the Indian/yoga tradition feel that they have to embrace the Gita in the same way that they have to embrace the *Hatha Yoga Pradipika*. But is it disrespectful if you think that these texts are unclear and not relevant to you (at that time)? Am I being disrespectful to a tradition I myself am so immersed in? If you think I am disrespectful, then consider the irony! Why should I believe in Krishna? Should I be a passive Arjun and just stay quiet and go along with what is being said, or should I be brave like a Krishna and uphold the responsibility I have to myself? Being dismissive of parts of the Indian/yoga culture is not rude if it does not agree with your way of thinking, who you are and how or where you were raised. Look at the huge irony of lost and confused Westerners in India learning about the science of self-realisation, yet they all no longer have a sense of their real self. If you believe in Krishna, then believe in his words when he tells you to stand up and be brave. Stand up and say that in the logic of the Western mind, Krishna is not God incarnate who came to Earth in human form for man's salvation.

Will it come across as rude to a believer in Krishna when I say that due to my upbringing and my own education (be it limited!), I cannot believe in his existence? Therefore, it is for these reasons that I dismiss some parts of the Gita, and you should too, if that is how you feel.

Just because something is "yogic" or part of the Indian culture does not mean that you, as a yoga student, have to accept it or agree with it and believe it to be true. You have your own judgement, your own mind, your own conviction, your own faith and your own rationale. Do not insult your own intelligence and your own authentic self by assuming that everything that has the label "yoga" on it has to be authentic or true. That is not to say it is not true, it is just not true to you.

*"Indiana was such a devout disciple of 'Shakti' (another name for Parvati) that she had once considered taking her name until her father, Blake Jackson, managed to convince her that a Hindu goddess's name was not appropriate for a tall, voluptuous blonde American with the looks of an inflatable doll."[9]* - Isabel Allende, Ripper.

This is the ludicrousness of the Western seeker.

*Disciple: Phew. Ok. I won't get my Krishna tattoo done just yet then. So, one last question on the Bhagavad Gita. It is a summary of man's inner conflict, correct? The battlefield is a metaphor for life and the central characters are different aspects of one's mind?*

This is my Bhagavad Gita summary, which also brings us back to the overall subject matter. The subject of man and mind.

Man is in such a confused state of mind that we are finding it near impossible to find the answers on our own. The answers we have for our own questions just create more confusion. I remember hearing how an Eastern philosopher once set out to find all the answers to life and existence itself. He dedicated his life to searching and seeking knowledge. Upon his deathbed, his wife asked him if had indeed found all the answers. The philosopher replied, "No. All I found where more questions".

Our minds are many. As many stars as there are in the galaxy. We have mini-minds that collectively create the phenomena we call "mind". So, is there any surprise that we get so befuddled when we are told to quieten our minds? Which one of the hundreds of thousands of mini minds are we supposed to quieten? So, what we do as an instinctive response to understand our minds is create (in our minds) alternative versions of ourselves that will represent certain parts of our mind. To give you an example, the confused and puzzled part of my mind I have lovingly referred to as my "disciple". This is my alter-ego. The very alter-ego that has been bombarding me with questions throughout this book. The less muddled part of my brain is my consciousness. If I wanted to understand the paradox of my mind, I could create an imagined conversation between the two. Between the disciple and the master. Between the confusion and the certainty. Essentially, this book.

   If I wanted to dramatize this conversation, in a movie perhaps, I would give them characteristics that would help the viewer better understand the reason for their confusion and/or knowledge. The confused part of my mind could be an everyday warrior who, although brave, gets confused and caught up in the harsh realities of the modern world. In order for you to better understand the authority figure, my consciousness, I may represent him to you as a god-like figure so you cannot question his judgement. Do you see where I am going? I believe that Vyasa (the supposed author) of the Bhagavad Gita (very cleverly) simply describes what is going on within his own mind.

He is desperately trying to understand and get his head around the ancient Hindu texts the Upanishads (the Bibles of Hinduism). The vast information that flows from these books has left him feeling overwhelmed. The author is drowning in the sea of knowledge. His mind is conflicted as to the ins and outs of the text. To help him make sense of it all, the author has then presented this conflict in the elaborate setting of the Mahabharata. Essentially, the Bhagavad Gita is his very clever commentary on Hindu dharma/law as the author has understood it from reading the Upanishads. Maybe Vyasa was losing his mind, and the only way for him to save his sanity was to split his mind into two characters and have a conversation between them. If it was not for this exercise, Vyasa's overactive mind may have resulted in him going insane. The collective "wisdom" of the Upanishads was too much for him to fathom. This is why man creates his harmless alter-ego. So the answers he gets from his own questions appear to be from someone else. They can appear more rational and less complex. It becomes easier for us to understand ourselves when we can separate the squabbling mind and listen to both sides. The dialogue within this book is testament to that. My alter-ego, who wants to learn about yoga, is asking questions that my more confident alter-ego is more the capable of answering. The "master" illuminates my own awareness. This conversation, which is essentially between myself, helps me better understand, and more importantly, de-clutter, my mind. If I am ignorant, who can shine a light on my ignorance? Maybe I can find the answers for myself? Maybe the answers are located in my own mind. All that is required is a little introspection, a pen and a pad and the willingness to have a conversation with myself. I think it was Carl Jung who said, "In each of us there is another whom we do not know". Try forging a relationship. Try it. You will be utterly amazed.

This could have been the case with Vyasa, the author of the Bhagavad Gita. Maybe the characters of Arjuna and Krishna are projections of his mind. Arjuna loosely means "wavering". The insecure and wavering part of Vyasa's mind could have been imagined as the warrior – Arjun. He is confused and introverted, but Vyasa does not want people to think that he is weak. So, he has given him the title of a warrior. This way, when we view Arjuna as a reflection of Vyasa's mind, we see a vulnerable hero, not a totally weak one. The confident and more assured part of Vyasa's mind is the confident extrovert – Krishna. To give his alter-ego the authority he needs to extinguish his own ignorance, he adorns him with gold and jewels and makes him an incarnation of the great Hindu God, Vishnu. Vyasa's imagined characters then have a conversation, which succeeds in allowing Vyasa to understand his own struggle. Vyasa must have concluded, by the end of the text, that the answer clearly lies in his own lack of faith towards god. If he can surrender his will to his god, maybe he will no longer be in conflict? The Bhagavad Gita is just the story of one man and his conflict.

The mind is never satisfied. The mind will always be uncertain. The mind is looking for more and more uncertainties. This is our conflict. To avoid schizophrenia, we must create these different alter-egos that can talk to us and show us the different perspectives and paths our lives can take. If it wasn't for this built-in system, our minds would be inundated with thoughts and ideas, all coming from the same place that can slowly drive us towards insanity. There are too many voices to try and follow.

In my opinion, the author Vyasa would have sat down, closed his eyes and "meditated". He would have been in a silent reflection where, rather than his mind and his thoughts driving him towards insanity, he very cleverly imagined this scenario that involved the two conflicting parts of his mind in dialogue with one another. Arjun represents the nature he fully associates with himself, introverted, brave and loyal. And Krishna represents the voice of his reason. Remember, Krishna is supposedly the author Vyasa's first name. He has named his consciousness after himself. This shows us how much the author wishes to be like Krishna. Deep down, he is someone like Arjun, but he is longing to be someone like Krishna.

So, the created Krishna tells Arjun that he is capable of anything and everything if he keeps faith in God. The extroverted, highly intelligent part of his mind that is Krishna, his pure consciousness, reveals himself to be god itself. So there is no argument to be made from Arjun. He has to accept. This is the battle we have with our own minds. We need a voice of reason. We need to create or imagine a voice in our head that can counter the sometimes timid and paranoid parts of our personality. This could be just another method in not necessarily defeating the mind, but simply dealing with and understand one's mind. A Sufi teacher once told me that you cannot be mindless. There is no such thing as no mind. If we fight the mind, our loss is imminent. The art of living blissfully is to understand the mind.

In a slightly darker spin on creating an alter-ego, in the movie True Romance, Christian Slater's character, Clarence, is in the bathroom washing his face and is in somewhat of an emotional struggle. He has fallen in in love with a "call girl" and wants to free her from her pimp. Sound ludicrous, but it's actually a great movie. While thinking of his next move, Elvis Presley himself manifests in front of Clarence and talks to him of his responsibilities.

Clarence does not want to kill the pimp as he doesn't want to end up in prison, but his consciousness, his inner torment that is Elvis Presley, explains that this is his responsibility and it is what he must do for love. Elvis leaves the scene by saying, "Clarence, I have always liked you. Always will".

This is essentially Clarence telling himself, via his alter-ego, that he is not a bad person. He is a good guy simply in torment over what to do. In the same way, Krishna replies to a question from Arjun and starts the sentence with, "O Sinless Arjun…". The author Vyasa is using the elaborate creation of Krishna to tell the passive part of himself that he is not a sinner and, that deep down, just like Clarence, he is a good person. His only "fault", if you could call it that, is that he is in conflict. But we cannot feel guilty for feeling that. There is no sin in having a conflicted mind. Clarence needed to clear his head as his overactive mind was giving him a headache. He was confused about so much he just needed to get up and go wash his face. His mind was a theatre. So, Clarence imagined his consciousness, the reasonable and intelligent part of his mind, as his hero – Elvis. Someone he would wholeheartedly listen to and trust. In the same way, Vyasa created Krishna. He created someone whose logic he could not argue with. Upon hearing the wise words of Elvis, Clarence is now more certain of his own dharma. He has clarity. All it took was a reflection of himself. Eventually, Clarence does kill the pimp, and he and Alabama live happily ever after.

*"Out of clutter, find simplicity. From discord, find harmony. In the middle of difficulty lies opportunity." – Albert Einstein, The Quotable Einstein*

On a slightly lighter note with less death and pimps, think about Carlton from The Fresh Prince of Bel-Air. Carlton is an emotional wreck. His cousin Will has just been accepted into Princeton, while Carlton himself has been rejected. He sits around the Banks mansion feeling sorry for himself and questions if he even should have been born. The mansion is his comfort zone and he wishes to just wither away on the sofa and let life pass him by. Such is life, it no longer makes sense to our square-headed friend. His dad, Uncle Phil (RIP), is extremely disappointed with him, and letting his dad down is perhaps the hardest pill for Carlton to swallow. In order for us to understand Carlton's struggle, the writer Benny Medina very cleverly introduces Tom Jones into the scene. Tom Jones appears in a puff of smoke and glides into Carlton's world. Tom Jones is nothing but Carlton's guardian angel. The voice of reason. Carlton's consciousness.

Carlton: "It's not unusual to have dad be proud of me... When I see dad hanging with Will instead of me... It's not unusual to see me cry. I wanna die."

Tom Jones: "It's not unusual to mess up at any time... When I see you down and out it's such a crime."

Carlton: "Did you ever want to be loved by anyone? Then you let them down — I blew it yesterday, my trust funds gone away."

Tom Jones: "My friend, it happens all the time. And life will never do... What you want it to. Don't give yourself, such a hard tiiiiiiiiiiime."

After that wonderful rendition of Carlton's favourite song, Tom Jones then shows Carlton what life would be like for the Banks family if he had never been born. He tells Carlton that maybe you won't be what your Dad expected you to be, but that doesn't mean that you aren't somebody or won't be somebody significant. Life is not perfect. Learn from the pitfalls. Stop using every mistake you make as an excuse to stop living.

After this spiritual intervention from Tom Jones, Carlton is able to see the bigger picture and we, as the audience, have a much clearer understanding of Carlton's struggle. It's all down to the clever way in which the writer Medina wanted us to visualise Carlton's emotional battle and how Carlton feels about letting his dad down. Without this wonderful setting, how much could we gather from Carlton's expressions? More often than not, as the audience or the person directly involved, it takes the intervention of someone else to help us see the bigger picture. This is how man can grow and evolve without resorting to seeking genuine divine intervention.

*"That's how I felt when I came to Bel-Air, like everybody had two skates and I was trying to keep up with one... Thanks for my other skate, Uncle Phil." – Will, The Fresh Prince of Bell Air*

The mind was once just a brain; tiny specks of grey matter waiting for life so it could develop into a mind. The mind has developed as a consequence of life. What we tell our mind, it becomes. If we tell ourselves we are sinners, we remain sinners and we waste our lives feeling guilty for who we are, and we even create images of hell. In many respects, we are already in a hell of our own making. But if we can tell ourselves how good we are, or can be, we can slowly convince the mind that this is our nature. We create a conflict in our minds between the passive and the aggressive. Between the good and the bad. We cannot allow them to clash and actually go to war, as this is what leads to anxiety and anguish. We just act as the intermediary. This is reflection. Not ignoring the mind but acting as an intermediary as Clarence and Elvis have a conversation inside your head.

The character of Clarence, Carlton or Arjun simply represent the comfort zone of our minds. This is a psychological state where one feels familiar and safe. Although conflicted, we can feel at ease. There is security. Deep down, Clarence does not want to remain in his comfort zone. He knows that true love only awaits him if he can break free. Great things for man cannot develop from the security of our comfort zones. What a rubbish film it would have been if Clarence played it safe and didn't kill the pimp! He would never have found love.

If I was to play the same scenario in my own head, before I met Laura I was in my own conflict. I was resting in my comfort zone, a trap set up by own mind. I knew it to be true, but we like to live in ignorance as it can provide security. Like Arjun, I had a few options. I could remain as I was and be trampled upon. Just because I refused to take part in the war doesn't mean the war would not start without me. I could not be a coward and remain in the safety parameters I created for myself. I could not be an ostrich and bury my head to hide from my problems.

I had another option, and that is to step aside from the war and just be an observer. This is my comfort zone. I could simply watch as life seemingly passed me by. This is the general state of one who is miserable and unhappy with life. They have created barriers from problems but also barriers from joy. They remain deeply miserable. At least the ostrich is involved in life, the observer is lifeless.

The third option I had was to listen to my voice of reason. Listen to my consciousness. For Arjun it was Krishna/God. For Carlton it was Tom Jones. For Clarence it was Elvis and for me, perhaps it's Amitabh Bachchan. Using my imagination, he appears before me and, in his distinctive tone, he asks me to take a leap of faith and step out of my comfort zone. To be a warrior and to fight life head on. "Reach out for what enchants you", he says. "Extend beyond your comfort zone and heaven awaits. Believe in yourself. Believe in your resolve and that which you desire (love), will surely come to you. Take risks, explore, live, love, laugh and be happy. Your comfort is the only enemy to your progress".

In return, I would look at Mr Bachchan and say, "Who the hell are you?" He would reply, "Rishtey mein hum tumhare baap hote hai…" (That line may only work on the Indians!)

The step out of what I believed was my comfort zone is what allowed me to see myself for who I really am. What I thought was my comfort zone was simply a prison. What I though was safety was nothing but chains. I simply freed myself from myself. In doing so, I was able to meet the love of my life, my wife. Like Clarence, I would not have met her had I stayed within the comfort zone of my inner conflict. Perhaps the answer to our problems and unhappiness is that we think that talking to ourselves is a sign of insanity. Psychologist Linda Sapadin says, "Talking with yourself not only relieves loneliness, it may also make you smarter. It helps you clarify your thoughts, tend to what's important and firm up any decisions you're contemplating.

We all need to be receptive like Arjun and take time to listen to the voice of a Krishna or an Elvis that exists inside our heads. Ultimately, what is an author? What is a filmmaker? They are just individuals who just want to share the workings of their mind with the rest of the word. In many respects, Vyasa would have been the greatest filmmaker of his time, with Krishna as his biggest star.

Once, the conflict in the author's head was the basis for his potential madness. Through introspection, he was able to turn this into his own form of meditation.

*"One way to think of religion is as a projection of the fears and longings of our subconscious mind onto the screen of life. Religion seems to be out there and to have a life of its own. But it actually comes from the depth of our own imagination. It's an entirely human production." – Author, Richard Holloway, A little History of Religion*

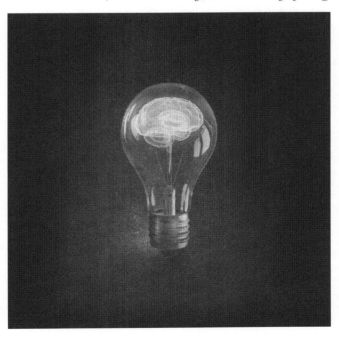

# Understanding the Mind via The Gita of Ashtavakra

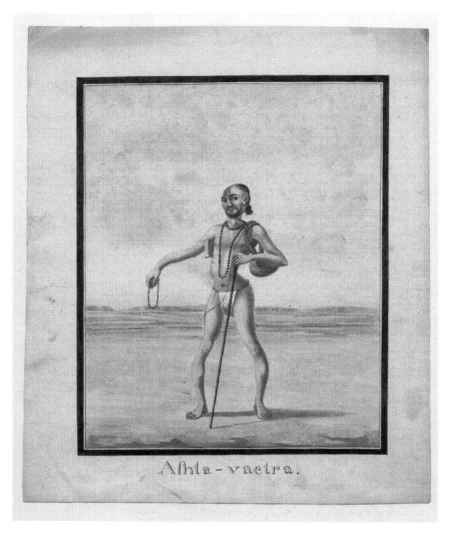

*above - An early 19th century painting of Ashtavakra. Used with permission from the British Museum.*

Another charming "Gita" that is available and more absorbing (in my opinion) is "the Gita of Ashtavakra". Ashtavakra as in, yes, the "arm balance".

Here's a little mythological story to set the scene.

It happened (the story is a re-telling and unless accompanied by a footnote, the dialogues are imagined by me - based on what I believe would have occurred).

Once there lived a holy man named Asita. He did great penance to please his Lord Shiva so the three-eyed one would bless him with a child. This is a wish Shiva would ultimately grant. Asita and his wife were blessed with a beautiful son named Devala. Legend has it that baby Devala was born crying as all babies are, but a holy man commented that in this instance, baby Devala was crying because he knew he had just entered a world of fools. It was prophesied at this moment that he would become exceptionally wise sooner or later.

Devaloka, where Asita and his family lived, is a plane of existence where gods and demi-gods all exist in sync. Rambha is the queen of Devaloka; she is a ruthless queen who leads with fear, but deep down, she longs to love and be loved. One fine day, Rambha notices Devala, now a teenager, and fell in love with him instantly. Previously, the queen used to shake her head and chastise anyone who talked about soulmates or love or marriage. She mocked the poor deluded peasants who were lost in such an extra-terrestrial notion of love. But then, she saw Devala. He had a cavalier smile and the posture of a prince. He was a polished man; the finest Rambha had seen. Thus, the cynic is converted - Rambha was deeply in love. She sent her guards to make a proposition of love, but Devala rejected it. Feeling spurned and having had her pride destroyed, Rambha cursed Devala and made him into one with eight crooks. Thus, Devala came to be called "Ashtavakra", which literally means "eight bends".

*Disciple - Poor guy. "Heaven has no rage like love to hatred turned/Nor hell a fury like a woman scorned". So, they say.*

Yes, in these "Vedic times", everyone seemed to have the power to inflict a curse (*shraap*). But perhaps, the meaning is not meant to be taken literally? Maybe the deformation is a reference to Patanjali's eight-fold *Ashtanga* system? (there is more on that in the Meditation chapter). Let's get back to the story.

A body that was once made of granite is now fragile as glass. Ashtavakra's body has become unsightly. So ugly is his appearance that mirrors shatter in his presence. His body is so crooked that he struggles to stand upright. His cane became his companion as did his hopelessness and gloom.

Ashtavakra does penance and practices Bhakti Yoga (the yoga of devotion) for many years. He prays to god hoping a miracle would mend his crippled body as well his broken heart. Krishna from the

Bhagavad Gita is his chosen god and on one auspicious day, he feels the warmth of Krishna's hand as he wipes the tears from Ashtavakra's face. Ashtavakra immediately looks up but Krishan is gone. It dawns on Ashtavakra that the only way he can free himself from this suffering is acceptance. He is living his *karma* and although a devotee of Krishna, all prayer would be fruitless if this is a consequence of his karma. Maybe he is suffering the reprisals from a previous life? Even the gods in Hindu mythology are incapable of fighting the laws of nature. Maybe the eight crooks in his body are symbolic? Maybe the answer is not in devotion but can be found in a more scientific and methodical approach. Perhaps each crook needs mending in the way each rung of the eight-step *Ashtanga* system needs ascending? This became a time of much soul searching for Ashtavakra. So Ashtavakra steps away from the temple and takes his search within. He starts meditating and seeking knowledge. He is soon lost in his books. For Ashtavakra, a book is like a lotus flower, a mountain, a glacier, a temple and a god. His books are his freedom and his salvation. With each new book Ashtavakra finds a more profound search within. He soon learns that man's greatest treasure is his knowledge and with each passing day, the ignorant part of his mind is defeated by his thirst for wisdom.

One day, Ashtavakra's mother asks her son to go and tell his father that a visitor has arrived. His father is at King Janaka's palace where he is debating other learned men - holy men, sadhus, pundits, scholars and gurus - about religion and philosophy. Ashtavakra makes his way to the palace and the guard allows him to enter. When Ashtavakra enters, there is silence. After an awkward moment or two, the silence turns to amusement as the educated visitors erupt into laughter. The tears roll down the cheeks of the "knowledgeable" as they point and laugh at the sight of Ashtavakra. Some even mimicked the way in which his hands are crooked, the way his knee is bent in an inhumane manner and most of all, his hunchback appearance. Ashtavakra's father is deeply embarrassed and stormed out of the palace. The only man who is not amused is the king himself. He instead looks intrigued by Ashtavakra who despite not being a normal man, radiates self-belief.

Ashtavakra looks at the king and says, "Why are you in the company of these shoemakers?". There is then pin drop silence in the assembly. "*Chamars* (shoemakers) work on shoes. They see leather. They see what is on the outside. That is all they see: what is outside. These idiot so-called scholars and swamis present at your assembly are of the same mold. At least, a shoe maker is honest. These men gathered here have no cognition. They know not of love, of compassion. They cannot see beyond the surface. Like a thief outside of your palace doors, they are too afraid of what they may find inside.

They only see the superficial. They are men without depth. Their ideas are not even fully formed. How can such men make claims of teaching you about self-realisation? How can such blind men who judge me based on my appearance teach you O noble King anything about self-knowledge and the mysteries within?"

Hearing this, the pundits and babas all bow their heads in shame. The king is left open mouthed at the maturity of this young man. "I am only here to fetch my father", continues Ashtavakra. "We have guests, so my mother has called for him to return to our humble abode. I am not here for any other reason".

"My apologies for troubling you O King. I am not rude or blunt nor am I abusive or vulgar. I only speak up when I see an injustice. These men are dishonest swindlers no better than pickpockets. They take advantage of your thirst for knowledge by filling your mind with distortions and inaccuracies. And they know exactly what they're doing. I only honour the truth, and I cannot stand for such wrongdoings. Remember O King, we are not of our bodies. I am not my body. Since my curse, men have stared, and poked and so-called wise men have laughed at my appearance. These same men who roll in amusement at my physical presentation are the same spineless pretenders who, stand in your presence, wish to teach you of enlightenment".

The assembly then ends as the king sends everyone away, except for Ashtavakra. The King drops to his knees and asks if Ashtavakra would become his master. Thus, begins the Ashtavakra Gita -The Song of Ashtavakra.

King Janaka asks him the following question:
"How can I acquire knowledge (on life, the soul, yoga, meditation)? How can I learn more on the subject of liberation (ultimate freedom)?"[1]

Ashtavakra replies that if one is seeking liberation or nirvana, one must firstly recognise that there is no difference between man and his destination. If you want to experience ultimate freedom, freedom from pain, stress, anxiety, etc., then one must know that they have always been free. There is no destiny to seek. Only the true nature of man can be discovered. Our mind has created a barrier between us and our true reality. Ashtavakra says, "The one who feeds on tranquility is never ever tormented"[2]. All suffering, Ashtavakra says, is simply an illusion created by the mind. The overall message of this Gita is a Guru (Ashtavakra) asking his disciple (the King) to try to understand a very basic question: What are you seeking? How can you seek that which you already are? If he was speaking to a sadhu, a man on the verge of giving up his life in search for his liberation, Ashtavakra would say, "What do you want to renounce? Put the complexity to rest, you are PURE as you are". Thus, no seeking is required. King Janaka, upon hearing these wise words, has a realisation: "Within the infinite ocean of my mind, the so-called world is all just imagined". Ashtavakra then tells the King to not live according to other people's expectations and observations. Don't simply renounce life and give up on life because this is a tradition that has been passed down from generations.

I believe Ashtavakra would give the same advice to the modern day "yogi" and yoga teachers. We cannot be puppets in search of some mysterious "oneness" that we think we will find in India. We are perfect as we are. The newly qualified teachers do not need to compare themselves to their favourite yoga teachers (who themselves have no idea who they really are). Why the comparison? Why the competition?

An old Zen saying goes, "The wise man does nothing while the fool is always tying himself up". This means that you should stop trying. You are already perfect as you are. The King is then told to avoid the company and the so-called wisdom of saints and seers and meditators (as I often say, avoid the so-called "yogis").

Our own consciousness is our guru and our teacher. Today, you are trapped in illusion, tomorrow you will rise and be free. Ashtavakra says, "Today you stand against popular opinion (which is to renounce, meditate, seek, and other such aspirations). Tomorrow, in the future, what will be the popular opinion?" The idea of liberation, renunciation and seeking god or freedom etc. are all activities of the mind. Ashtavakra says these thoughts are the very bondage that enslaves man. Stop searching for that which you already are. He says the real you, the joyful, blissful and happy you does not seek liberation, this is just the distraction of man's mind.

There is much to comment on this dialogue between the king and the man behind our favourite arm balance. The questions are very straightforward and of a philosophical nature. They seek philosophical acknowledgment, and this is what Ashtavakra wholeheartedly lavishes on the king.

Ashtavakra however speaks so directly and so matter-of-factly that it becomes easier to understand what it seeks to explain. And to be honest, Krishna (in the Bhagavad Gita) talks of enlightenment from the perspective of 'god'. 'God' is telling us what we should do and how we should live. My response to Krishna is that it's easy for you to say. You are 'god!' How can I relate to you? Ashtavakra on the other hand is not god and makes no such claims. He is a seeker himself who has found his way through knowledge. Ashtavakra even says that "God is not the creator of all. In the times of problems and fortunes, certainly, gods and goddesses have existed"[5]. But more often than not, belief in an almighty figure like a Krishna has created more suffering than how much it is has helped man in fighting for liberation. On the other hand, you alone exist as pure consciousness according to Ashtavakra.

Through his own misery, Ashtavakra has found a way to find peace within himself. Despite his physical appearance, Ashtavakra was one of the most beautiful souls the king had ever met. Ashtavakra used his physical limitations as a device to attain a state beyond the mind. His own odyssey has to have been incredibly arduous due to his almost crippled body. How hard must it have been for someone like Ashtavakra to go beyond the attachment to his body? Most people turn to alcohol and drugs to create a barrier between the body and the soul. Ashtavakra turned to introspection and thus he found that the moment he was no longer attached to the physical (the body and mind), he was free. Ashtavakra realised that all men are the same, once we go beyond the body and mind. The saying that yoga is the "union" of mind, body and soul would be inaccurate to a man like Ashtavakra. He would say that there is only the union of his true self and his consciousness when he is finally free from mind and body.

Ashtavakra says that we should all just be happy! "For you are joy, unbounded joy. You are awareness itself. Just as a coil of rope is mistaken for a snake, so you are mistaken for the world".

The great Swami Vivekananda has profoundly said; "It is our own mental attitude which makes the world what it is for us. Our thoughts make things beautiful; our thoughts make things ugly. The whole world is in our own minds. Learn to see things in the proper light. First, believe in this world — that there is meaning behind everything. Everything in the world is good, is holy and beautiful. If you see something evil, think that you are not understanding it in the right light. Throw the burden on yourselves! ... Whenever we are tempted to say that the world is going to the dogs, we ought to analyse ourselves, and we shall find that we have lost the faculty of seeing things as they are"[4].

Krishna, in his Gita tells us what is expected according to the words of 'god'. Ashtavakra speaks from the mind of man. He tells us that he himself has struggled as we all have and continues to do. He tells us that he knows the emotional torment that is a consequence of our physical pains. He speaks to us not from the lofty perch of the heavens but from the same level of an everyday man. We can relate to Ashtavakra because he is one of us. His message is within our understanding. When he says that "happiness and sorrow are attributes of the mind", he is speaking as someone who has scratched and clawed and fought his way to such a profound conclusion. These words are not the same cliché words from another almighty figure or words passed down from his guru or teachers. We can trust Ashtavakra because he feels our pain and knows our conflict.

It is the same as a modern-day yoga class. The perfect yoga teacher with the perfect posture tells us how to do a pose yet struggles to relate to why we cannot either do the pose or why we are stuck. Sometimes, they cannot relate because they themselves have not experienced the struggle. We relate better to someone who, when we battle with our posture, sits next to us and tells us why they think we are in conflict with our body. If a teacher shows human vulnerability by telling us that they have been through the same struggle or shows us that they are battling with something of their own, then we are able to build a bond of trust. Through this trust, we are more receptive to guidance. This is why man has created prophets. Man has always known that we need an intermediary not because the words directly from god would makes our minds explode and obliterate our bodies but because we wish to relate to it. We want to know that what is being shared are not just empty words but words that are coming from involvement, experience and participation. This is why men are often (not always) more drawn towards male teachers. They want someone who will perhaps relate to their own insecurities and/or restrictions in a pose.

The overall message of the Gita of Ashtavakra is so powerful. The wisdom (and there is plenty of that) comes from a man who, for once, is not of divine origin. He is someone who has experienced "stillness of mind" and in doing so has come to the conclusion that our fear is a product of our minds. Ashtavakra calls for equanimity. He asks for calmness and composure, especially in difficult situations. He asks us to detach and become a witness and not a doer in events that can create chaos, fear and such varying emotions. He tells us to not be attached to such fears because they are man-made. They are manufactured by the neurons within our brains. Our minds are the architect. And remember, these words are not coming from a divine being. They are coming from a man who has been tormented by words his whole life. Ashtavakra understands the value of being a witness as barrages of cruel words are fired at you like arrows - each with more venom than the next.

Ashtavakra asks that these words should not enter our hearts and if they do, we should not allow our thoughts to dwell on them; even years after they've been callously thrown at us. Each reflection in our minds ignites a sense of remembered pain. This is all manufactured by the grey matter inside our heard. This is part of their collective activity and their expression. This is the mind. Don't allow negativity to enter and if it does, let it pass through you.

Ashtavakra says that meditation is an act that appeals to the ego – it is an "act" that appeals to man in the absence of knowledge. This act of trying to experience self-realisation (via meditation) is a bondage. "Place of rest or without rest; meditation or self-searching of consciousness. This should be avoided. Performance of action is due to no-knowledge"[5]. The very act of meditation is against the teachings of Ashtavakra as he asks what is it that you are actually seeking? It is the same as prayer. Who do you pray to when the universe is already within you? And what is it that you ask for in your prayers when the answers are already within you, embedded in your cells. It is the same in modern times in the west when many so-called yogis say that they "meditate" but all they are actually doing is gratifying their egos. I have often asked the question of the modern individual in meditation, what are you seeking in your meditation? If it is a genuine search within themselves, then I have no problem with it. But more often than not, it is just an act – the same as performing on stage. When an actor plays a specific role in a play, they do so with full awareness that the stage, the play and the role they are playing is going to appear very real to the outside world. But it is just a show – it is only a performance. With regards to a person who is "meditating" to find themselves or to find their "destination", Ashtavakra says, "Detach yourself from the subject of liberation. If you are interested in that subject, then this is your bondage."[6] He continues, "Practicing meditation and stopping thoughts, that is what stupid people try to do"[6a]

Ashtavakra also says that when we do try to "meditate", all that happens is that our mind begins to destroy this mode of thinking by replaying old memories to disturb our peace. But what if there are no thoughts to replay? What if the cruel words were never allowed to enter the consciousness? This is why Ashtavakra tell us to just be a witness. You should create an armour and be impenetrable. Words cannot hurt as it is what we attach to these words and our own minds that create pain. Ashtavakra says that all is within our minds. "So, give up meditation completely. Do not let your mind hold to anything."[7] He goes on to explain to the king that the man who tries to "control" his thoughts and mind via meditation is ignorant. You cannot meditate as this is an action. You cannot DO meditation and you cannot practice meditation – you can only arrive at a state of meditation.

Ashtavakra says that we should not allow words (people's opinions and thoughts, etc.) to enter our consciousness because the state of meditation is not from the outside. How can we learn of who we really are when there is so much of ourselves that belongs to the outside world? When we lose our awareness of the outside, when we become a silent witness in our "meditation" just like a Buddha, when we are free from tension and when all that is outside cannot affect us, all that remains is what has always been inside. That which is left inside of us is who we really are: our true reality. This is meditation. It is our identification with what has always been inside of us at the core of our being.

Strictly speaking, in the West, what we think we do when we are "meditating" is not actually "meditating". When we close our eyes and "meditate", all we are trying to do is remove outside influences. Ashtavakra would call this practice "showing heart". Once all obstacles have been removed, we are "meditative". Until we are actually "meditating", all we are doing is showing heart. Our heart creates our armour. With regards to "meditation", Ashtavakra once said…"I didn't come to meditation. Meditation just happened".

Ashtavakra's finishes by telling the King that he is not what he thinks he is. He is not a Brahmin (member of the higher caste). Ashtavakra says that life has no religion. Religion is a product of a mind that needs attachment. He is attached to his way of being. You cannot be free if you label yourself with a religion. Humanity has no religion. If Janaka wants wisdom, emancipation and freedom, he has to know that he has created a self-imposed barrier by calling himself a "brahmin". So, his caste, an attachment to a hierarchical system, must be dropped. Ashtavakra also says, "you are not in any of the four stages of life"[9]. The "four stages of life" is a reference to the Hindu way of thinking: the student, the householder, the retired and the ascetic (the one who renounces life). So according to the wisdom of Ashtavakra, renunciation and the life of the ascetic is not required. You do not have to seek salvation at a temple because you are a temple. The divinity or freedom you seek as a begging sadhu exists already inside of you. "Know this and he happy" says Ashtavakra. So, anyone of any faith (or lack of faith) can be inspired by the words of Ashtavakra. In the same way that anyone of any faith can attempt the methods that Shiva taught to Parvati. Real yoga, which is an understanding first and then a state of no-mind, is for all religions and faiths. It accommodates any type of mind because that is the only requirement: Have a mind of your own. Make the enquiry of yoga a discipline and then over time, that very enquiring mind will experience the stillness of no-mind. This is ultimate freedom.

The king upon hearing and absorbing Ashtavakra's wisdom finally replies, "Yesterday I lived bewildered. In illusion. But now I am awake. Beyond the world".

After delivering his discourse to the king, Ashtavakra set off back to his home. He returns to his hermitage and pursues his thirst for worldly knowledge.

Sometime later, when the time came, Ashtavakra felt that his time on earth was drawing to an end. He knew this to be true because he felt nothing: no fear, no anxiety and no thrill. These are all of the mind and he was no longer a slave to the mind. Ashtavakra was all heart. His heart had conquered the mind, and he was ready to leave his body because he also knew that his true self would exist long after his physical body had turned to dust. So Ashtavakra sat quietly and waited patiently to unite his consciousness with that of the universe. He was ready to be free.

The mythology part of his story has it that after some time, Krishna himself, accompanied by his consort, Radha, appeared before him. Krishna was Ashtavakra's chosen deity as someone symbolic of the higher reality. To him, Krishna symbolised ultimate freedom from life, pain, sorrow and fear. Krishna's partner, Radha, was shocked by the ugliness of Ashtavakra. The myths say she was uncomfortable when she saw him as she had never seen such a grotesque being. Krishna, however, stepped forward and embraced Ashtavakra and held him firmly. At once, Ashtavakra lost all his crooks and returned to the beautiful man that he was before the curse. At that time, a chariot descended from Krishna's heavenly abode, and all three of them left for heaven.

The end of the story, which is purely mythological, has been passed through generations to try to inspire the people of India with the hope of instilling that God, or the higher reality, does not care for your physical appearance and only cares about what is in your heart. And it is what is in your heart that will inspire you to ascend to the heights of your existence (whatever that may be). Your heart will ferry you across the river of ignorance and defeat the manufacturer of all your fears, doubts and frustrations – the mind. Even though this is based on mythology, imagine the state of man if we had all been taught this underlying message of Ashtavakra as children.

*"Many of us fight for and boast our freedom of what is ultimately the ability to prove ourselves to other people. It is unfortunate that only a few of us are so free in our joy, we no longer feel the need to prove ourselves to anyone."*[10] –
*Criss Jami, Killosophy*

*Disciple - Ashtavakra says "listen to your heart". How do we know when it is our heart that is 'speaking' to us and not still our minds?*

It is difficult to know what is talking to you when you are not struggling, let alone when you are in anguish. Is it your mind or your heart? It can be near impossible to know the difference. Ashtavakra asks that we just be a silent witness. Just let the words and the thoughts pass. Let the clouds pass so to speak. When the voices die down (if you can allow them to), just be observant to the gentle voice - the quiet voice of reason. Ashtavakra says that this is your heart. It is the softness in the core of our being, and the gentleness of the voice simply shows us the depth of our souls. So, be a witness and just let the thoughts pass until you can hear the melody of the heart. If we are not witnessing we are over resistant. Ashtavakra implies that "meditation" is just silence. Just be an observer until all arrives of its own accord. Let the truth reach your heart. The Sufi's also say; "Show your readiness to receive by your silence". This does take time and patience. But this is how the mind is to be defeated according to the wisdom of Ashtavakra.

*"To find out what is truly individual in ourselves, profound reflection is needed; and suddenly we realize how uncommonly difficult the discovery of individuality is."[11] -*
*C.G. Jung*

*Disciple: Why is Ashtavakra's Gita (and the earlier mentioned Vignana Bhairav Tantra) so relatively unknown compared to The Bhagavad Gita and other more famous yoga/Hindu texts?*

I don't really know the exact answer but of course I do have a theory/opinion of my own.

We Westerners have always been fascinated with the yogis and the mystics of the East: Krishnamacharya, Iyengar, Patabhi and even as far back as Vivekananda, Yogananda and Maharishi. However, they are, first and foremost, deeply religious men. Their religion is in their blood and bones. They live and breathe their "gods". They are "Hindus" primarily who use yoga as a means to reach their god. This has to be understood. The men we have been learning from and sitting next to and praising so highly for so many decades now are men who have been raised to believe in god and believe that their sole purpose in life is to return to the source from which they have been formed.

When the British first went across to the mesmerising land of India, they became fascinated with the "spiritual" rituals and belief systems of these holy men and yogis. They sat next to them and learnt from them. They read their scriptures and even visited their temples. In a stark contrast to the way the British treated the country and its culture generally, they observed and then absorbed their religions and found themselves fascinated at everything these gurus and priests said and taught. They respectfully went to the yoga gurus and asked what books or scriptures they would recommend. What publication can they endorse? The British scholars where fascinated at this mystical, esoteric, divine system of realisation. Fascination aside, the British where also probably quite aware of the political and economic benefits they would gain via their quest for knowledge of ancient Indian texts.

What book/text on yoga is this guru likely to advocate? It will be a book he himself has perhaps been brought up with. A book that was sung and recited in his home ever since he was a child, a book that his family, who are all also deeply religious, would have embedded into his brain. It is the Hindu scripture of all scriptures. Of course, we are talking about "The Bhagavad Gita". This was the first work that was translated from Sanskrit to English and was the foundational event in the history of Sanskrit studies in the west[12].

The first translation was from a man name Charles Wilkins. Wilkins was widely acknowledged as the first Englishmen to learn the classical Indian language that is Sanskrit. His translation, published by the East India Company in 1785, was the first of over 300 translations of the Bhagavad Gita. And more translations followed with each passing year. The translation was done alongside an Indian gentleman by the name of Kasinatha Bhattacharya. An esteemed pundit (brahmin priest) from Benares.

I am just speculating here, but if Charles Wilkins had gone to this pundit and asked him what the sacred text of the Hindus was, Bhattacharya would have replied the Bhagavad Gita because this text, from a Hindu perspective is all the wisdom man will ever need. But the problem lies with the fact that Wilkins was asking the question to a priest. A priest for whom Krishna is god. Not a metaphor for god. But god itself. So, what other text but the Song of God would he recommend to Wilkins? It certainly would not be the Gita of Ashtavakra because this text can be seen as anti-religion and not consistent with the Brahmin system (the priestly cast system).

The westerner intrigued in yoga philosophy is still reading the 'Bhagavad Gita' today some 230 years on because this was not only the first translated text but is also the most widely translated and commented upon. What else is there that has the same authority? Even today if you ask the locals in India and the pundits what the most revered and respected text is in all of India, they will reply the 'Bhagavad Gita'. If you ask them what the most religious text is in all the country, they again reply with the 'Bhagavad Gita'. If you ask them for the quintessential read on yoga, most will reply with the 'Bhagavad Gita' again. To the people of India, it is all encompassing. Very few people in India are likely to mention the Yoga Sutras of Patanjali and no one is likely to recommend the Gita of Ashtavakra or the Vignana Bhairav Tantra.

The Gita of Ashtavakra, is not as "famous" or as well read as Krishna's because it rebels against the dogmatic teachings of orthodox Hinduism that tell us we must believe in the existence of god and that we must free ourselves from a cycle of rebirths. Ashtavakra says that this is nonsense. He aims to empower man while religion aims to enslave man. Empowerment does not work for the Hindu establishment: The priests, the sadhus, the gurus and the pundits. They want their seekers in chains so that they can give you the Gita and tell you that your salvation is through Krishna alone and without god, you can never be free (this is the same in all religion-dominated countries). They teach you that without the guru and the pundit, you can never be free because it is, they who lead you to God. They are Gods 'representatives' and if you don't believe in a God there will be no need for them. So, their insistence that you believe in God is actually all about their own self-preservation. Ashtavakra message of freedom does not appeal to parents and the local pundits because they don't want people to feel empowered. This is the harsh reality. When you are free you are not reliant on anyone. What would the parents and the school teachers and the pundits do if man was free? What would be left for them to do? Thus, Ashtavakra's Gita has never been taught in schools and at home by parents. It would possibly have been set aside just like a Quran or a Bible because it "corrupts" their establishment.

How different, how independent and how free would people be if rather than being taught the holy scriptures in our schools, we were taught books like Ashtavakra's Gita or Kahlil Gibran's Prophet? All they do is teach man about empowerment and love. Would Pakistan and India be on the brink of war today (as I write this) if that was the case?

As a summary, for the past few hundred years we have been learning about yoga from yogis and gurus from India who have been raised as strict Hindus. We only read, study and pay attention to that which they have recommended to us. Luckily for us, there have been rebellious yogis and gurus who have embraced the Tantras as well as the Ashtavakra's of this world. They have embraced their world and vision and simply want to be free - free from dogma, free from imagined gods and free from a culturally conditioned slave mentality.

Summary of the Mind Chapter.

The human species are trapped in a maze of our own creation. It may take a lifetime for us to be conscious that the maze has been created by our own minds. The remedy for this is a little introspection through which, one day, we can penetrate the unexplored depths of our self and hear the soft and gentle tone of our heart. Yoga is either madness or meditation. It is up to us to decide what we want it to be.

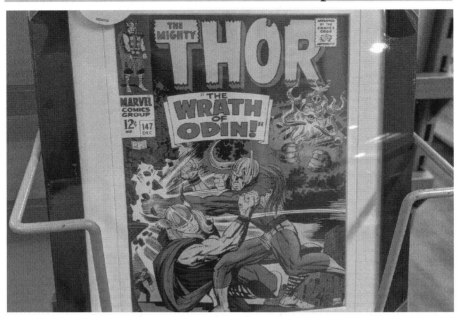

*Disciple – A state of no-mind is the goal for a traditional yogi. This is where one merges or unites with the highest reality. Is this highest reality "god" itself?*

For some, this state of 'no-mind' was said to open the doors to the divine. You become a witness to god. Your consciousness and that of the divine consciousness come together. They yoke. They join. This is yoga. So, the idea of 'no-mind' just opens the door to an even greater dimension of life and being. This is why some religions have, in the past, used yoga techniques. Because of the way modern politics have played out in recent years (Team Mohdi), yoga has been presented as a very Hindu culture and it may appear surprising that other faiths and in particular Islam had previously embraced elements of it. Around 1,000 years ago, one of the greatest scholars of the medieval Islamic era, Abu Al-Biruni translated a version of Patanjali's sutras as well as travelling to South Asia and authored a study of Indian culture after exploring the 'Hindu' practice of Yoga. He did so from his idea that religions should be treated objectively, striving to understand them on their own terms rather than trying to prove them wrong. In doing so he became fascinated at the concept of this higher reality that would have matched his own faith in 'Allah'. It has also assumed by some scholars that the path of 'Sufism' (Islamic mysticism) itself has been influenced somewhat by Yoga. This was the assessment of Sir William Jones in the

18th century (a curious claim and hard to prove but just a theory anyway). Ultimately, Yoga is a pathway or an avenue to a higher dimension of life that has fascinated many great religious and non-religious leaders over the centuries[1].

Many yogis and yoga books do refer to this higher dimension/consciousness or higher reality as god. There are numerous mentions of god in B.K.S Iyengar's "Light on Yoga" of our ultimate union with god. This our ultimate freedom he would say. But this is only his or a yogi's interpretation of god. A Hindu believes the highest reality is their god. There is nothing higher or greater. So, they may refer to infinite space and reality as god. A Muslim who does yoga may say the highest reality is Allah. Nothing is higher. A Christian would say they wish to create unity with Jesus. Some might say their highest reality is Morgan Freeman. You never know. But if you don't believe in a god, or the existence as god itself, then you may just let the notion go and consider what exists simply as a higher reality. Remember, Shiva didn't tell us of a god. He gave us no concept of god. Buddha who attained enlightenment and experienced this reality also did not speak of god. The highest reality is beyond even their vast minds and intellects.

Personally, the more time I have spent reading and studying the complex science of yoga, the more I have become put off by the word "god". Not god itself, but just the word "god". The word "god" itself is now a lazy, lost and redundant word. The word has become so contaminated through history. The word "god" has become tainted with our pre-conceived ideas of god, and these ideas and perceptions of ours cannot be god. As soon as we say "god" to someone, they have created an ideal of god in their heads. This cannot be god. There are so many theories on god that god has now become lost in our theories. God, or the highest reality, cannot be presented or thought of. It cannot be described, drawn, felt or even imagined. Whatever is presented is only our desperate need to understand. We cannot even study god. We can study theories and concepts, but we cannot study god itself. We are limited by our imaginations and the highest reality is beyond our imagination. Our idea of god is limited by the limited workings of our mind. As we are, until we reach this state of 'no-mind', we cannot perceive god.

Friedrich Nietzsche once said, "god is dead"[2]. Apart from proclaiming that the western culture was outgrowing metaphysical explanations of the world, part of the idea I believe was to destroy our own ideas of what god is. Clean our slate. If 'no-mind' is ever experienced, only then can the true reality of "god" be revealed; "revealed" is a very important word in this context. God will be "revealed" to you as it is. It cannot be conceived.

The neurosurgeon, Dr. Eben Alexander, (who had an out-of-body experience) after contracting bacterial meningitis, was asked by Oprah Winfrey if he had met god when he had this near-death experience. He answered, "Yes". Oprah then asked Dr Alexander to describe him. He replied saying that he could not describe it. He also said that god is formless and genderless. You cannot describe it. You can only experience it. He realised that words fall short. You cannot do god any justice with words or poetry or imagination. Dr. Alexander went on to say that "While writing it all up weeks later (the experience), God seemed too puny a little human word with much baggage, clearly failing to describe the power, majesty and awe I had witnessed"[3].

I have asked many teacher training students the question, "Do you believe in god"? Very few students will raise their hands. Then I ask them if they believe in "something", "a higher reality" or "something that is not someone sitting on a throne with a long white beard". Most students will then raise their hands and say that yes, they do. But what is the difference? As soon as I use the word "god", you create a god with the imaginative part of the mind. Essentially you are limited by your imagination. And god is beyond this - beyond limitation and beyond imagination. So, as we are, we cannot possibly fathom its existence. IF, and that is a big if, one is to embark on a serious yoga journey and go beyond the mind, once may experience the true reality of what it is. From what I have read and understood, once this happens, there will be no words. So, words cannot describe god before a state of no-mind and then words fail to do justice when we go beyond the mind.

*"When the Great Reality is not known the study of the scriptures is fruitless; when the Great Reality is known the study of the scriptures is also fruitless."[4] - Shankaracharya*

This is why the realised yogis, and or mystics, talk very rarely about god. They prefer not to use the word that has created more violence than any other word in the history of man. What other word or concept has created as much hate, fear, violence and war as the word "god"? Shiva and the Buddha both never mention the word "god". Shiva only said that man, if willing, can go beyond the mind. He didn't say what was waiting for us once we can go beyond this mind. Even Shiva could not explain.

There is a mythological story of how Parvati was satisfied intellectually with Shiva's response (to her questions on the higher reality) but wanted to experience higher consciousness or reality for herself. Parvati wished to breach the boundaries of existence and go beyond the physical creation. She wanted to experience the reality that Shiva himself was constantly immersed in. So, she asked Shiva if she too could realise this higher dimension of life. Shiva then embraced Parvati "limb-to-limb" and both their physical bodies merged. Shiva accommodated his beloved in his own body and what was experienced was a perpetual state of ecstasy. It is believed culturally that the moment Parvati embraced Shiva, she became one with him. Shiva could not explain it in words, he could only share the experience with her. What is experienced when in "no-mind" is thus beyond our intellect.

Before we move on, again, I am not against god at all - far from it! I am personally just against that word "god" as it no longer universally represents "peace" and "love". Debates and argument over the meaning of the word "god" will forever continue and so will the destruction and violence that accompanies it. There are a few certainties in life but man arguing over god is definitely one of them. Why does man think it his eternal responsibility to fight for his "god"? Is it because deep down psychologically, he is simply defending his own creation? Those who truly believe in what exists do not need to fight. That which is the source of creation and the creator of the vast universe and cosmos does not need our help to defend its honour.

If you don't believe in god, each time the word "god" is mentioned in this book (or the Bhagavad Gita), replace it with "ultimate freedom".

*Disciple - You have mentioned that yoga believes in a higher reality. Yoga is the union with this phenomenon. How can we know for sure that this reality exists? If I dedicate my life to yoga in search of the higher reality, will I find it? Does it even exist?*

Firstly, you don't have to do yoga for any other reason than to just stretch. I want to make clear that is it okay not to believe a word of what I am saying and just do yoga because your hamstrings are tight.

So, to answer your question, let me use Love as an analogy. Up to when I met my wife Laura, I can say with certainty that I had yet to experience actual love. I had many experiences where the immature mind perhaps convinced itself of love, but the heart would eventually say no. That was not love. So, what is love?

Rumi, the great Sufi poet, once said of love, "The garden of love is green without limit and yields many fruits other than sorrow or joy. Love is beyond either condition: without spring, without autumn, it is always fresh."[5] The Lebanese poet Khalil Gibran who wrote the wonderful The Prophet says, "Life without love is like a tree without blossoms or fruit."[6] Are these poetic responses likely to convince me that love exists? Can they adequately describe love? Will these quotes convince the doubting mind of love? Probably not. These words, as wonderful as they are, would give me a poetic understanding of love, but nothing can ignite love in me but the experience of love itself.

I had not experienced love. So, based on this, am I to convince myself that love does not exist? How can someone convince me? What would you say to me if I asked you if love really exists? You would probably say, "You don't believe because you have yet to experience it. But one day you will." You would tell me to not bother myself questioning love. You would tell me to just be. Just be yourself and trust in life. One day you will experience love and when you do it will be your own experience. So, don't worry about questioning the existence of the divine, or the higher reality (or any of the many words chosen to describe it). Just be. Maybe one day the higher reality will find you the same way love found me.

My wife Laura reminded me about a scene in the movie I Origins. The scientist Sofi asks Ian (her fellow scientist) about worms. She asks Ian; "how many senses do worms have?". Ian replies that they have two. Smell and touch. Sofi then comments that worms live without any ability to see or even know about light. They cannot see. The notion of light to worms is unimaginable. But humans know that that light exists. It is all around them. Light is right on top of them and yet they cannot sense it. This is the same as God or the higher reality in yogic lore. We simply do not have the senses to perceive its existence.

It happened. Seriously.

A man, an ordinary man was a seeker. He was seeking God. Or, the answers to life's questions. He was a sage, a holy man, but he needed a master. A guru to help him find the light.

One day he saw a mystic, an old man who looked homeless. The seeker approached this old wise man and enquired about a guru, a master. Did this wise man know of a guru who could show him the light? The wise man was Shiva himself dressed as a beggar as he was trying to hide from all his devotees. Shiva needed some space. Upon seeing the eyes of this seeker, Shiva's heart sank. He could never turn down his devotees, but he still needed some space. Perhaps he was still grieving the loss of his first wife.

So, Shiva said to this seeker: "You have to find a man with certain characteristics. He will have a particular way of being and behaving. He will be sitting under a tree, with a serpent as a companion. A bull will be keeping guard. He will be wearing a robe that looks like the skin of dead mammal and his eyes will look like this (pointing to his own eyes)".

The seeker thanked Shiva, thinking he was just a fakir (religious ascetic) and set off on his search. Forty years passed and the seeker had roamed all over this earth, but he could not find this guru. Tired and exhausted, the seeker came back to his home town. Upon arriving, he saw the wise old man in the exact same spot where he had left him forty years earlier. As the seeker approached the old man, he noticed the tree and the bull. He noticed the serpent and the robe. He looked at the old man and he noticed the eyes! The seeker was overjoyed and immediately bowed and touched Shiva's feet.

He then asked the old man why he had tortured him for forty years. The old man revealed himself to the seeker as Shiva and explained that this is the tragedy of man.

Shiva had told the seeker what he was looking for, but the seeker remained blind. He was blinded by desire. His desire for God meant he was never alert. "I was here all along," Shiva said, "In your home where you left me. I was closer to you than your siblings, your parents, your lovers and you still didn't notice me." The journey is long and arduous, so Shiva was pleased that at least the seeker didn't lose heart.

The moral, as is obvious, is that God, or the higher reality, or Zen, or bliss, or peacefulness, or happiness, are all present within us. Or, they are closer to us than we realise. Throughout life, we will lose track and we will convince ourselves that this happiness is something we need to chase or to gain. But it is always close to us if we can be alert.

Many holy men never find God. They die in pain, physically and spiritually because they are always seekers. In certain yoga philosophies, there is nothing to seek, only to discover. It is within you this whole time. Enlightenment, or freedom, or bliss, or this state of 'no-mind' is already within us. It is closer to home than we know. The Buddha, or our own Buddha, our own realised soul is our actual nature. We are all Buddhas with our eyes closed. When Buddha was asked what he found through meditation, Buddha said nothing. Nothing was gained. Only negative impressions had vanished. He said everything was here in front of me this whole time. The enlightened mind, the state of no-mind exists in us all.

Menaka Desikachar, a senior student of the lineage of Krishnamacharya, told this story about the search within.

"My father-in-law used to tell me, God is always inside you, so you do not have to go to the temple to find him there. I liked that very much. He also told a story to accompany that idea. Long, long ago God was moving like us in this world. But because people knew he was God, they used to chase him everywhere. And even though he was providing everything, they were so greedy, they only asked 'give me this', 'give me that'. So, he got fed up and he said I have to hide myself from these people, so that they don't find me. So, he went inside the heart of each one. And only those who don't look for more outside, but start looking for God within, will find him."[7]

If you don't believe in God, don't think of the highest reality as God. Look beneath the story. Look for the spine of the story. Happiness, bliss, is your reality. This has always been within us. It is our nature. The Sufi's say, "I look into you…and I don't see any other barrier than yourself. You are standing in your own way. And unless you understand it, nothing is possible towards inner growth." If you don't believe in god, then you must believe in something. Call it love. Read the story again and replace god with love. The story will have a whole new dimension. But, remember you are not asked to believe in anything. Religion requires belief. Yoga does not. Science does not require belief. Science is concerned with knowledge, with knowing. This is why yoga is a science and not a religion in my opinion. But religion and science can exist together. To the holy men of Indian subcontinent, the sadhus, yoga is a religion. This is based on their faith, their unbreakable faith that Shiva (or Krishna. Or Ram and so on) is god and, through the discipline of yoga, they will ultimately be united with him. Yoga, for these orange robed sadhus, is very much a religion. Our yoga, the yoga for the modern western student is in search of something else. We are unsure of what that is. Because of this uncertainty, our yoga is not religious. You can be a Muslim and do yoga. You can be an atheist and do yoga.

Those of multiple faiths have been doing yoga for centuries. Yoga is not bound by religion. Our yoga is concerned with knowledge, knowledge that is gained by doing. Knowledge gained through our own experience and not the experience handed down by others. This is our own journey. This will be our own unique reality.

In F. Yeats-Brown book printed in 1937 – 'Yoga Explained', the author (a believer in Christ) explains to his readers that yoga is not related to the belief in god. Yeats-Brown (1886-1944) was one of the first proponents of yoga in Britain and wished to clear a misconception that yoga was a religious system. He goes on to say; "Yoga sets up no god or gods, neither does it deny this existence of god. It is, I repeat, a method of physical and psychic culture. You may be a Christian, a Buddhist, a Moslem, or a Hindu, and yet a student of yoga. You may also be an atheist. If you are, you will probably be impelled to establish a new religion"[9].

Yeats-Brown has further said that yoga can be a servant of religion and not a rival[9a]. So, to reiterate, you are not required to believe in God, or a higher reality. Believe in infinite love. Believe in immeasurable happiness. If you ever reach a state of no-mind, this will be your reality.

*Disciple - You have answered the questions and helped me understand reality and enlightenment from a yogic perspective. What do you believe in? Do you personally believe in this reality? In enlightenment?*

I do believe in an enlightenment in that I do believe that this yoga enlightenment exists. Or, can be found. Or, discovered. However, very few people in our times actually experience this. A Shiva and a Buddha appear once every 10,000 years. Over the course of time, I have come to understand that the words enlightenment and true reality can create too much of a barrier for us. The words are too confusing. Too unclear and not logical enough for us to understand. So, we dismiss the idea or spend too much time in debate or discussion regarding the subject. I believe there is not just yogic enlightenment, but other types of enlightenment. If we look at the word itself, it means the action of enlightening or the state of being enlightened via education, insight, interaction, instruction and even experience. I think that, throughout our lives, we will have many enlightening moments or experiences. This is important for us in the modern world (especially in the west) to understand. These moments collectively shape our lives, our consciousness, our personalities and the lives of our loved ones. These factors affect our happiness in life. This is discovered through immersion in yoga, and we can learn how to be more peaceful within. This is known and proven. Yoga works. This is not a stretch or an exaggeration. We know that yoga can slow us down and that it can slow down our breathing, which, in turn, has an effect on our minds. Our monkey minds can be still for a moment. Sometimes, that moment, in itself, is a mini moment of enlightenment. We will have many of these moments in our lives. Meeting our life partner for the first time. Having a child. Making big life decisions. Achieving our handstand. These moments, when reflected upon in later life, are the moments of enlightenment that shape our character and who we are. We don't always know this at the time, but we only realise upon reflection later on in life.

Recognising these moments of enlightenment is more important for us in the west than aimlessly chasing the enlightenment set out by Shiva. These moments are relevant in our western lives and can be seen as safe and accessible. The key, I believe, is not to overly desire these moments and not to chase them obsessively. But, let them happen. Let them flow like the law of nature (or Tao). Don't fight the tide, don't resist the tide. Just go with the flow. One day you will look back on life with a smile as you remember all those mini moments of enlightenment. Before you die, you will be smiling and laughing about life. Remember the song from one of my previous chapters? "Everyone arrives (in this world) crying, but the one who exits laughing is the conqueror of his destiny." This, for me, is enlightenment.

What about the other reality? The reality that Shiva and the Buddha are immersed in. Is this for us? Can we western practitioners ever experience this? Hmmm. I am not sure. We are trying to become one with the highest reality, the universe, the stars. One with the cosmos. Is this viable? Is it attainable?

We live on such a small planet in the grand scheme of things. We are so tiny and irrelevant within the cosmos. Apparently, there are 10 billion galaxies in the observable universe. The number of stars in a galaxy varies, but assuming an average of 100 billion stars per galaxy means that there are about 1,000,000,000,000,000,000,000 (that's 1 billion trillion) stars in the universe. That is a figure beyond ridiculous. The stars, the universe, this reality is so far from our reach I do not think we will ever know it's true grandeur. All that you see above, the cosmos, is so large in scale our brains cannot fathom it. Yet, we feel that somehow, we are so special in this cosmos (you could arguably call this God) that may not even know we exist. Can we create union with something that is not even aware of our reality? I suppose we could. Only in our minds.

At his talk at the end of a week-long intensive meditation retreat, the great Zen master Xuanhua concluded, "Now we have finished. Everyone stand and we will bow to the Buddha three times to thank him. We thank him because, even if we did not have a great enlightenment, we had a small enlightenment. And if we did not have a small enlightenment, at least we didn't get sick. Well, if we got sick, at least we didn't die! So, let's thank the Buddha."

I think we should be thankful for what we have and who we are.

"Instagram provides us with endless distorted versions of what beauty, love, relationships, friendships, and happiness look like in real life."[10] - Orge Castellano.

The day that we can collectively understand that the reality in which we find ourselves is all an illusion, the more enlightened we will become. The day we realise that someone like Krishna is just a figment of our imagination and that true salvation and realisation come from invincible belief and faith in oneself and not an imaginary blue skinned deity, we will become free from delusion. Maybe this is what Iyengar meant all along by ultimate freedom. We are free from the creations and the nonsense of man. We are liberated unique and self-reliant beings who are free to roam and free to soar. Our happiness is dependent on our freedom. Our freedom from our gurus and our pundits and our chains and our insecurities, our social media, our anxiety, our fear, our destruction and our self-pity. All it takes to be free is to be brave. This is our enlightenment. This is our meditation.

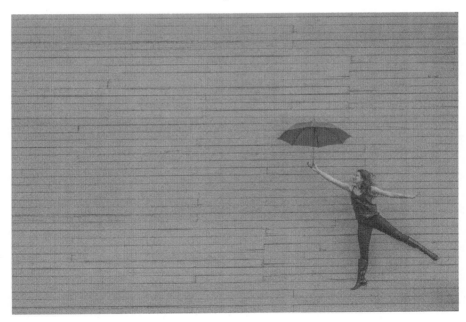

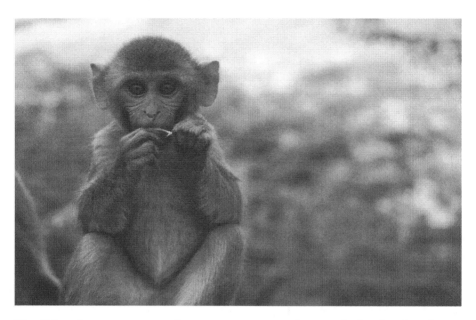

Traditional yoga, as we have come to understand, is simply about taming the monkey mind. Or, sending the monkey into a deep sleep. B.K.S. Iyengar said, "Everything we do in yoga is concerned with achieving this incredibly difficult task (controlling the mind). If we achieve it, Patanjali said, the goal and the fruit of yoga will be within our grasp."[1]

When I teach yoga today, in the west, I am not just trying to stretch and challenge your body but attempting to stretch and challenge your mind as well. I often tell the students in the studio that yoga is psychological. Understanding this not only helps us better understand the subject, but it helps us in our quest of mastering the yoga poses. We start to realise that restrictions and our inability to do poses are not always physiological, but that they are psychological. Our yoga practice exists in another paradox, somewhere between physiology and psychology. For some weeks or months, our yoga can be dominated by our physiology. This would be the case after an injury or setback. Then, after time, our yoga is dictated by our psychology. Perhaps still as a result of the same injury or hindrance.

The very first pose that Mr Iyengar would teach, the mountain pose (just standing upright) would deal with this arduous task concerning the monkey mind. This creates a pattern for the rest of our class or classes. If we go into class, as we often do, thinking the class is all physical, we may stretch and loosen our bodies, but our minds remain as they were, and, deep down, part of the appeal of yoga, even for those who just come for physical reasons, is to calm our minds. Calm our thoughts. Just to slow down the frantic pace of life.

So, our modern-day yoga should be both physical and psychological. We have to overcome barriers within our bodies that create so many movement restrictions (our muscles and nervous system) and overcome the barriers in our minds that create so many additional obstacles for us in other parts of our life. If we can tame our monkey mind in class, can we transfer this to everyday life?

I could give you many examples of how this is possible. I had a student who wanted to go for a promotion at work, but who lacked belief in her skill set. She avoided putting her name into the hat on many occasions through fear of failure. Part of this is also the ego's cunning trick of not wanting you to fail. The ego does not like failure. We cannot bear the feeling of rejection. On one random afternoon, this student, seeing that a more advanced position had become available at her work, decided to hand in her CV and go for this post. She felt that her efforts should have been rewarded by this promotion with months ago. She got the promotion, and it was one of the most satisfying achievements of her life. It was a mini-moment of enlightenment. She told me about the promotion and, at the same time, gave me some chocolates. I asked her, "Why the chocolates?" She insisted that her new-found belief (in herself) is the result of her ongoing practice of yoga. She imagined what I would say to her when she was contemplating handing in her CV. She imagined her headstand scenario. She thought, "I never in a million years thought I would do a headstand. Zahir told me that I am not a miserable little creature. I can do anything I want if I show enough heart." So, she did. She was brave and she sought the job she felt her skills deserved. This is her dharma, her responsibility to herself. She deserved to be the best version of herself. Anything less is the biggest crime we can commit on ourselves. So, the practice and discipline of yoga will change your life in ways you cannot imagine if you just go with the flow and do not shy away from poses that you think are too advanced for you. They may be too advanced for you today. And that is fair. But they won't always be. You have to believe this.

Recently, a relatively new male student was nice enough to email the following:

"Hi Zahir and Laura,

I hope that you are both well!!

I really just wanted to say a huge thank you to the both of you (also Kate and Sheree too as I have been to their classes too). I started my yoga journey late last year after a good friend convinced me it would be a good idea as I had never been to anything like yoga before. You may not be aware, but I have had a tough few years on a personal level and was feeling a little underwhelmed with me personally and also generally with the world around me. Having started on my journey to a better emotional and physical well-being, I feel that I have become stronger as a person, more mindful about the amazing world around me and I feel so positive about life in general. Yes, I am still single (LoL), but happy with me...finally! I feel that your classes and the comments you make (yes, I do listen to them...ha!) have helped a great deal and look forward to continuing my journey with you and also my personal journey with me.

Thank you!"

Although, we in the west won't completely rid ourselves of our monkey minds and find the 'Nirvana' of the Buddha, or the 'Bhairava' of Shiva, or the 'Samadhi' of Patanjali, we will, through immersion in yoga, experience a better quality of life as happened for the two students above. This is our enlightenment. This is our freedom. It is freedom from the reality of fear, nerves and anxiety that we have created for ourselves. Only we can find this freedom for ourselves.

So, although our turning inwards isn't the same as the turning in of the Buddha, in many ways we are trying to achieve the same thing.

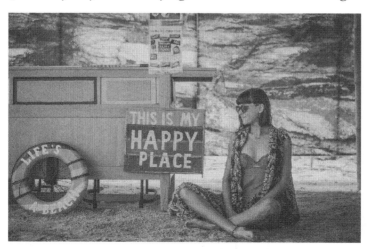

# Chapter 11 – Modern Day Yoga

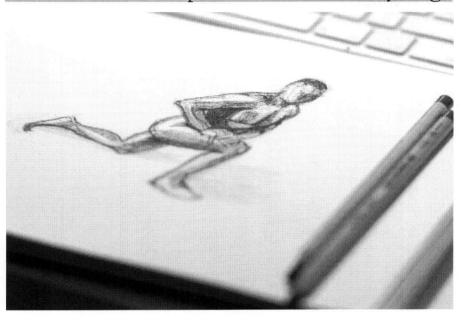

*Disciple: How about modern-day yoga? When did that begin?*

A little closer to modern times, a great yogi by the name of Gorakhnath or Gorakhsha is said to have "invented" *hatha* yoga in and around the 12–14th century. He may have done so alongside his guru, Matsyendranath. The origins of *hatha* yoga can also be traced back to another yogi, someone who was supposedly the incarnation of all three main gods of Hinduism (Shiva, Vishnu and Brahma), his name is Dattatreya. Perhaps, rather than originate or invent, both "men" played a part in the ascension of what we call *hatha* yoga. This is, however, debatable and a constant source of exploration. There is much academic research that goes into understanding the origins of *hatha* yoga. The last time I checked in with academics, *hatha* yoga's origins can also be attributed to tantric Buddhists and a text called *Amrtasiddhi*, which was composed around the 11th century[1].

The most simplistic explanation of the goal of *hatha* yoga is to create physical purity: Cleanse your body and the body may one day be able to bear the burden of meditation. One of the key texts on *hatha* yoga is the "Hatha Yoga Pradipika". Not a big fan of the text myself but it does play an important role in helping us understand the advancement of yoga through the years.

The direct translation of "ha-tha" is "sun and moon" while the indirect implied translation is "forcefully" or "willfully". Thus, the accurate description of *hatha* yoga is a forceful union of your sun and moon energies. A union between these two energies creates an equilibrium that, in turn, prepares your body for meditation. *Hatha* yoga unlike the other forms of yoga asks us to take care of our bodies and keep them pure. So, you could say that in the pre-eighth century, yoga was very "spiritual" and "meditative". And since Gorakhnath, yoga has become more physical. We have begun to understand that unless we first take care of our physical bodies, nothing "spiritual" can be gained. We cannot attain to the reality as discussed by Shiva and Parvati until we first take care of our physical bodies.

*Disciple: So physical yoga started from Gorakhnath. From what I understand, a lot of the yoga poses in those days were seated (as a means to prepare for meditation). When was the birth, invention or introduction of the poses we are familiar with today?*

Yes, many were seated but not all. There is evidence of many non-seated poses going back hundreds of years. Bahr al-Hayat (or Ocean of Life) was a Persian book printed in 1602 by Muhammad Ghawth. Ghawth was a Sufi saint. This was his Persian translation of the original Sanskrit text - Amrtakunda, the Pool of Nectar[2]. This was probably the first illustrated book on yoga and showed many poses we are familiar with today[3]. This included *Kukkutasana* (the cockerel pose) and the yogic headstand. The original Sanskrit version was lost, and word has it would have been composed anywhere from the 12th to the 15th century. Interestingly, for me anyway, Ghawth states that the personal mystical experiences of yoga and Sufis are very much alike making this text, "the most unusual examples of cross-cultural encounter in the annals of the study of religion".[4]

Other non-seated 'earlier' poses include the arm balance posture, *Mayurasana*, The Peacock Pose (an image in a temple in Jodhpur, India 1810[5] - which you can view on Wikipedia) and the 15th century hatha yoga pradipika text that again describes the *Kukkutasana*. There is a fascinating and wonderful 18th century manuscript called the *Jogapradipika* that shows eighty-four postures. Of those we see what we know of today as shoulderstand and headstand. At that time shoulderstand is called *viparita karani* and headstand was called *kapali asana* (the head posture). The standing postures are however completely absent. This manuscript is at the British Library and has been so since 1861 having been taken from the Indian Library of the Rani of Jhansi in 1858 during British rule. You can see these wonderful images for yourself in Gudrun Buhnemann's book; 'Eighty-four Asanas in Yoga. A Survey of Traditions'.

In general, the answer is yes. Most of the 'classic' yoga pose were seated, somewhat designed to prepare the aspirant physically for the demands of meditation and/or penance.

Modern yoga, or the yoga we are all familiar with today, the more physical postural form, owes its formulation and even creation to a mixture of characters and influences. Shri Yogendra (1897-1989) was a yogi and poet who was the founder of the 'The Yoga Institute' – one of the oldest yoga centres in the world – opened in 1918. It is said that after learning yoga from his guru, Yogendra decided to share his teachings with everyday householders as well as the average Joe taking yoga, from a strict guru to student practice to the masses.

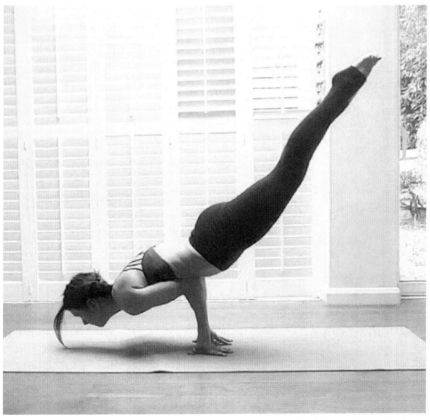

*above - My wife Laura in a variation of Mayurasana, the Peacock arm balance posture.*

Swami Kuvalayananda is also another pioneer (1883–1966) who was known for his research into the scientific foundations of yoga. One of the swami's students, though, arguably played the biggest part in the revitalization, or even "creation", if you will, of physical yoga, and that was Tirumalai Krishnamacharya, a 5'2" Brahmin born into a small village in Southern India in 1888.

*Disciple: Hang on . . . is this the man from the Bhagavad Gita that you mentioned earlier?*

No. That is just Krishna. This is Krishnamacharya. I imagine Krishnamacharya was named after Krishna. This is like the Brazilian Ronaldo. His heir apparent was someone lovingly named after him, Ronaldinho or 'little' Ronaldo. The same is true of Krishna and Krishnamacharya – they are both trailblazers in their own ways but very different people.

*Disciple: So, tell me more about Christian Macharya.*

It's Krishna-macharya. At his birth in late 1888, yoga as a philosophy was dragged out of the wilderness by the great Hindu monk, Swami Vivekananda, but the physical side of yoga was still overlooked. Vivekananda's focus was on philosophy and the promotion of a better understanding of dharma (duty and/or righteousness).

However, the physical side of yoga - the asanas - was not commonly practiced. If you did asanas, you were considered unhinged or unstable or as B. K. S Iyengar says in The Breath of the Gods, "In the early days, yoga was an alien subject to the Indians also. It was not respected by scholars or the pundits (wise teachers/priests) or anyone else. Only they were interested in the philosophical aspect but not in the practical aspect at all. There was a feeling that those who embraced yoga in the early days, they may be mentally disturbed, or they must have quarrels with their parents. That was the imprint people had in those days that yoga was meant for those who are half crooked or half cracked people"[6].

Asana (the poses of yoga) was associated with madness or the circus, certainly not the art of healing. This was Krishnamacharya's mission in life: To awaken the art of physical yoga from its slumber to use it as a healing method to first expose it to the masses and then to make it accessible to anyone and everyone.

Krishnamacharya realises that this was his fate in around 1920, after completing his studies in Tibet. From that time onwards, he developed, refined and formulated most of the asanas we are all so familiar with today. They may not have the specific alignment details that Iyengar later pioneered in the 60s, but these asanas provided the framework for everything Iyengar would later do.

In the Yoga Makaranda, on the subject of asanas, Krishnamacharya wrote the following:

"How many asanas are there? It is said that there are 8.4 million asanas as there are so many varieties of living beings. Ramamohana Brahmacharya (his guru) had 7,000 asanas, and I have learnt 700 from him"[7].

Around 1925, Krishnamacharya got a job as the personal yoga teacher/healer and counsellor of Sri Krishnaraja, the Maharaja (king) of Mysore (and his family). With the help of the Maharaja, Krishnamacharya opened his first yoga school (yoga shala). Krishnamacharya taught boys, girls, men and even athletes. Two of these students would become famous later in their own right: Pathabhi Jois and his wife's older brother, B. K. S Iyengar.

According to Krishnamacharya's children in the Breath of the Gods[7], the young men and boys were taught a vigorous style of yoga to enhance their speed and strength. This was just before the partition of India, so it was imperative that the youth were strong and active. Initially, the yoga poses being taught were static. However, upon the Krishnamacharya's development of the vinyasa method, asana was transformed. It went from a static "exercise" to a dynamic one. The development of vinyasa allowed the exercises (as they were being taught) to become a flowing sequence, integrating movement with breathing. The idea being, if the young boys went to war with Pakistan as was expected, they would have the strength and vigour that could perhaps not be gained by practicing static poses.

Krishnamacharya's long time disciple, A. G Mohan has said that Krishnamacharya's favourite vinyasa was centred on the warrior pose. He loved challenging his students' co-ordination and balance. Mohan said, "When I did the warrior vinyasa, Krishnamacharya recommended that I bring into my mind a feeling like that of a bird. This is particularly appropriate in the devotional tradition in which the principal devotee of god is depicted as an eagle named Garuda. The eagle Garuda would also function as a vehicle carrying the lord on his back. As you do the warrior vinyasa, keep in mind that you are in service of the divine. Krishnamacharya would say. 'Extend your arms and look down, bring the feeling that you are above the world its various concerns and that you are close to the divine. Feel that the feet of the divine are resting on your hands'. To this, I once replied, 'This is relevant for me, but what if a practitioner has no religious beliefs?'

Krishnamacharya replied, 'Still the imagery is valuable. Instead of thinking of the divine, bring the feeling that I am without fear or burden. I am not troubled by the future or the past, flying above worldly pressures."[8]

With his vast learning in yoga as well as other systems of Indian philosophy, Krishnamacharya emphasised that the practice of yoga must be adapted to the individual and the other way around. This deeply held view was one of his most significant contributions to the field of health and healing through yoga.

Around the 1940's, Krishnamacharya always counted in Sanskrit, yet in the 70's, the grandfather of modern-day yoga began counting in English[9], adapting his teachings to not only accommodate changing times, but to accommodate his audience which now included more westerners. Some food for thought for modern day yoga teachers who insist on counting and chanting the names of poses in Sanskrit. The idea that counting and saying names of poses in Sanskrit because it contains something mystical and spiritual is all nonsense.

The period of success and great achievements for the great man came to an end in 1940 with the demise of the Maharaja. His successor did not have as much interest in yoga. A desperate Krishnamacharya, now in his late fifties, had to struggle to earn a livelihood to feed his family. He was offered a job as a lecturer in the Vivekananda College in Madras. He migrated and lived there for the rest of his life. At the age of 96, Krishnamacharya fractured his hip. Refusing surgery, he treated himself and designed a course of practice that he could do in bed. He continued to live and teach in Chennai. Even though the accident prevented him from performing full asanas easily, he still practiced and performed his pranayama daily. His mind remained sharp and crystal clear up until 1989 when suddenly he slipped into a coma. Shortly after, Sri T Krishnamacharya passed away at the age of 100.

German filmmaker Jan Schmidt-Garre asked Krishnamacharya's son Sribhashyam the following question when interviewing him for a documentary:

"What is the essence of yoga that he (Krishnamacharya) taught his students?"

Sribhashyam replied, "If I remember well, he was giving three reasons to do yoga. One is physical health. Second is mental health, that is purity of thought, courage and perseverance. Very good objectives for his students. The third is concentration, mental concentration, almost like preparing them for examination."[10]

Krishnamacharya had a number of students. Two of these men would go onto further influence and inspire modern yoga practice many years after his death. Those two students are his brother in law B. K. S Iyengar and one of his star pupils, Pattabhi Jois. Pattabhi continued to teach the vinyasa and the more dynamic ashtanga practice that his guru pioneered. Mr B. K. S Iyengar moved away from the dynamic style of yoga being taught by Pattabhi and create what became known as "Iyengar Yoga", a slower, methodical and more alignment-based yoga.

Both systems of yoga, the Iyengar method and the Ashtanga Vinyasa method are both essentially hatha yoga with different interpretations. They both have great emphasis on bodily "postures" and the same ideology that suffering can be reduced or even removed by exercising the physical body and keeping it active. Both systems also believe that in order to have strength in the mind, one must have strength in the body. The physical body is understood as being a temple where your soul resides. So nothing "spiritual" can be gained unless the physical body is first attended to. A huge priority is placed on our bodies by both systems, which was not really emphasised before. It existed before 1920 but not with the same importance as it does now.

Most modern yoga teachers teach a hybrid of the Iyengar and Ashtanga Vinyasa system (almost unknowingly sometimes). They are essentially the original schools of modern physical yoga. Everything you see today has been influenced in some manner by them.

So, as a brief summary, yoga was created by Shiva 12,000 years ago (culturally speaking) and then defined by Patanjali some 2,000 years ago (as the stillness of the mind). It was then given a different dimension by the great Gorakhnath around 1,000 years ago. It was then made popular by Krishnamacharya between 1920 and 1940 with a much greater emphasis on the physical body and yoga postures/asanas. It was finally refined and redefined by the late great B. K. S Iyengar in the 1960s.

Additional teachers who have paved the way for teachers like us include the inspiring Indra Devi (1899–2002), who was an ex-dancer of Russian decent and the first foreign female student of Krishnamacharya studying alongside B.K.S Iyengar and Pathabhi Jois. Indra Devi was instrumental in creating the worldwide appeal of physical yoga, having taught the first ever physical yoga class in China in 1939. Indra Devi once said, "Yoga is a way to freedom. By its constant practice, we can free ourselves from fear, anguish and loneliness"[11].

T.K.V Desikachar (1938–2016, Krishnamacharya's grandson) developed viniyoga (a more individual-adaptive form of yoga rather than a class-led one). On the subject of yoga, Desikachar has said, "Yoga is a mystery. It does not mean the same thing to each and every one. In spite of the vast field it covers curing chronic ailments, extra-sensory perception, etc, hardly anyone is able to define it in simple terms. Where is then the hope of experiencing its true significance?"[12]

Bishnu Charan Gosh (1903–1970) was an ex-bodybuilding champion born in Lahore, Pakistan (pre-partition). Gosh was the younger brother of Paramahansa Yogananda (1893–1952, Author of the *Autobiography of a Yogi*). Gosh opened his college of Physical Education in India 1923 and taught not just bodybuilding exercises but, at times, a hybrid of bodybuilding and yoga poses. Gosh would later train someone in a very physical and strength-based form of yoga, and this student would himself go on to popularise physical yoga internationally. The student is none other than the infamous Bikram Choudhury.

Choudhury, controversy aside, placed such a huge emphasis on physical fitness and aesthetics with his form of heated "hatha" yoga that he gained for yoga huge mainstream and worldwide attention.

There is obviously a huge gap between Shiva and Patanjali, and this is no way a complete history of yoga or physical yoga. I have kept it short and sweet to keep it simple and accessible. Once the fundamentals are understood and a foundation settled, it becomes easier to build upon.

*Disciple: So, the poses we do in class - the triangle, the warrior 1, the lotus and the like - are all poses derived from hatha yoga?*

Correct. The degree of their authenticity and when they originated is an ongoing academic examination that we will not discuss but in general, the answer is yes. Are the poses we do part of the original 8.4 million yoga poses Shiva taught his wife? (more on that in the next chapter) I very much doubt it but it's nice to say yes, as a romantic notion.

*"The complex transformative practices that we know as yoga today is itself the product of some four thousand years of transformation"[13] — David Gordon White, Yoga: The Art of Transformation*

*Disciple: Then why are there so many different versions of the same pose? Why is warrior 2 for example taught so differently by different teachers? What is the right way to do it?*

Shiva and Parvati's children where in a deep discussion.
Kartakeya: "There are so many different paths, so many competing and sometimes contradictory philosophies. How do I know which one is the truth?"

Ganesh replied; "Who says anything is the truth?"

This is for the same reason that there is no one way to get to any destination. Say your destination is your place of work. You may have your preferred route to get to work, and it is this very route that you will recommend to others. This is the tried and tested formula that you prefer. Someone else may however prefer to take a different route to your workplace. The destination is the same, but the journey is different because they do not come from the same place as you. They may live in a completely different area. Nevertheless, if they were asked for directions, they would give their preferred route, especially if they are not even aware of additional routes.

Most teachers teach in a way that has either allowed them to get into the pose themselves or in the way they were shown, which they think is the easiest way to teach. Thus, different and varying teaching methods exist. Another reason for why there are so many variations and different ways "to do" a pose is because our bodies are all so different. Teachers, over the years, have thankfully adapted their teaching to accommodate the various shapes and sizes. Ultimately, there is no wrong or right way "to do" or to get into a pose. Each way or variation is just that - a different way or another variation. One of the beauties of yoga is the fact that there is not a right way. There are multiple interpretations.

Observing the way students do their poses is also a fascinating look into the mechanics of the human body and why there is no one way to do a pose. When a student does not do exactly as they have been asked by the teacher, this is often for one of two reasons.

One: The student's body is seeking the path of least resistance. The student does not want to push their body for whatever reason. It could be because of an old injury, laziness, attention-seeking and so on. On a side note, what is the teacher to do? Should they leave them or nurture them? There really is no right or wrong answer.

Two: The other reason a student does not always do as they are asked is because they are doing something within the pose that will instinctively accommodate their own anatomy. To give you an example, let us consider the downward facing dog. Some students cannot have their feet hip-width apart. Some cannot straighten their legs or get their heels down. The hand position is rarely the same from one student to another. Interestingly, the only teacher (my wife aside) who has never tried to correct my downward dog is the yoga anatomist, David Kiel. He commented on it but did not correct it. My downward dog is wider than the average person's. My hands are at a much wider position, my legs are bent, and my heels do not touch the ground. My entire focus is on the integrity of my spine and not my legs. I have to do the pose in this way to accommodate the problems I have had in the past with my back and sciatic pain. David saw my longer stance and just moved on. I was convinced he would "correct" me and ask me to step in more, bring my hands closer together and make other such suggestions (as so many ashtanga teachers have done before), but he did not. After the pose, he asked how my back was. I said "fine". He said, "Good. Learn to listen to your body".

David Kiel saw my body and how I moved and correctly assumed that I was bodily aware. This was not my first saw yoga class. So, David gave me the freedom in the downward dog and assumed I was doing the pose a little differently to accommodate my unique anatomy. Without over instructing me, David gave me the freedom to explore and independently arrive at my "destination". This is what real teaching is. He found the simplest and most effective method of getting me into the final posture. David was not telling me how to do downward dog in the way his teacher taught him, he was allowing me (under his guidance) to arrive at my own conclusion. This mirrors what Shiva did with Parvati. He offered guidance, but Parvati had to arrive at the destination for herself. Thus, David Kiel may be the most yogic teacher of them all - What a revelation!

Teachers who, in the past, have told me to walk my feet in and straighten my legs more are demanding that my anatomy fit into what they think is the ideal way to do the pose. This caused me physical pain each time. We are all so unique that we cannot always accommodate a pose the way a teacher prefers it. We have to find a way to make the pose fit around us. For this reason, no downward facing dog looks the same. Each person will and should do the pose slightly differently. David's approach was the perfect approach for my body, What David was doing allowed me to begin my own enquiry regarding my body. Kahlil Gibran once said, "If he is indeed wise, he does not bid you enter the house of his wisdom, but rather leads you to the threshold of your own mind". This is what David did. While he remained quiet on the surface, it was real teaching that allowed me to do more than just a pose; I was able to have an experience.

These experiences change the way a teacher approaches and teaches a pose. A teacher can only share his or her own experiences in class. Some give freedom while others do not. Yoga teachers have different techniques in the same way a personal trainer at the gym does. It is all so subjective. Each trainer thinks they know better, so they will have a slightly different take on something that you may have done a hundred times before.

Every yoga class presents a new opportunity to grow, understand and move forward as well as to become more aware of the very subtle sensations throughout your body. Stay the course because you are still moving in the right direction. Ultimately, the right path and teaching points for you are the ones that agree with your own logic and make you happy or at ease within yourself. The art is to try all the methods until your own conclusion is reached. Do not just do something or believe something because your yoga teachers say's so. For all you know, you may know more about the human body than they do. The key is to listen and then absorb what is logical to you and disregard the nonsensical. So, if a yoga teacher says your hands should be wider in downward dog, then take them wider and see how it feels. The class is your laboratory to experiment. Is yoga not a science after all? If another teacher says the hands should be narrower, then give that a go. Then after some time and practice, draw your own conclusion. The wrong way is the hand position that creates pain. It is that simple. Contrastingly, the correct way is the hand position that feels comfortable yet difficult in a non-nerve stabbing sort of way. Over time, you will work it out, and you will learn to ignore the various teaching points that are thrown around so often.

My wife has a hand position in downward dog and in handstand that I think is too narrow for her frame. The proud teacher in me wants to "correct" her as her hand position is not 'textbook'. It does not agree with the aesthetics I have come to understand. So, should I correct her? I know, it would be brave to do so. But apart from fearing for my life, there is another reason I have not said a word. Laura's hand position is only incorrect according to my own understanding of the aesthetics behind the pose. This does not mean what Laura is doing is wrong. It only means that I think it is wrong. Is it not better to just ponder for a while? Laura has been doing downward dog for longer than I have, and there is no obvious pain or noticeable postural distortion as a result. So, is she doing it wrong? Also, as much as it pains me to admit it, her handstand is ten times more graceful than my own. As she moves into the upside-down position, you are instantly hit by her beauty and elegance. All this, with her hands in a position that Zahir, the teacher, thinks is wrong. So who is right - the angelic students on her hands defying gravity with her grace or the know-it-all teacher who thinks he knows best?

The art, in a long-term sense, for the student is to embrace the fact that each time you are told to do something differently, do not see it as the teacher saying his or her way is better - it is just different. You will learn to disregard nonsense and observe the useful. This is part of the journey.

*Disciple: So, modern yoga, the yoga poses, can you tell me why we do them again?*

*"The result of this branch of physical Yoga is to make men live long; health is the chief idea, the one goal of the Hatha-Yogi. He is determined not to fall sick, and he never does"[14] — Swami Vivekananda*

The poses are all designed to remove stiffness from the body and restore your energy levels. If there are restrictions in our bodies (tight muscles), the body seeks the path of least resistance. This means that muscles work when they should not or some muscles overwork. This creates a pattern of muscle overuse, which leads to fatigue and injury. The idea is to preserve muscular energy. Thus, training your body in a certain way ensures that it learns to switch muscles off when they are not needed and to not over-stress the muscles that are being worked.

Yoga poses work because they can, with time, restore the elasticity of muscles - muscles shorten over time and with overuse. The tight muscle in question can then make the relevant joint stiff, which then impairs movement. For example, think of the hamstrings on the back of the thighs. If these muscles stay tight and short, perhaps from playing sport or sitting all day long, they can limit the movement of your knees and hips. This can then create a cumulative effect that can even go so far as to affect your breathing and posture. If you can stretch the hamstrings in a yoga class, you can restore their elasticity and give them back the freedom they crave. The hips and knees now do not feel the pressure of tightness, which ultimately means you can move better, more freely and without pain - this is the theory. If you can move and feel better physically, you can think more clearly too.

Yoga is thus psychological, and we just use our bodies to influence or alter our psychology.

*"When the body is sufficiently controlled, we can attempt the manipulation of the mind." - Swami Vivekananda*

*Disciple: Okay, I am starting to piece it all together now. So, what type of yoga do you teach?*

I teach *hatha* yoga. All teachers today teach *hatha* yoga. Most people who ask me this question get this usual response. Then they say, "*hatha*? What . . . like slow n' shit? And I reply, "err . . . not really". Most people think *hatha* yoga is slow yoga. But all yoga today is *hatha* yoga. The difference is just in people's interpretations. The philosopher Susan Sotag once said that interpretations are the intellectuals' revenge on art. I see her point. In the case of *hatha* yoga, the earlier interpretations were needed to make yoga more accessible for modern man. However, the newer types of yoga you can practice now owe nothing to intellect but instead ironically, a lack of it. We are in the age now of gimmick yoga where every teacher and their down dog has a trick or a unique selling point. This is the reality that we live in. One day, I fear that the systems of Iyengar and Ashtanga will no longer hold any authority or credibility. Both will be in a hostile takeover situation by modern yogis trying to invent something "cool": Bollywood yoga, spin yoga, face yoga and so on. I could go on, but it is very painful.

Do not get me wrong, I am happy for people to move and exercise. I am happy that people do things that help their health and minds. But the line has to be drawn somewhere because the yoga of the future will eventually no longer resemble the yoga that is being done today.

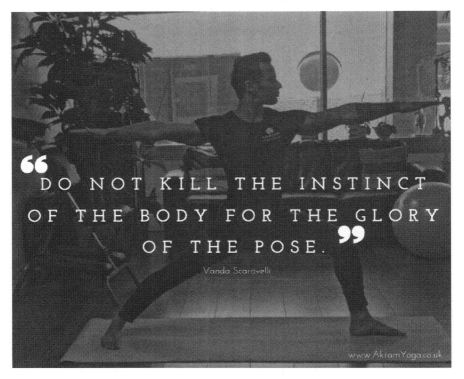

**DO NOT KILL THE INSTINCT OF THE BODY FOR THE GLORY OF THE POSE.**

Vanda Scaravelli

www.AkramYoga.co.uk

The earliest meaning of *"asana"* was not in reference to a "physical posture" as it is today. It is more likely to have been just a seated posture or it could have even been referring to the seat itself. The word *asana* could also just mean "to exist" or the "manner of sitting (gracefully)" or even just "observance".

In modern day Hindu dialogue, I have often heard the word asana be used when referring to a couch, a sort of high chair (signifying authority) or even a throne. *"Aap asana me behat jaiye"* – which means "You should sit on your high chair/stool" or in the context of this dialogue, "a throne" (it was said to me very sarcastically). Today, in modern yoga, when we say *asana*, we refer to the physical poses of yoga – here, *asana* means pose or posture: the triangle and the warrior 2s of this world.

# Mythology of Poses
## The Dancer

The cultural view is that the cosmic couple Shiva and Parvati created the concept of these "*asanas*". In a further conversation with his wife Parvati all those thousands of years ago, Shiva taught the love of his life 8.4 million yoga poses! There are as many poses as there were species at that time on this planet. Some poses where created and added to yoga folklore as a result of the ongoing cosmic dance between the two. Think of the modern-day dancer pose as an example (image below). Shiva and Parvati, being the ultimate yogis, spent most of their time practicing together or immersed in each other's arms.

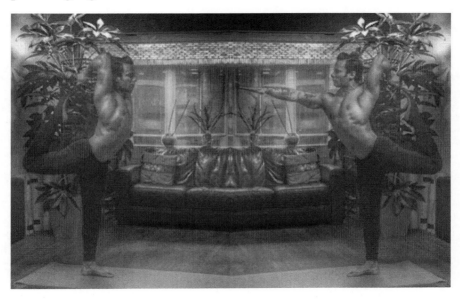

*above - Attempting my Natraja posture using a sock. I keep telling Laura I am catching her up. Of course, this is far from the truth.*

Shiva once lovingly challenged Parvati to a dance contest knowing Parvati's competitive but playful nature. Parvati had to imitate all of Shiva's poses and perform them as perfectly as he did. The theatre in Parvati's heart was about to begin. She danced and performed the poses with gentleness and grace as the moon adoringly looked on. Nature also came to a standstill. It was impossible to not be mesmerised by a woman who displayed the grace of a goddess. Shiva himself was hypnotised.

In order to tease her, Shiva took up the difficult posture known as "*urdhva-thandava*" (*urdhva* loosely means "upward"; *thandava*, means "the divine dance"). In this pose, Shiva, from a standing position, lifted his foot straight above his head with elegant simplicity. Shiva radiated masculine elegance. Parvati tried but was unable to imitate this particular posture, so she responded with an equally beautiful feminine pose. This elegance under pressure was the epitome of divine beauty. This is supposedly the modern day "dancer pose": *natraja-asana*, called the lord of the dance. However, this could just be Parvati's interpretation – the goddess of dance.

After the dance "contest", Shiva hailed his glorious wife saying, "Your magic spreading, it is making my heart go a little crazy. You must be born of fire such is your will. What can this heart do but love? To experience the dancer (*Nataraja*) in the pose, we must get so immersed in the pose that we become the dance itself. So, when we practice, we don't just do the dancer pose, we immerse ourselves in it as if we are the dancer. *Nataraja* is the dance of Shiva. Thus, when we make the shape of the pose, we embody the fearlessness of Shiva and/or the grace and elegance of Parvati – we become so immersed in what we are doing that we become the pose itself.

So remember, we don't do the dancer pose, we become the dancer in the pose.

The language within our souls is expressed only, at such a time that we become immersed in the posture. We should ideally feel the dancer in every part of our bodies, our skin, our nerves and our muscles. The pose is not about the bendiness of the spine or the perfect balance, its more about the vitality and energy you parade. The final posture becomes the most upright, elegant and graceful pose that we can perform. Only through the intensity of the pose can we experience the enchantment of *nataraja-asana*.

Nietzsche once said, "We should consider every day lost on which we have not danced at least once."

## The Forward Fold

There is another story with reference to the birth of *Paschimottana-asana* (the seated forward fold). Before Parvati made her glorious enquiry of Shiva's nature, she observed Shiva's meditation with much curiosity and noticed a cluster of stars above Shiva every time he was absorbed in his meditation. Parvati was spellbound at such beauty. Once Shiva was out of his meditative state, Parvati asked Shiva if she could see those stars up close. Shiva said yes but that it would not be fair to the stars as they would lose their lustre in the presence of Parvati's beauty. "All this is of you O radiant one," Shiva said, "Your smile is brighter than the moon and your eyes could decorate the cosmos. The stars will hide in the far galaxies upon knowing your grace". Overcome with shyness, Parvati asked her husband to stop teasing her. Shiva then said that before she could touch the stars, Parvati must do something for him. Parvati agreed. Shiva asked her to sit on the ground with her back and legs straight. Shiva then asked her to reach for her feet. When she could not, Shiva then lovingly laughed at Parvati and said, "How can my exquisite wife reach the stars when she cannot yet reach her toes?" Parvati, feeling embarrassed, got up immediately and stormed away. Shiva then chased his lover down and reminded her he was just teasing her as he so often did. Shiva then promised to one day bring the stars to his beloved: "O radiant one, the sky will turn to darkness as the thousands of stars will be presented to you like lotus flowers. Your every wish is my desire".

Romance aside, this is an interesting metaphor. We often have the desire to do and master certain poses but as Mr. Iyengar once said, "How can you reach god if you cannot even reach your big toe?" We should thus start our practice of yoga with short-term goals. Reaching your toes for the first time could be a minor moment of enlightenment as it was for me.

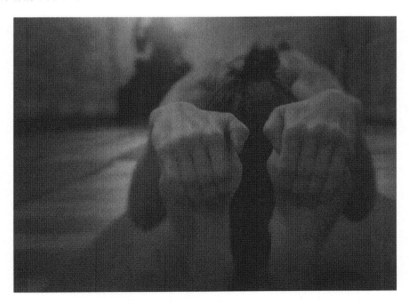

*above - My friend and fellow yoga teacher Emma Talbot in her forward fold posture.*

# Archers Pose

Continuing with the "mythology" of the poses, let us look at the archer's pose (*Akarna dhanura-asana* - below) that most of my students perform so enthusiastically in class.

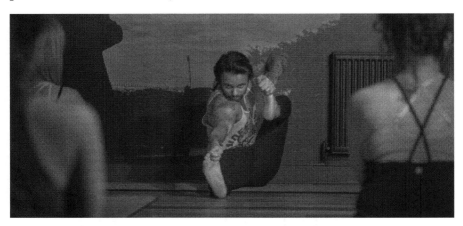

Long ago, a demon named Taraka, who was proud of his invincible might, was causing much havoc and terror in the world. Even the kings where afraid of him because many years before Taraka turned evil, he had received a divine gift that only Shiva's son would be capable of killing him (in Hindu mythology the demons were always good before they turned "bad", and they always seem to have convenient "boons" or gifts given to them by a god).

This was during the time when Parvati, the future wife of Shiva, was performing penance praying that Shiva would awaken from his years of meditation and notice her. Think of this story as a prequel to the Shiva and Parvati love story. Shiva has not yet noticed her, and they are not married.

Indra, the king of the heavens, also became desperate to awaken Shiva as he was convinced that Taraka would soon overthrow the heavens. He also knew that the only person who could stop Taraka would be Shiva's unborn child. He was desperate for Shiva to open his eyes and fall hopelessly in love with the divine Parvati. But Parvati's penance and prayers were fruitless as Adiyogi's meditation was impenetrable – there was no awakening him. In a final attempt to awaken Shiva from his samadhi, Indra desperately called upon Kama, the Hindu cupid, the god of love and desire. Indra pleaded and begged with Kama to use his arrow made of heavenly flowers and scent to rouse the passion of love in Shiva's mind. "Go and fill Shiva's heart with desire for Parvati. Force him to give up his meditation and embrace the entrancing princess," Indra said to Kama in a trembling, fearful voice.

Kama replied, "*O tere baap ka nokar hoon kya?*" (do I look like your father's servant?). Okay, he did not really say that. Kama actually said, "Are you insane?" as he had no intention to interrupt Shiva who sat with the skin of a dead animal over his shoulders, protected by ghouls, goblins and snakes; there were also skulls scattered around him with smoke arising from them all. Kama was more sensible than to incur the wrath of someone no one knew much about.

Finally, after being guilted into saving the earth and the heavens, Kama agreed. He proceeded to the place in the Himalayas where Shiva was in his meditation. He stood and patiently waited for the perfect opportunity to strike Shiva with his arrow of love. His body perspired, his heart was beating at three times its regular pace, his mind was anxious, and his knees trembled.

After a while, Kama observed Parvati approaching Shiva and placing flowers at his feet. Too impatient to wait any longer, Kama decided now was the right time. If the arrow of love was to strike Shiva, his eyes would open, and he would notice Parvati. This was the perfect opportunity. Kama shot the arrow of flowers from his bow. Time appeared to stand still as the arrow made its way towards Shiva. Parvati noticed the fragrance of the flowers and turned her head. She saw Kama and the arrow of flowers and observed as the arrow approached Shiva's chest.

As the arrow made its way towards Shiva, Shiva awoke from his samadhi (deep meditation). Adiyogi saw the arrow approaching at a great speed and was furious; "*Kutteh, main terra khoon pee jaaunga*" (Bollywood dialogue – props to Dharmendra). This means "You dog/rascal, I am going to drink your blood!" So Shiva didn't really say that. I am just interjecting for dramatic effect. Shiva then burnt the approaching arrow with his eyes. The ash-covered yogi was furious at being awakened so he incinerated Kama instantaneously and turned the Indian cupid into ash.

Usually, even if Shiva opened his eyes for a split second, it was his practice to close them again and return calmly to his meditation – such was his control. But this time, thanks to Kama's intervention, he was unable to tear his gaze away from Parvati's enchanting form. He stared at her as if spellbound, and Parvati, who had been longing and waiting for this day, gazed deeply into his eyes. Shiva's anger at Kama, however, was short-lived: Kama's spirit would be reborn as Pradyumna (no one ever really dies in Indian tradition. They are always reborn).

Shiva and Parvati were then united as per the story at the start of the book. Parvati's beauty and wit conquered the heart of this great yogi.

They fell into each other's arms, their love enrapturing the universe. Their love then created balance in the cosmos. After marriage, the cosmic couple would have their first child, Kartakeya. In due course, Kartakeya would slay the demon Taraka and bring peace once again to earth. And thus, everyone lived happily ever after.

The pose we assume when in the archer's pose resembles Kama readying himself to fire his flower arrow at Shiva. If the bow is too tight, the strings will snap. If the bow is too loose, the target will not be met. Therefore, the pose is about finding the correct balance of effort and relaxation. If you pull on your foot with too much force, you may snap something. If you don't pull it enough, nothing happens. So next time, you are in this pose, think carefully. When you are at full draw, the tension in the "string" will force the bow to align itself in a certain direction – straight ahead. Subsequently, when you "release", the arrow will hit the intended target.

The idea of balanced effort is not just relative to our bow pose but is transferable to many and all poses. Our nature is to do the poses via either of the two extremes: extreme effort or extreme non-effort. We don't try enough for the poses we consider too challenging, and we work too hard for the poses we can do with our eyes closed. Thus, the middle path is the preferred way. It is a harmony between the two opposites. When I was young, my mum used to always say don't laugh too much because you will soon be crying. This logic appeared absurd to me at the time, but it is true. We can't laugh or cry all day long. We cannot stay at the end of these extremes. We cannot be too positive or too negative. We have to be realistic. We cannot stay and gaze into the sky all day and just be spellbound by nature in the same way that we cannot sit all day at our desks. Life is about seeking a balance.

*"Your hand opens and closes, opens and closes. If it were always a fist or always stretched open, you would be paralysed. Your deepest presence is in every small contracting and expanding, the two as beautifully balanced and coordinated as birds' wings." - Jelaluddin Rumi[2]*

## Parvati becomes Mastya

On another occasion after marriage, Shiva watched enchanted as Parvati was flowing through her daily yoga routine. Shiva couldn't keep his eyes off his beloved, so he interrupted her practice. "O divine lady, I have never seen one beautiful as you, where has my heart been before this? I'm starting to live more than ever, more than ever, I am dying for you".

Parvati was flattered but wanted to really test Shiva. She knew he was poetic, and he always said the right words but spent more time in meditation that he did with her. Although married, she was starting to feel lonely. So, Parvati told Shiva that his "*jhuti muti baatein*" (his sweet words) were no longer enough. She wished for Shiva to show her how he really felt. Parvati shocked Shiva by saying she was leaving him, and he should not follow her. If their love was real, he would one day find her. Shiva was devastated. He may have presented himself in such a way that some felt he was of divine origin, but under the surface, Shiva's insides were tearing him apart.

Parvati left, and Shiva was lost. In the valleys of his daydreams, all he could see was her. From the earth to the sky, Parvati's fragrance was everywhere. Shiva felt like the earth was burning around him, and he was helpless. The moon had lost its splendour. Nature no longer danced to the vibration of the cosmos. There was a storm in the heart of this great yogi, and he was restless for his companion.

After only a few days, Shiva decided enough was enough. He yearned for one of Parvati's sideway glances. He had taken the goddess for granted, and now he was going to win her back and bring her back to the icy peaks of Kailash.

Shiva set off in search for his beloved hoping she would once again accept his words of love. After many months of searching aimlessly, Shiva noticed a woman in the distance who he believed to be his wife. He hid and observed her. She looked like Parvati and had the same angelic glow. Wherever she walked, flowers would blossom, and whenever she smiled, birds would sing. Shiva could taste her fragrance in his breath. Shiva's heart began to pound as he yearned for Parvati's gaze. But at that moment, Shiva noticed something peculiar. Parvati was surrounded by fisherman, and she herself was dressed as one. Shiva became intrigued. Upon listening further, it transpired that Parvati was now living as Matsya (which means fish). She was living as the adopted daughter of an elderly fisherman. Shiva took the disguise of a regular man and approached Matsya. She noticed him immediately but continued walking with the rest of her adopted family. Shiva smiled to himself knowing that his love would not give in so easy – this was part of why he adored her so much. Shiva had to come up with a plan for his wife to once again accept his words of love.

Shiva stayed at the village for a few days to make a plan. But it was not going well. He didn't know what to do. Then in his moment of anguish, Shiva heard a commotion. He went to see what the problem was and noticed that all the villagers had gathered around. The head fisherman announced that the great shark had returned and was making it impossible for them to fish and earn a living. As the head of the village, he was desperate for a solution. With his *izzat* (reputation/ego) at stake, the head fisherman announced that if anyone could capture the shark, they would be rewarded with his daughter's hand in marriage. This daughter was Matsya or Parvati to you and me. There was a huge eruption as all the men, even those who were already married, rushed to their homes to collect weapons of any description, so they could catch this shark. There may be plenty of fish in the sea, but none quite like Matsya. She was considered the most alluring and beautiful person the village had ever seen. She was the messiah of love and grace, which is why even the married men set off to look for their tools.

Many brave and soon-to-be single men tried. Many courageous men failed. This shark was not to be captured. The villagers grew desperate and prayed feverishly to Narayan (one of the main gods). Narayan observing from his heavenly abode just laughed. He was enjoying this cosmic dance between Shiva and Parvati and knew what would transpire.

Soon, the villagers' prayers were answered. A stranger entered the village with the lofty promise of capturing this shark. No one had seen this man before. The villagers looked puzzled but hypnotised at the same time. This man was an enigma with an alluring appeal. It appeared as though nature had been kind to him as his handsome features made the normally timid women of the village giggle like schoolgirls. The village elders normally so uptight with their wives no longer cared. They pleaded with this man to save them and their village and slay this shark. The beautiful stranger replied that he was only here to get rid of the shark and not kill it. Desperate, the villagers agreed. Matsya upon hearing the commotion the village ladies where making peeked over a few shoulders and saw this stranger. He was devilishly handsome with eyes that looked like a tiger's peering out of the forest. Matsya sensing something fishy looked closer and beyond the disguise of the beard and garments. Upon looking intently, she was left open-mouthed. It was our hero: Shiva.

Did anyone see that coming? He gave Matsya a flirtatious wink (that set off a flutter of butterflies in Matysa's stomach) and set off to capture the shark. Matsya kept her composure but was secretly delighted. She had missed her husband severely. A few moments later, Matsya heard an outburst of loud cheers. She made her way to the banks of the river to see what had transpired and who would have guessed it? The stranger had already captured the shark. The Aquaman of Indian mythology caught the shark and set it free someplace else so as not to bother the villagers again. There was a huge celebration and the villagers drank and sang to the early hours. For the first time in many months, the locals rejoiced – they had a whale of a time. Their community could once again flourish now that the shark was no longer eating all their fish and making their lives difficult. All the while the valiant stranger spoke to the village elder and asked if he would honour his promise. The village elder was so happy that he said the stranger could also marry his own wife if he so wished! The stranger laughed and said that something told him Matsya would be more than enough for him to handle. Matsya was presented to this stranger and was asked if she was happy with the arrangement.

Matsya lifted her veil and asked the brave stranger, "It is you who wishes to make the mistake of falling in love with me?" The stranger replied, "I have been falling since I saw you for the first time. The matter of my heart that was so tucked away is now like an open book. O divine one, I ask that it is you who makes the mistake of again falling in love with me. I ask that your love be medicine as I was poisoned the moment you left. I have come upon hearing your name. O radiant one, my life is only complete with you". Matsya upon hearing these words revealed herself to all as being Parvati, the wife of Shiva. The stranger revealed himself to be Shiva, the Adiyogi. The villagers were ecstatic as the world once again rejoiced in the love of the cosmic couple.

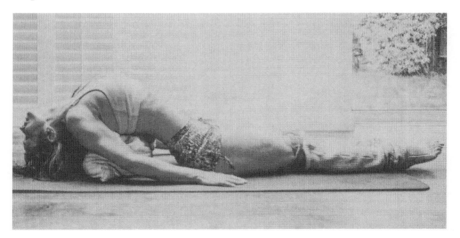

*above - My Laura in the Matsya fish posture.*

*Disciple: I didn't have you down as the romantic type Akram! So, is that why we do the fish pose, Mastyasana – to encourage us to not hide behind our alter egos? Or when we lift our chests in the pose, are we opening our hearts and being more receptive to love?*

What? No. It has nothing to do with anything like that. More often than not, the pose has no "spiritual" meaning at all – such as when it is named after a fish or a cobra. Most of the time, the pose is just about taking the shape of something. It has no hidden meaning. We yoga people desperately want to psychoanalyse a pose and its history and find a context. With anything to do with India, we are always look for a hidden meaning. It never ceases to surprise me how our enthusiasm and imagination always tries to place spiritual significance on nothing. We ask ourselves; "What is this pose telling me about me"? My answer is it is telling you nothing. It is just a pose. There is no philosophy. Sometimes our drive to seek meaning in something makes us miss the obvious truth.

Sigmund Freud has said, "Sometimes a cigar is just a cigar".

*Disciple: Oh, so why tell the story?*

I just like the story.

*Disciple: Oh. Okay. So, 8.4 million yoga poses? Is there a mythology behind the "Bird of Paradise" pose?*

I imagine some former dancer (in the past ten years or so) with very pointy toes just made it up, and someone decided she looked like a bird from paradise. Then other students said, "Wow that's so spiritual". Oh, I don't really know

# The Poses

*Disciple: So the poses kind of tell the story of Shiva and Parvati? I have heard from my yoga friends during our many vegan brunches that most of the poses we do today are a modern invention and have just been 'made-up' over the past few decades.*

The modern physical yoga culture is not a modern invention as such. Although many poses continue to develop to this day owing much to the 'creativity' of the modern yoga teacher. Or more like the fickle attention span the teacher feels the students have. But in any case, yoga has always been an adaptive culture. Hence why it has survived for so many centuries. At the time of the big exercise boom in India during British rule, yoga adapted and found a way to survive. This may have involved borrowing or taking ideas from wrestling and or gymnastics or perhaps the physical yoga poses that already existed where given a new lease of life or a more modern interpretation.

As for how these more modern day (non-seated) yoga poses developed - An 1899 article "Anatomy of a contortionist" shows what would many years later, become yoga poses (including foot behind the head pose, chin stand and hanuman splits)[1]. How or who merged these exercises or movements into the existing yoga poses handbook is anyone's guess.

Scandinavian gymnastics was also a huge influence in what we know of today as the modern yoga poses. A 1944 Danish text shows what would later become the Warrior poses, downward facing dog and the reclining thunderbolt pose[2]. Traditional Indian dance and Indian wrestling was also hugely influential in yoga adapting and becoming more popular. From the 1850s onwards, a culture of physical exercise developed in India to counter the colonial stereotype of supposed "degeneracy" of Indians compared to the British[3].

Physical fitness was not just an Indian fascination, in early 1900 the fame of the bodybuilder Eugene Sandow (1867-1925) also made it internationally, very much in vogue to look after one's physical appearance. It is said that Sandow deserves the credit for the international craze for physical fitness. In his book; 'Yoga in Modern India: The Body Between Science and Philosophy', the author Joseph Alter suggests that Sandow is the one person who had the most influence on the development of modern-day physical yoga. Sandow visited India in 1905 and made such a wave with his physique and popularity, being referred to as the 'fakir of physical culture', that physical yoga borrowed many of Sandow's exercises and routines. Much of Sandow's influence owes to his approach. Rather than play up the gritty iron side of weightlifting, Sandow presented his approach to Calcutta as a kind of 'meditation with muscles'. In a Bengali newspaper, Sandow said; "It is the cooperation of the mind with the body that makes the system so unique and explains the great results which have been attained"[4].

This boom in the physical culture is perhaps the key reason why you and I are so fascinated in yoga today.

Some poses such as 'bridge' and 'wheel' may also be, dare I say it, 'inspired' by the Kama Sutra. There is a position called the turning posture and chakra asana (wheel pose). These sexual positions are paintings found on the exterior of many temples in India. This particular one that may have inspired wheel pose (or upward facing bow pose), is called 'the wheel posture' and is from a 19th century painting in Nepal[5]. I have heard it be said that the Kama Sutra inspired various yoga poses but it could also easily be the other way around.

Are the modern-day yoga poses, the same poses from all those thousands of years ago? Like I said previously, chances are slim. But this does not mean they are all modern inventions. Maybe the poses have just evolved like so much of the Indian culture has. Perhaps being an adaptive culture is what defines yoga tradition. Change is reflective of the modern period of life and sometimes, your need to adapt is what ignites your imagination and creativity. For physical yoga to flourish and for Krishnamacharya to survive and even earn a living, yoga had to evolve from a culture where one was readying the body for meditation, to becoming one where physical vitality was more important. The seeds for success and longevity are flexibility and adaptability. No pun intended.

There has been a bit of an outcry from western yogis (over the past few years) who feel 'let down' that so many of the poses they have been doing over the years are not 'authentic' or have been 'made up' in recent times. Their disappointment stems from their original belief that the modern-day yoga poses are 15,000 years old. I feel these practitioners are missing the point and don't fully understand the culture they feel they are so immersed in. Hinduism, yoga tradition and India itself has continually grown and adapted to the demands of modern times. Throughout history, anytime orthodox Hinduism was under threat, it took that threat and somehow weaved it into their own culture. When Gautam Buddha arrived and dismissed the Vedas, the Hindu establishment was threatened yet they somehow years later adopted the Buddha as their own and as an incarnation of their own Lord Vishnu. The crafty so and so's.

Hinduism is the world's oldest religion and is perhaps so because it has evolved and embraced change. Yoga as a 'branch' of Hinduism (or the other way around to be fair) has followed suit. It has adapted and then adopted various contortionism, gymnastics and wrestling type exercises into its repertoire and if it had not, I doubt I would be writing this book now and I doubt that any of us would be doing physical yoga postures today.

*Disciple – How did we hear about Shiva's yoga poses according to the traditional view-point? Did he scribe them on tablets and pass them down to his devotees from a mountain top?*

It happened. You may want to suspend your belief for a second. As with all stories that start with… 'It happened'.

There was once a holy man or sage, who was in meditation on the banks of the river Ganga. Suddenly, mid-samadhi, the sage was swallowed by a giant fish. The sage was stuck inside the fish as the fish swam upstream. For many days, this sage sat hopeless in the stomach of this big fish. But one day, the sage overheard some people talking outside. The fish must have swum all the way to the abode of Shiva in Kailash as the voice he heard was that of Shiva! The fish was now taking a nap from the long swim, so the sage was able to overhear Shiva and his wife Parvati in conversation. The sage overheard as Shiva taught his beloved wife a number of yoga poses (including the ones above). The sage memorised them all and knew he had heard this discussion for a reason. He was blessed. Sometime later, the holy sage escaped the jaws of death and raced away with this divine knowledge and shared it with whomever would listen and thus was born the system of yoga *asanas*. The sage was then called Matsyendra (which means "lord of the fishes") and is highly regarded in yogic lore.

This story must be taken with a pinch of salt. Like I said earlier, there is perhaps a metaphor that is probably far too advanced for me to fathom.

The following also happened.

Mullah Nasreddin, the wise fool from the Sufi tradition, while passing by a cave, saw a yogi in deep meditation and asked him what he was seeking. "I am contemplating the animals, and I learn many lessons from them which can transform a man's life", said the yogi. "Teach me what you know. And I will teach you what I have learned, because a fish has already saved my life", answers Nasruddin.

The yogi is surprised as only a saint can have his life saved by a fish. He decides to teach him everything he knows. "Now that I have taught you everything, I would be proud to know how a fish saved your life."

Nasruddin replies, "It is simple. I was almost dying of hunger when I caught it, and thanks to it, I was able to survive three days".

What is the relevance of the above story to me? Add a fish to the conversation with an Indian yogi, and they will believe anything you say. So I have come to discover.

*Disciple: Why do you are start each story with "It happened"? Are you mocking the mystics who start each story this way or are you just being sarcastic?*

It is a bit of both. Psychologists say sarcasm is hostility disguised as humour. I think I'm just amusing myself.

So, continuing our study of the history of asana, this sage Matsyendra (the lord of the fish) then passed this knowledge down to his students, who passed it down to their students who continued that lineage (the guru to student oral tradition called "*parampara*") for thousands of years until it fell into the hands of Krishnamacharya who, if you remember, passed this down to his student B. K. S Iyengar who would go on, in 1966, to show us around 200 of these poses in "Light on Yoga". Are the poses in "Light on Yoga" the very poses Shiva taught his wife all those thousands of years ago? The chances are slim. But you never know. Like I said earlier, there is much academic research that is being conducted in discovering the true origins of physical yoga poses. There is no doubt that this research will continue for many years to come. Not that their findings can make the yoga poses any less effective, but it at least gives academics something to do.

*Disciple: Why do these bendy and crackling yoga poses (asanas)?*

The *asanas* (yoga poses) are designed to eliminate physical and psychological suffering. They are a means to balance the body energetically until one is ready to sit still for long periods of time. In the West, however, we use this branch from the tree of yoga to just help us move with more freedom and think with more clarity. The *asanas* help us to either advance or preserve our physical flexibility as well as address, correct or maintain a balance of opposite forces within our bodies. The philosophy behind this is that an increase in flexibility and mobility allows your joints to move the way nature intended and with less stress around them. The lesser the stress on your joints, the more freely you move. And the more freely you move, the less pain you suffer. The less you suffer, the happier you are and the more likely you are to preserve your mental faculties. As Dr. Dre profoundly says in "Express Yourself", "You ain't efficient when you flow, you ain't swift, Movin like a tortoise, full of rigor mortis". This in a nutshell is why we do yoga. I appreciate that the Doc is talking about someone else's "rap flow", but you can easily apply that to modern man and the way he moves or doesn't move.

Our salvation from physical pain and psychological suffering are the poses of yoga.

The poses have been very intelligently designed to create balance within the body. This means that if followed and practiced correctly, the muscles on the right side of your body will be just as able, moveable and flexible as the muscles on your left side. The idea is to strive for symmetry and not flexibility. However, perfect symmetry can never be attained. We have so many unique differences in our bodies that aiming for perfection ahead of progress will only leave your body floating in an altogether different yoga paradox: not one that exists somewhere between madness and meditation but between stiffness and dislocation. Thus, perfection shouldn't be prioritised ahead of progress.

The yogis in the East say that asana is a way to channel and/or to drive energy into various parts of the body – parts that become redundant through everyday life. The idea is to nourish even the cells in our body with this dormant energy. Through discipline, we can learn to direct and even feel this energy influence our bodies.

The Western yogi (like me) says that I do various yoga poses because ultimately, it will make me breathe better, move better, think better and be better.

# The Warrior Poses
## The Tragedy of Sati

*Disciple: What about the Warrior poses? Legend has it that these poses tell an interesting 'mythological' story. Seeing as you love a story, what are the adventures behind the three Warrior postures?*

The three warrior asanas/poses are named after the mythological warrior, *Virabhadra*. The postures tell a story of an almighty battle of wills between an arrogant father, Daksha, and his unconventional son in law, the first yogi, Shiva.

I have provided more context in the following paragraph to set the tone:

Although I have previously referred to Shiva as a man and simply as "Adiyogi", in this story, he is "god incarnate". So, Shiva, in this mythological story, is one of a plethora of Hindu gods and arguably one of the most dominant and surely the most compelling. The woman in question, Sati, is also of divine nature. Sati is an incarnation of the supreme Goddess. Like her male counterpart, Sati herself is all powerful and dynamic. In some trains of Indian thought, the highest reality or god is made up of the masculine energy of Shiva and the feminine energy of the goddess. They are two sides of the same coin. One completes the other. When they arrive to earth in human form, although of divine energy, they are very much like us. They experience the same trials and tribulations as the rest of us but just with a little more flair and fantasy.

*Disciple: Sati? Who is she? And what happened to my favourite character of all – Parvati?*

Oops My bad. I didn't explain that part. This story is a prequel to the earlier stories involving Shiva and Parvati. This is even earlier than the story at the start of the whole book. It is important to remember that this is a prequel. You see, before Shiva fell for Parvati's celestial charm, he was a lonely hermit. Word is that the great yogi spent aeons on earth just wondering or sitting in deep meditation in what is now Kashmir. Many years before he met Parvati, he fell in love with and married another woman by the name of Sati. Here is the potentially confusing part. Sati and Parvati are the same person – sort of. They are both the same soul of the great goddess, *Adi Shakti*. At first, she was on earth as Sati and later, she returned as Parvati. Nevertheless, they are the same soul.

*Disciple: What?*

Just listen. And like a Tarantino movie this will all make sense by the end.

It happened many, many years ago.

Daksha was the lord of the people and the father of the princess Sati. Sati, after much family drama and squabble (which would need to be seen to be believed), was married to the wandering yogi Shiva. Daksha was at odds with Shiva because he found it very demeaning that the daughter of a man of his stature was married to a "vagrant beggar". Daksha as the emperor of the people wished for his daughter Sati to be married into royalty. Ultimately, he gave in to his daughters wishes but with each passing day, Daksha grew more and more frustrated at his decision.

Daksha really ought to have appreciated what a great honour it was for his daughter to be married to Shiva, but he was foolish and vain and could not see past initial appearances. Despite Shiva's grandeur and his position as a god in this story, he is frequently depicted in the scriptures as a wild untamed character who hung out with goblins and ghouls. He eschewed culture and refinement and lived in burial grounds, covered in ashes and wearing garlands of snakes and serpents. Nevertheless, the true devotees of Shiva see through these unprepossessing first impressions and give him the honour that is his due.

The more time that passed, the more Daksha's fury increased at the thought that his daughter was still married to such an apparently oafish wastrel. He was further incensed that Shiva refused to pay obeisance to him. Daksha had become so very arrogant in his position as the emperor of the people, he wanted to show the world that he was far greater than the yogi Shiva. So instead of honouring Shiva, he cursed him and to add insult to injury, when he conducted a fire sacrifice, as was the tradition during the Vedic age, Shiva and Sati were willfully omitted from the guest list. This was considered an extremely shameful act at that time in India, considering that Shiva was a god, and Sati was his daughter. It was the ultimate insult. This act of ego was seen by Sati as being the ultimate indignity towards herself and more importantly, her husband. She confronted her father on his audacity, but Daksha reacted with venom and insulted her and her husband Shiva in front of all the guests.

"Your husband Shiva is a vagabond and a lunatic. That gent spends his days inebriated in dance and his nights howling like psychotic untamed animal. I have heard via mere whispers that he is divinity in human form, yet I see no gemstones and no grandeur. All I see is the carcass of a desolate refugee. He has no majesty like Vishnu. No crown like Brahma. He adorns no gold like Indra, no diamonds like Chandra. How can he be a god? He looks impoverished. He dances with snakes and sings to the dead. Did you think of what would happen to my reputation after you married such a brute? I no longer wish to associate myself with the both of you. I have a reputation to defend as a king and a god among men and I cannot allow this fakir (yogi-mystic) to be part of my entourage!"

Sati became overwhelmed with shame and fury at her father's insults, "You are heartless and immoral in every way. I will have nothing to do with this body born of you. I curse that I was ever born from you as you are as ignorant as you are wealthy. I shall discard this body born from your seed like a corpse because the very idea I was born as your daughter nauseates me. This body born from you is now only worthy of contempt".

Tragically, Sati could take no more. She threw herself into the sacrificial fire and killed her physical body. Her mother, sisters as well as the guests tried to save her, but they were unable to get to her in time. Sati was thus no more.

Upon hearing about the traumatic events that had transpired, Shiva was devastated. The news broke Shiva's heart. The pain was that of a thousand arrows all piercing through his once impenetrable heart. Pain soon turned to madness as Shiva created a savage warrior "Virabhadra" from a lock of his matted hair and instructed him to kill Daksha and destroy his army.

"Find the palace of Daksha and destroy all in your sight. No man should walk free and show no mercy to the ones who sat around and watched unbothered as my love leaped into the flames". The warrior Virabhadra was Shiva's rage manifesting itself as a half-human – half-monster. Virabhadra was thus the vengeful and terrifying form of Shiva himself.

*"Sometimes human places, create inhuman monsters." - Stephen King*

Powered by rage and out of love for Sati, Virabhadra let out a huge roar. The stars fell from the sky and the earth shook in fear. The entire earth rumbled as tornados and tsunamis where unleashed by the rage of the mighty warrior. Virabhadra was on a blood thirsty rampage and would lay waste to anything that got in his way. He ripped the hearts out of the demi gods and drank the blood of his victims. He broke bones and tore limbs and destroyed Daksha's kingdom. The air was filled with the howls of ghosts and ghouls, and the frightened gods could do nothing but wail in fear. The women and children were allowed to flee, but no man in royal garb was offered the same mercy.

Finally, on the claret-soaked marble floor of the king's palace, Virabhadra dragged Daksha by his hair and laid him on an altar. He dragged him like Daksha would himself drag the goats to slaughter to make his own sacrifice. The irony of the situation was unnoticed by the terrified King. Virabhadra then raised his sword in honour of Sati and proceeded to decapitate Daksha. Again, the irony is that often as a symbol of his greatness, the king would dance around the skulls of his favourite victims. Today his own skull, empty of benevolence, humility and love was made as an offering to the very sacrificial fire that Sati herself had killed herself in.

Shiva then arrived at the dwelling of the king and found it to be drowning in blood. Shiva howled in agony as he mourned his beloved wife. He removed her lifeless, charred body from the fire and held it in his arms for what felt like days to the loyal devotees.

*"Only in the agony of parting do we look into the depths of love"* - George Eliot

After agony beyond compare, Shiva carried Sati's soulless body around with him wherever he went. At times, Shiva roared in sorrow and at other times, he just sat and gazed at Sati's empty frame, but the cruel feeling of anguish was slowly dining away at his heart. Before Sati, the great yogi had not experienced Love. Now without her, he was, for the first time, experiencing pain. Soon Shiva's very heart was dead. He felt like he was drowning. Pain was like water that was pushing its way through every minuscule part of his body. There was no way to stop it. Shiva was drowning in the ocean of distance that was now between himself and his beloved. So overwhelmed was he with grief that he felt like he was fending for his life and yearned for Sati to bring him back to the shore. Shiva was beginning to understand the human condition that one cannot experience love without pain – both are inevitable.

Shiva spoke to Sati's body as his tortured voice echoed in the icy peaks of mount Kailash.

"The last time I felt alive I held you in my arms. I was looking into your eyes as the seasons seemed to pass us by. If I had known then that this would be the last time I would be breathing your air, I would have never let you go. Your gaze has been lowered so now the sun cannot rise. It is impossible to imagine a world where the sun only rises when you awaken. But this is what you have spoilt me with. I will hold you firm even as your charred body begins to burn my skin. The hour at which only your bones remain, I will still be here holding what remains, quite simply because I cannot let go. What pains me most is I have such divinity, yet I cannot follow you. I know not of where you have gone."

For what seemed like an eternity, Shiva suffered the cold-blooded pain of love. The days passed and the seasons changed, yet Shiva remained nursing the remains of his companion. Consumed by the fire buried in his heart, Shiva was shattered. His body was devoid of life, and his heart was bare. Although it was only one person who was missing, to Shiva the whole world was empty and barren. The sphere of life that once pulsated with nature was slowly drowning in Shiva's grief.

Let us examine the poses:
Legend has it that the warrior 1 (image below) position represents Virabhadra holding his sword in the air, arms reaching up and gazing upwards ready to destroy Daksha and all those who witnessed the events. He is channeling the divine strength from his guru, Shiva.

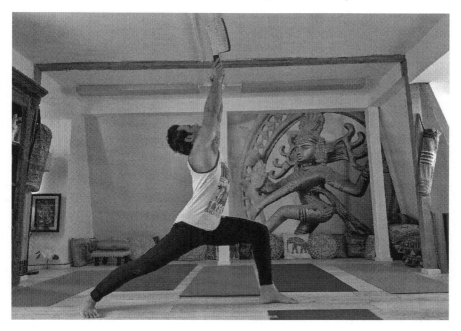

Cultural folklore has it that the warrior 2 pose (next page) represents Virabhadra as he readied himself, drawing his sword. His front arm reached forward as his finger pointed towards the petrified king. His sword was held exquisitely in his back hand. Or in my case a plastic meat cleaver

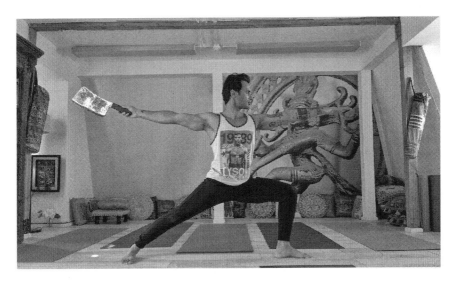

And finally, the Indian tradition says that warrior 3 (below) is the position that Virabhadra would assume after decapitating Daksha and offering his head to the very fire sacrifice that was the catalyst of the entire event.

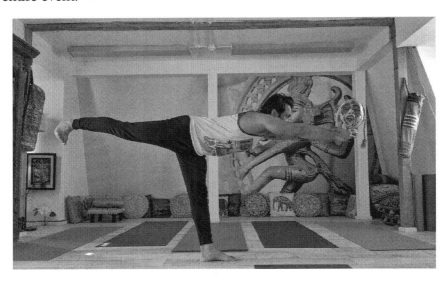

*Note – No actual human heads were severed in this recreation. You never know when various Halloween props can become handy.*

*Disciple: This is a gruesome tale. Am I supposed to be inspired in my yoga practice by this? This is a lot for my delicate yogic sensibilities to handle. Plus, I am a vegan.*

Calm down. Let me tell you about the next part of the story. The next part has nothing to do with the warrior poses but does finish the story with a happier ending. Let us digress slightly.

So Shiva didn't take Sati's lifeless body to a crematorium. On the contrary, he carried the corpse of Sati all over India in search of some physician or shaman who could bring her back to life.

*Disciple - Oh man, if only he had heard of Deepak Chopra's chakra mist spray.*

When Shiva first carried her, Sati's body was still hot like fire. Soon, Sati's body began to burn Shiva, but he wouldn't let go. He held her even tighter. The tighter he held her corpse, the more it burnt. The legend tells us that Shiva carried Sati for twelve long years. During this time, the world was drowning in Shiva's sorrow. He carried her in the hope that somehow, she would return to life or that some magician could heal her. He was clearly deluded, yet no one would dare say anything to the impenetrable yogi. Shiva was in chaos. He had lost control of himself and no longer had any perspective on life. Love and loss had left him with the inability to even protect himself.

In those twelve long years, parts of Sati's body started falling off. Because of the way Sati died, her body was part ash. Parts of her body slowly began to fall off – first her hand, then her leg and then her head. Shiva knew that parts of his beloved had fallen off, but he was too afraid to look. He couldn't accept that she was gone even though so little of her now remained.

Shiva was afraid to look at her because deep down, he knew that she was dead. But his mind convinced him there was hope. His mind wanted to believe that she was alive. His heart was mourning, but his mind lived in illusion. Shiva holding onto a lifeless body even though it was burning his skin was testament to his love and to his human side. Is this not what we do? Gautam Buddha one said, "Holding on to anger is like grasping a hot coal with the intent of throwing it at someone else; you are the one who gets burned". Shiva was a great yogi, and when he sat silently, his mind was at rest. But during this time, his time of sorrow, his mind resurfaced, and he was now a slave to the mind. But Shiva wanted to be blind. He didn't want to accept that his beloved was gone. Shiva knew that Sati was dead, she was in the past. But he held on, clinging to this past and the more he did, the more the future and his reality become increasingly darker.

So finally, the last parts of Sati turned to ash. The ghost and ghouls that were Shiva's previous companions were now replaced by grief and misery. The more Shiva mourned, the more the world sank in his sorrow. The gods Narayan and Brahma had to intervene as the balance within the cosmos had been lost. Shiva needed his spiritual energy, Sati, to maintain the balance of life. She breathed life into the wandering ascetic and without her, he was almost inert and incapable. The universe was a reflection of Shiva in this mythology. The universe had lost its "*shakti*", its source of energy. The rivers dried up, the sun would no longer shine, and the birds could not sing. The world and its creations were dying a slow death.

In Hindu mythology, Shiva and Sati are considered to be the primal principle of everything that exists and everything that does not exist in the universe – Sati is the energy force of Shiva. Shiva is consciousness and Sati is energy. The universe exists as a result of balance between the two. Without energy, Sati, the universe as we know it would come to an end. So, the gods, Narayan and Brahma, prayed to the great goddess. They asked her to once again take human form and be one with Shiva. They begged the goddess to return to Shiva and restore the balance within the cosmos. The goddess deliberated and was, at first, unsure of what to do. She had taken human birth previously and suffered terribly as a result. The human life was not something she wished for again. As she looked down onto the earth, she could see Shiva lost in meditation. The world seemingly crumbling around him. Shiva was at a loss. Without his shakti, without his energy, without his wife, he was *Shava*, which means "a corpse" or "someone who is lifeless" (as in *Shavasana*). The goddess could not stand the grief of seeing Shiva this way any longer, so she took human life once more and was reborn as the princess Parvati. Shiva and his consort would be together again, and the universe would find its balance. It is a story with a roller coaster ride, but I believe it was Shakespeare who once said, "The course of true love never did run smooth".

*Meaning:*
It is obvious that this is a mythological story. And with all or most mythologies, there are deep and often hidden meanings. So, what can we make of this story? And how does this relate to the warrior poses? I will elaborate on this point later in the chapter.

The entire story of Shiva and his wife Parvati revolves around one question . . . Can one exist without the other?

170

*"According to Greek mythology, humans were originally created with four arms, four legs and a head with two faces. Fearing their power, Zeus split them into two separate parts, condemning them to spend their lives in search of their other halves."*
*– Plato*

Can Shiva survive without Sati/Parvati? The conclusion is that he cannot. They have always been together and always will be – one balances the other. The universe is an ongoing dance between Shiva and Parvati. The male energy cannot survive without the feminine and vice-versa. They are two aspects of the same reality. They create universal balance.

There are many versions of the above story, many hidden stories and many prequels, but they all send us the same message. No matter what happened, no matter who interfered, no matter who the villain, Shiva and Parvati would always come back together. Their love was a divine love that couldn't be ripped apart as consciousness and energy cannot survive without each other. Everything that is non-physical in the universe is Shiva (consciousness) and everything that is the physical dimension is Parvati (energy). The universe cannot survive without them, and their stories cannot survive without them either. They create balance within the cosmos, and the universal equilibrium is created by a balance between consciousness and energy (Shiva and Parvati).

## Consciousness & Energy

*Disciple: Are Shiva and his wife "real" people, or are they just metaphors to explain the yogic science of consciousness (Shiva) and energy (Parvati)?*

That is a great question. It depends on who you ask. Did Shiva and Parvati really exist? If they did, have they been elevated to the status of "gods" to get the scientific message across? Is the Shiva in the mythologies the same Shiva or Adiyogi who created yoga? Are all of these just metaphors? Is Indian culture itself entangled in these metaphors? Again, it all depends on who you ask.

I have learnt to separate Shiva (or the Adiyogi who created yoga) from the mythological Shiva (who stars in these stories). It is just a personal method that helps keep me sane. In India, you will find that many people find the words "mythology" or "metaphor" insulting when referring to the various ancient stories. Many believe them to be genuine truths passed through generations. As with religions all over the world, in India you are also raised to believe that everything mentioned in your holy books are true. They are part of your DNA. You are raised to never question them. They are your blood and bones.

So, many Indians believe the stories of Shiva and Parvati to be factual. Many Indians believe that the cosmic couple did indeed walk this earth many thousands of years ago. There are also some, many more so in modern times, who believe that these stories are purely fictional and designed simply to express a moral code. These stories help people understand their place in the world and the code that governs existence. In India, life can be summarised by the conflicted views of the river Ganga. The logical Indian is disgusted by the idea of leaping into one of the most polluted rivers in the whole world. The holy man dives in with zero hesitance. The logical man drowns in the same Ganga that the sadhu will bathe in with joy. The logical man will say the holy man simply escapes reality by immersing into a life of metaphors. The holy man will say the logical man needs to look beyond the metaphors. If you penetrate enough, you will find the truth. Both are right but in their own unique way.

Logically, we can use Shiva and Parvati to simply understand yogic science. The world is made up of consciousness (Shiva) and energy (Parvati). The cosmos, the ever-expanding universe, the entirety of existence is a constant interplay between the two – an ongoing dance. They are two aspects of the same reality. In some Indian schools of philosophy, this dynamic dancing interplay is referred to *parusha* (consciousness) and *prakriti* (energy). In this school of thought, Shiva signifies *parusha* (consciousness). Parvati signifies *prakriti* (energy). All these stories and mythologies do is help us understand the dynamics between the two.

In yoga philosophy, our left side is our feminine, Parvati, and energetic side – our *prakriti*. Our right side is our masculine Shiva side – our *parusha*. This does not mean biologically female and biologically male rather this is energetic. A balance between these two seeming opposite energies is what creates equilibrium within our bodies. Spiritually, when there is the meeting and then balance between Shiva and Parvati, there is no longer a distinction between man and woman. Both are now as one. This balance between the two energies creates liberation. This is universal liberation, and it is this same liberation that we seek in our lives and also our warrior poses.

*Disciple: Can this understanding of Shiva and Parvati help us in our warrior poses or yoga itself?*

Yoga says that humans are made in the same way as the cosmos. We mirror it. We are a reflection of creation. We follow the same laws of nature. We, just like the cosmos can only exist if there is a harmonious balance between our own masculine and feminine energies. We manage to exist, but if balance is not discovered, we often end up agonised and lost. On a more physical note, we can end up injured.

When we do the warrior 2 pose (or many modern-day yoga poses), we are attempting to create a balance between these dynamic opposites, our left and right sides. Some of us are much more dominant on one side. This is not abnormal but in fact, very normal. So, when we create the pose, if we have a more dominant side, energetically this shows up in our warrior 2 pose. Maybe the body leans too far to the right or the left. The idea is to search for and find that dynamic interplay so that the energy is balanced. When the energy is balanced, you are balanced.

# Balance

*"Perfectly balanced, as all things should be" – Thanos to Gamora*
*(Avengers – Infinity War)*

Balance can be defined as follows:
– a situation in which different elements are equal or in the correct proportions
– put (something) in a steady position so that it does not fall

Balance is the key ingredient to life. Without balance, the earth would crumble, and the stars would fall. In the story, as soon as Sati the feminine energy left the world, the world and the universe drowned in Shiva's sorrow. The universe was engulfed in Shiva's darkness. He needed her light as did the universe. His madness was a result of his blindness. How can you expect to see anything in the cold dark universe without light?

Shiva carried her lifeless body around for centuries. The universe lost its balance and had no opposite to Shiva's masculine energy. The world remained lifeless until she was to return. Everything has an opposite. There is universal conflict as there is within us - a conflict of body and soul, matter and mind, love and hate, cold and heat, materialism and spirituality, science and religion, day and night, West and East. In all of these opposites, a balance is required for spiritual and physical sanity. Think of the "yogi" trapped in her Western body who wants to be an Indian yogi and live in India. She is lost and wants to escape to the fresh air of India. But she leaves behind her own roots, family, identity and friends. Surely a balance must be found? If balance is not found, we remain lost in our minds, in turmoil, and never really find happiness. The balance as the Buddha would always say is in the middle path.

To find the middle path the practitioner must first experience both the *dukkha* and the *sukkha* of their physical practice. *Dukkha* loosely means "suffering". *Sukkha* is best defined as "the absence of *dukkha*" The entire structure of our life is held together by the tension of its opposites and so are the warrior poses (and all the other poses when we think about it). Thus, the suffering or discomfort in your asana cannot be ignored. It was Krishnamacharya who once said that *dukkha* is a gift. You must learn from the suffering you have experienced. It is this experience of pain that helps you understand your limits.

The great Lao Tzu once said that opposites are not really opposites but, complementary. He tells us not to divide them as they are interdependent. How can love exist without hate? How can life exist without death? How can heaven exist without hell? Hell is not against heaven; they are complementary and exist together. They are two sides of the same coin. Be open both, and Lao Tzu says life will become a symphony of the opposites.

The warrior pose (and so many others) are a symphony of opposites - an orchestra of opposite notes, a harmony of opposition and contradiction as well as a balance between our Shiva and our Shakti. We constantly search for this harmony as the ingredients for both darkness and light are equally present in all of us. Thus, without balance, life is no longer worth the effort and the warrior poses are no longer worth your time.

So, to answer your question, don't look for an increase in flexibility in your warrior poses. Look to find balance between the left and right side of your bodies. In warrior 1 for example, try to remember the sensation and the depth of the pose when your left foot is forward. Create a subtle awareness of what your body is doing and the try to recreate this sensation on the opposite side. Mr. Iyengar has said before that our outer world is a reflection of our inner world. Our warrior 1 pose only looks as good as the way it feels inside. Thus, no mirror is needed, but just an acute inner understanding of what each part of your body is doing and the role each part plays in your equilibrium. If we can apply this to all our poses, if we can create a balance of opposites, we can slowly start to master our poses and discover this physical balance we all seek.

*Disciple: So although many people including myself are attracted to yoga as a means of increasing flexibility, you are saying it's not ALL about that? The key is balance and a constant search for this balance? Is this correct?*

When I say finding balance, I am not referring to the balance that you seek in a one-legged pose. I am referring to the balance between opposite forces in your body - the balance between the left and right side or the front and back of your body. If balance is created (in terms of flexibility/strength and so on), then flexibility can be a by-product of this new-found balance. But balance is not a by-product of flexibility. So, it does not work the other way around. If you think of a standard forward fold as an example, I don't want to feel more of a stretch or sensation in my left hamstring as I do my right. This is referred to as a muscle imbalance. In this scenario, if I do feel more of a stretch in my left hamstring than I do in my right, it would be fair to assume that my left hamstring is tighter than my right. If I continue to stretch further, I only exacerbate this imbalance. We have to create that feeling of symmetry. We need to create an even sensation in the back of our legs.

*"Remember the story of Shiva and Sati/Parvati? We want a harmonious balance between the left and right side of our bodies to create optimum physical health" - Guru Zee*

A hamstring that is tighter on one side is a muscle imbalance and is more likely to cause me an injury than both my hamstrings being equally tight. Muscle imbalances tend to refer to the strength or flexibility of contralateral (right versus left) muscle groups. The late Dr. Vladimir Janda, an expert in chronic musculoskeletal pain says, "Muscle balance is necessary because of the reciprocal nature of human movement, which requires opposing muscle groups to be coordinated"[6]. Muscle imbalance occurs when the length or the strength of opposing muscle groups prevents normal movement. So, my first approach when doing yoga for myself and in teaching is to address the balance within my body - is my body symmetrical?

*"Optimum physical health is an expression of the balance within your body. When balance is compromised, so is physical health." - Baba Zee*

The following is excerpted from B. K. S. Iyengar's Light on Life: "Through yoga one can begin to develop a perfect balance between both sides of the body. All of us begin with imbalances, favouring one side or the other. When one side is more active than the other, the active side must become the guru for the inactive side to make it equally active. To the weaker side, we must apply attention. We must also show more care. We show keener interest to improve a dull and struggling friend than for an eager and intelligent one. In the same way, you have to show yourself this same compassion and act on the weaker side of the body while taking pleasure in the achievement of the active side."[7]

Let us examine what is considered a "scarier" pose - the handstand. We know from "The Mind" chapter that the biggest barrier in this pose and other such advanced poses is psychological; however, let us consider the physical side for a moment.

In the handstand, what, in my experience of doing and teaching this pose, is the biggest barrier? It is not lack of strength or flexibility. Although I won't deny that a lack of both can cause some problems. The real barrier is a lack of balance or more specifically, it is not knowing where your centre of gravity is. So a more accurate explanation of the barrier is our lack of awareness of how to find our balance. Unless we come from an athletic background, we are unlikely to know where our centre of gravity is. When I do my handstand, I position my hands as I would in my downward dog, or my arm balances (this creates consistency for me), and the first thing I do before I attempt my handstand is ensure that I am pushing both hands equally into the ground. Even someone who has not done this pose before can tell me that unless I use both my arms equally, I will fail in my attempt. So, I look at my hands and ensure that they are both stretched and in equal contact with the mat. I then take a few hops (not yet trying my handstand) but just creating that feeling that both my arms are going to do equal work. I am essentially sending messages to my brain, via my nerves, telling my brain and body what it is I want to do. When I transform my hop into handstand, both sides of my body need to work equally. If one legs falls behind, I lose the pose. If one-foot kicks more than the other, the pose is lost. If there is more weight in my right arm, I lose the pose. So, the key in getting up and maintaining my handstand is balance.

Strength and flexibility play a much smaller role in this pose than people realise. This pose is about self-exploration and really digging in until you discover that mini moment of enlightenment. When you discover that moment in a class, you will look at me with pure animation. A big cheesy grin will be plastered across your face, and your eyes will be as big as your chakras. It is that look that I see so often when I teach that makes teaching yoga so rewarding. That look tells me that you may not be able to do the pose as well as you would like, but you fully understand the theory behind what you are attempting, and you even felt that centre of gravity while you were upside down - even if it was for split second.

# Handstands

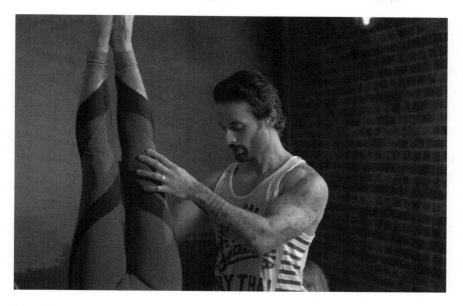

*Disciple: So all that is required to do my handstand is balance?*

No. Understanding the idea of balancing opposite sides of the body is the foundation for your handstand. Something else that we need to understand is the concept of muscle memory. The muscles that are required to work in handstand will adapt, over time, to the demand being placed on them. Through repetition, the right and left sides as well as the front and back of the body will sync and work together to create the pose. This creates a balance between the opposites. Still using handstand as an example, it requires conscious muscle movement and muscle activation to attempt and create the pose. But with time and practice, the handstand movement will become an unconscious movement. To rephrase, initially, the pose requires lots of thought, focus and awareness, but with practice, none of this is required. The pose then happens almost automatically.

*Disciple: How is that exactly?*

Picture my Laura doing a handstand. I am reliably informed that she was not born like this. She had to create a memory of the handstand movement within her brain before she could do the pose so effortlessly. This is similar to learning how to walk or ride a bike. We must first create a pattern of movement. When Laura first attempted her handstand, there is every chance she did not have the arm 'strength' or core control to do her handstand. Even if she was able to get up, the more dominant muscles in her upper body would have taken charge (and overworked). This could have been her left shoulder, for example. Because this creates an imbalance, Laura would have failed in her attempt to do her handstand. It isn't that Laura is not strong enough, her muscles just don't know what to do when she tried to go into an upside-down position. So, her dominant muscles (we all have them) worked overtime and the other muscles required to perform the task did not work at all. Unless she has a background in gymnastics, why would some of her muscles know what to do when she is upside down? They would have no muscle memory of the task at hand.

Laura must have wobbled on her first dozen or so attempts - there were perhaps hundreds of them. Before each handstand attempt, Laura needed to think consciously about what she was doing and the movements she needed to make. She needed to think about her hands, her arms, her core and so on. She needed to repeat the action of her handstand attempt a number of times until her brain understood the demands being placed on the muscles and adapted accordingly to create muscle memory. Now, the dominant muscles would not overwork as they would have before, and the other muscles now understand their duties within the pose (whether to relax or tighten). Now all the muscles of the hands, arms, shoulders and core work in unison. But how many repetitions are required to create this muscles memory? How long is a piece of string? Several hundred repetitions are required.

So, what is going on in Laura's brain as she attempts a handstand? The hundred billion or so neurons in the different parts of the brain are all firing and active as the brain slowly with each repetition understands and memorises the stresses or demands being placed on the body. Once both sides of her body work together, the brain fully memorises the movement and the good stress Laura is constantly placing on her hands, arms and core in a handstand. Once her brain knows what she is doing, Laura can almost unconsciously create her handstand. She just lifts up without a pause or even a thought. What was conscious is now unconscious. What required minutes or seconds of thought, awareness and patience is now done in an instant. This is muscle memory - a phenomenon that occurs after continual repetition of a particular action. These repetitive actions turn even a complex action (like a handstand), which requires conscious thought and effort, into something that is automatic and requires very little if any conscious thought and effort at all.

# Neuroplasticity

Let me introduce you to Neuroplasticity - This refers to the ability of brain neurons to continuously change and re-organise themselves so as to meet the demands of life.

We know that repetition is key in learning and mastering our poses. When we attempt a handstand, cells move to the part of the brain that is being used the most and as a result, new neural pathways are being created by the brain. This is neuroplasticity. Thus, the mastery of poses is actually a science. You create the positive intention and follow through with this intention, and science will take care of the rest. All it takes is willingness, repetition and a hundred billion or so neurons in your brain.

To summarise, Laura's brain adapts to the stress being placed on the body and sends messages to the muscles making them do what they need to do (tighten or relax) before she has even thought about it, so she can create the pose. This action takes place in her cerebellum, the back part of the brain. The memory of the movement that is stored in Laura's cerebellum allows her to create a handstand almost with her eyes closed. It is not magic. This is science. It is not that Laura is lucky, she simply has the cognitive capacity to comprehend the task and then the iron will to perform it. Laura may have the face of an oasis to the observing student, but what isn't seen is her willingness and the character she has that allows her to keep on trying even in moments of gloom. Willingness equals repetition. If you have the character and you keep trying, science will take care of the rest.

The same could be said of me as I am typing right now. My nervous system has the memory of typing, and it does so without me thinking about what I want to do with my fingers. I create a thought, and the brain and its wondrous neural pathway tells the fingers to type. The same is true of driving or learning a musical instrument. You can sit in front of your piano having not played for months and still remember what to do. Think again of your yoga poses, you do your part, and science will take care of the rest. It is just like one plus one equals two. The science is that exact. This is the basic and most fascinating economics of yoga.

As my Laura pointed out, this is perhaps what Pathabi Jois was saying when he famously said, "Practice and all is coming". Along these lines, Aristotle once said, "For the things we have to learn before we can do them, we learn by doing them." This means that with regular practice, through repetition, the body will adapt. This is science. Be patient and trust in the process.

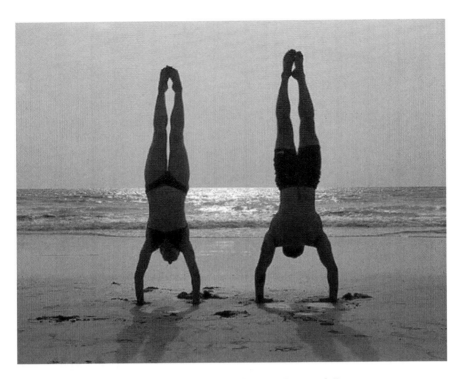

*above - Handstanding in Goa with Laura.*

If the science of movement can help those who have suffered brain damage from a stroke, then the science of movement and repetition can definitely help you. Many decades ago, the prevailing thought was that the brain's movement pattern was unalterable like the earth's orbit. We now know that is no longer accurate. Due to the stunning power of neuroplasticity, the brain can indeed be altered, retuned and rewire. It can activate wires that have been long shut down and run new wiring like an electrician[8]. There is a tremendous amount of plasticity and malleability in the adult brain[9]. Much more so than we realise. I have a client in her 60s who is learning patterns of movement in yoga she never believed was possible. This is yet another example of a mini moment of enlightenment.

The brain does not just change and adapt to new movement, it can also change as a result of the thoughts we have. The brain can be altered by pure mental activity. So, we can make our brains stronger and more efficient by creating positive thoughts and intentions[10]. As corny as it is to me, when a yoga teacher starts the class and asks us to "set an intention", maybe they are on to something.

Thus, the more repetition of a particular action (like the handstand, triangle, walking after rehab and so on), the more of the brain's real estate is zoned for that movement. If a movement is ingrained into the brain, it becomes second nature. There is a lot of evidence that shows how dynamic the brain is - more so than we ever realised[11]. The brain is constantly remodeling itself in response to an experience and repetition. Just be patient.

Let us further examine the handstand.

No other pose replicates the handstand in terms of the way it makes you feel - the negative emotions while trying and failing and then the positive emotions when you are successful. No other yoga pose summaries "madness or meditation" quite like the handstand. If you allow your mind to convince you that you cannot do a handstand, the mind defeats you. You become a slave to the monkey mind. In yoga philosophy, it is this that creates madness. Overcoming the mind and making your mind your slave is what leads to meditation. No pose is equal to a handstand. If any teacher tells you otherwise, it is because they cannot do it. When yoga teachers say that you shouldn't do or desire certain poses, it is because they cannot do that particular pose themselves. It is that simple.

So, ignore teachers who say handstands are not yogic. Ask any student who went from anxiety and fear to floating like a butterfly in their handstand; ask them how the handstand makes them feel.

When I first went "upside down", I felt my life doing the same thing, like it was turning on its head. I didn't have time to think or breathe. My hands where my instruments of balance keeping me in harmony. I felt like I could feel the earth rotating beneath me. I could feel my stomach muscles putting on the brakes and trying desperately to support me. I could feel my heart pounding in my chest. I realised once I came crashing back down to earth that the handstand and other "advanced" poses are not to be feared but understood. We fear that which we cannot perceive. Fear for me, had not left my body. Fear is infinite. It will always rise like a phoenix. Fear is one of the most crucial human responses, and it is essential for the survival of our species.

Thus, fear still existed for me, it just no longer had a hold of me in that pose. I realised that each time I was doing my handstand, fear was like the proverbial monkey on my back. It is no wonder that I had zero sense of symmetry. But to understand courage, I had to confront my fears. This was obviously the fear of falling or failing. This was the startling realisation for me with regards to the handstand. I cannot know courage without confronting my fear. Having broken so many bones in my exuberant youth, I had a fear for my body. What is there to be gained from a handstand I wondered? But this is the other problem I had. I was looking to gain something. Upon completing my handstand, I realised I had not gained anything, but in fact, I had lost something - the fear. It was after this that I better understood the meaning of courage. This was another mini moment of enlightenment for me. The first thought I had after my successful handstand was Rumi's famous quote: "You were born with wings, why prefer to crawl through life?"

So, don't be afraid to fall and don't be afraid to fail. When we fear failure, we withdraw ourselves from our practice. We can withdraw ourselves in other parts of our life too. However, action must overrule reflection. We may fail today, but we may also succeed today. We may fall but what if we fly? We will never know our potential and we will never know who we truly are unless we stop worrying and start doing.

*"The greatest teacher, failure is" — Master Yoda*

*Disciple: So, to get into and ultimately master the handstand, does it simply take willingness and repetition?*

Yes. To be willing is to have a certain attitude, a certain spirit and a daringness to fly. Willingness is a commitment that will ultimately set your soul free. Willingness is self-motivation. Success only comes from the willingness to never stop trying. Willingness, like courage, originates from the three-pound (or so) lump of corrugated flesh that we call our brain. We have been given a brain; the rest is up to us.

Willingness and repetition work hand in hand to create the full expression of the pose you wish to succeed in. But we must, at the same time, pause and not get too carried away with ourselves. Our commitment can also become food for our ego. We must learn to nurture our discipline so as to not let it mutate into an uncontrollable desire. We must learn and understand the difference between desire and discipline. Maybe the best way to learn this is through our own journeys and experience. So maybe there should be some desire or else how can one overcome something they know nothing about? Maybe the path to discipline is through the painful path of desire? Thus, I am not going to tell you to not desire and to not crave advanced poses. After thinking about it, I have realised that I actually encourage it. This is our greatest learning tool. We learn more about ourselves and the philosophy of yoga while battling with desire and discipline than we will ever learn from reading a book or from a 'wise' yoga teacher.

So 'desire' away. Experience desire and learn from it as have I and have all the other teachers who have advanced in their practice.

But consider some words of wisdom as well. A very wise man once said that the three greatest treasures for man are simplicity, patience and compassion. No, that wise man was not me, but Lao Tzu.

In the "Tao Te Ching", Lao Tzu continues, "Simple in actions and thoughts, you return to the source of being. Patient with both friends and enemies, you accord with the way things are. Compassionate toward yourself, you reconcile all beings in the world."

As for repetition, Patanjali introduced us to these concepts all those years ago. Way before science believed we could create new neurons (more on how the brain works in the meditation chapter), Patanjali had already emphasised the need for constant repetition. Patanjali uses the word *"abhyasa"* that refers to fighting old habitual patterns to create something new or igniting something old. *Abhyasa* is a Sanskrit word meaning "practice" and refers to a practice that aims to achieve a tranquil state of mind. Back when science believed that we had a better chance of altering the earth's orbit than we do of rewiring the brain, many would have looked at Patanjali's concept of *abhyasa*/constant repetition as an idealistic notion. It would have sounded romantic to think that we could alter the brain's biology and create a peaceful state of mind. If you are in anguish and in mental despair, Patanjali says, "Now the instruction in yoga". Now you are ready. You can alter your brain chemistry from one that is in anguish to one that is blissful. Science has had a different viewpoint - the remedy was to medicate. Patanjali's remedy was meditation.

The Nobel prize winning neuroanatomist Santiago Ramon y Cajal declared, "In the adult centres, the nerve paths are something fixed, ended and immutable"[13]. This gloomy assessment would have made people think that either Patanjali was an idealistic madman or just very impractical. They would have concluded that this "science" of yoga is not actually scientific at all. But today with our increased understanding of the brain and of the term "neuroplasticity", we know that we can indeed alter and rewire the brain. We can, like an electrician, rewire our brains. It can adapt to what we what we want it to do. If we want to become meditative and improve our mental health, we can indeed fix any short circuits in the brain. It begins with an intention. The brain will then create a new neural pathway simply based on an intention. Then, when we follow through with this, we can alter our brain and adapt[12]. Patanjali was no longer considered a madman but a genius scientist. We will discuss the brain in more detail later, but first, how does this relate to our poses? It is in exactly the same way. We create an intention to do yoga and improve on our poses. Once we commit to this intention, we are literally creating new neural pathways from our muscles to our brains. We adapt, and we do our handstand because neuroscience says we can change the physical structure of the brain long into adulthood. We have the ability to reshape ourselves, physically and emotionally.

We cannot place our hopes and faith in the outside world. The outside world is an illusion because what we see is all our brains will allow us to see. What we understand is also limited to the workings of the brain. We cannot trust the outside. The transformation comes from inside. Depression and the remedy for mental health does not come from looking out into the smog-filled skies. The remedy is inside of us and always has been. Patanjali says that constant repetition and practice will take you towards your promised land. We must show courage and have faith in science and the science of Patanjali.

One of my favourite quotes is; "Trust in God. But also tie up your camel"[14]. We must have faith, but we must also take the steps required to do what needs to be done.

*Disciple: What if I try a handstand and fall?*

In the Lion King, the wise Rafiki says, "Oh yes, the past can hurt. But you can either run from it or learn from it".

*Disciple: That's deep. What else affects our ability to master the poses?*

The Buddhists believe that we are slaves of memory and imagination. The same memory and imagination that is so essential to the survival of the human species may one day be its downfall. So, what can be used to create so much joy is more often used to create so much sorrow and suffering. Rather than use our memory to recall behavioral patterns and memories of loved ones and birthdays, we use memory to dwell on our failures. The imagination that we should utilise for our growth and success is used instead to picture failure and misery. The Buddhists say we dwell on the negative impressions of the past and overthink what lies ahead in our future. This is why they place such an emphasis on the here and now. Being present is such a trendy yoga word that it pains me to say it. But the idea is to apply this Buddhist philosophy even in yoga. Our inability to do a pose, at times, is dictated by our own memories and imagination. The idea is to not to dwell over a previous failure. The longer we dwell on our past behaviours and failures, such as our botched attempts at a headstand, the greater is their power to harm us. Remember a failure in a headstand attempt (or any other pose) is only a failure if one dwells on it. The Buddhists will tell you that if you leave what has happened in the past and simply be present, the concept of failure is redundant.

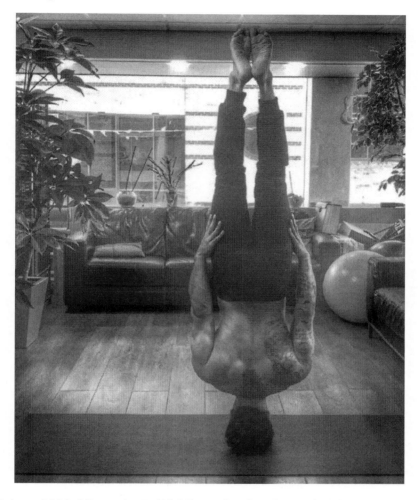

*A leap of faith. Neuroscientist V.S Ramachandran has said; "Any ape can reach for a banana, but only humans can reach for the stars."*

Further, we shouldn't stress about the future. What if we fail? What if we fall? The idea of being present is to just take advantage of the here and now. Letting go of memory and imagination and simply being present is a Buddhist principle and the same principle shared by Patanjali all those years ago. They are just negative impressions of the mind. These two "modifications of the mind" (as Patanjali called them) are additional factors holding us back in our *asana* (and everyday life). Once we let go of them, we release the anchor.

Another factor that has one of the biggest impacts on your ability to do and master poses is your anatomy.

Mullah Nasreddin was once boasting about his ageless strength. "I am as strong as I was when I was a young man." "How can that be?" asked people. "There is a big rock outside my house. I couldn't move it then, and I can't move it now!" said the Mullah.

There are some things you just cannot do and that you are not designed to do. So, what can you do? You should definitely do your best but accept that your anatomy and the way your bones are designed and shaped will affect how far you can go. To give you an example, let us consider the wheel pose. Does everyone's wheel pose look the same? From the perspective of the teacher who is looking at everyone as they enter the pose, the answer is no. There really shouldn't be a universal cue of feet pointing straight ahead or heels down and so on because each body is unique in how it will express the full pose. If there is pain, the students either stops or finds a way to reduce the discomfort. This may not agree with the aesthetics the teacher wishes to see but that is the reality of what happens to our bodies in the pose. The greatest learning curve for a teacher is to ask students to do a pose and then just be an observer knowing that if someone is doing something "wrong" (causing themselves pain), they will exit the pose for themselves. While in the pose, the teacher becomes a witness to the fascinating anatomy of the human body. Each body is doing something unique and different. Each body tells a story and, in some cases, the inability to do a pose has nothing to do with anything but your bone structure.

Consider the famous Lotus posture for which around ninety degrees of external rotation movement is required at the hip joint. But we have around 60-70 degrees of movement in general. Can we create that extra 30 degrees? That depends on so many other factors. I will not talk anyone out of not trying, I simply try to get students to make peace with their inability to do something. Can you increase this angle with time and flexibility like you can other parts of the body? That is a constant source of investigation for me. In my case, my hips (outside) and hamstring muscles are the most developed muscles in my body. So, can I at the age of forty make these muscles lengthen after sending them the opposite message for so many years? If for twenty-five plus years, these muscles have been generating force, can they now all of a sudden relax enough to become flexible so I can do the lotus pose and finally look like a yogi? This is the synopsis of my ongoing examination.

Further, what of the bones themselves? Do the ends of our thigh bones all look the same? Do they all have the same angle as they enter the hip socket? The answer is no. Each person has a variability. Over time, we learn to make peace and stop stressing at some of the things we cannot do. This is not a lack of will or courage, this is just the way your body is.

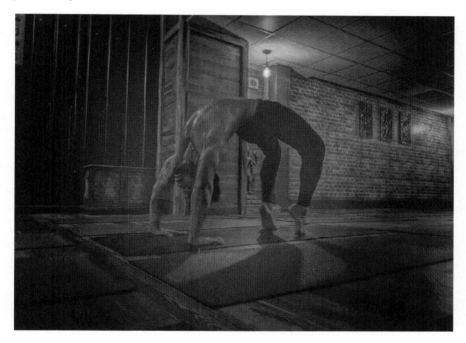

*above - Practicing the wheel posture at my studio in Addlestone. Many teachers say the feet must be flat. But why? Coming up onto my toes takes the stress off my lower back and makes the pose more accessible so how can this be 'wrong'?*

Before you do yoga, ask yourself, what have you been doing with your body until now? If you have been running your whole life, how can you expect to have flexible hamstrings? Don't worry. Just do what is best for your body. If you have been lifting weights your whole life, there is a reason you struggle with the wheel pose. Maybe your chest is too developed. Again, don't worry, just do your best with your anatomy as no one expects perfection. The small amounts of movement you are capable of may be enough to give you the balance of strength and flexibility that is required for the human body.

Interestingly enough, for me, the great mini moment of enlightenment was the day I stopped stressing over my forward fold. When I realised that my hamstrings would not get any more flexible, I stopped over-trying. I then just concentrated on my breathing and stopped fighting myself. This is what has allowed me to go further. It was "not trying" as absurd as that sounds. Not trying too hard is what has allowed my hamstrings to relax. When I was stretching them before, they were getting the same message they have been receiving for twenty-five years. They were still trying to generate force. Even though I want them to get more flexible, I instinctively try to achieve this by making them work harder. I am thus contradicting my own body.

*Disciple: If the pose remains just physical, just a stretch or just an exercise in balance, are you not missing out on so much? If asana is a branch on the tree of yoga, are you not missing out on something by making this about just physical exercise?*

That is a good question. You have been taught well. The pose should gradually move into a different dimension from a physical one like an evolution or a metamorphosis. So, the pose may be just physical for the first few years or decades (finding your balance) and then you may find yourself in a much deeper or further enquiry into yoga. You may find yourself asking questions and reading books you would not have been ready for all those years ago when you first started. The gradual mutation should be very natural and as a consequence of disciplined practice and not forced because the yoga community says you should be reading a certain book or doing something esoteric by now. This again is just our mind and insecurities that make us feel desperate to fit in. The reality is that it should not be forced. You cannot enforce dietary changes or spiritual changes on anyone or even yourself. After a while, you just go back to the way you were because this approach does not make you happy.

So, to reemphasise, the changes including the new-found interest in the deeper machinations of yoga and meditation should be natural and organic to you but never forced. Patanjali teaches that we should let go of desire and adopt discipline. If you desire spirituality and meditation, you will always be ignorant. You will always be unsure and feel lost. If you adopt discipline and just practice asanas as a lifestyle rather than a race, you mutate into the real you. You will discover who you really are. This never happens when you desire as the very desire to achieve creates a bondage and appeals to the mind. The mind has no concern and interest in discipline as discipline is a trait of the heart. This requires courage. But with desire, the mind reacts and finds an opening. It then feeds this desire until you are so fed up with desiring that you drop everything. You drop yoga and in resentment, you move on.

Thus, I would suggest when creating the discipline of yoga, don't rush, and yoga will change you in ways you never thought possible. These changes will be natural and genuine and not forced at all. Forced changes (we have all done them in some way) are not real. They are false and only create fake faces and facades. We create false identities because we decide we need to change. It may be a good, wholesome, new, more vital and healthier you. But if it is not natural, it is false. It is fake and will not last. Let us use the holy men of India as an example: They work their whole lives and have families and jobs and children. One day, a great realisation suddenly hits them that they have misunderstood life, and they should make a change so as not to be so orientated towards money or power. This family man, this householder, now becomes a wandering sadhu. He has replaced one identity with another. He is now a blind seeker. All he has done is one replace one ignorant man with another. The new identity is not real because it has been created as a counter to the old one. This is forced.

In the same way as the modern yoga teacher who qualifies and wraps herself in a sari and gets toe rings is trying to create a new identity. She "meditates" daily and becomes a vegan overnight. There is of course nothing wrong with this as long as it is a gradual metamorphosis of who you are rather than an emotional response to who you were. There was nothing wrong with the person we once were. It was that person who got us to the place we are in now, so we must have been doing something right. Both the sadhu and the yoga teacher now have new faces, but their new identities cannot and won't make them happy. Their new identity has no roots. It is as if the person they once were has been erased from time. But ironically, that person who you try to no longer identify yourself with is the real you. The new face, the new identity, is just a reflection of how you feel you should be. You cannot try to achieve the real you. It is something you have to arrive at. Again, our identity needs roots. If we want yoga to play a role in our lives and improve our health, we have to think of yoga poses as seeds that allow our real potential to blossom in its own time.

The following took place in a flower shop.

A woman was strolling through a shopping mall when she noticed a poster advertising a brand-new flower shop. She was ecstatic. When she went in, she got a shock; she saw no vases, no arrangements, and it was Shiva, Adiyogi himself, in person who stood behind the counter. "You can ask for whatever you want", said Shiva.

"I want to be happy. I want peace, money, the capacity to be understood. I want to go to heaven when I die. I want to master my handstand and I wish for happiness. I want to find my true nature."

Shiva, flinging the serpent around his neck to one side, opened a few pots that were on the shelf behind him, removed some grains from inside and handed them to the woman. "Here you have the seeds," he said. "Start planting them because we don't sell the fruits here."

The asanas are like the seeds of yoga. We have to accept and embrace them deep down in our hearts. Our hearts become soil for these poses. When nurtured, the seeds will sprout, and only then will yoga have meaning - only then will the seeds produce fruits and flowers. I once heard that the creation of a thousand forests is from a single acorn.

To fully understand yoga and for yoga to improve our lives and our health, the asanas that are the seeds of yoga must be done with the heart. There should be no airy fluffiness, no egotistical search for spirituality and no esoteric nonsense. You should just put your heart into your poses.

*Disciple: Many yoga teachers and websites say that yoga is more than asanas (which it is). And I am made to feel bad because I only started doing yoga to make my glutes look better or because I wanted less tight hamstrings. Is this bad? It is okay to just do yoga for physical reasons?*

You can do yoga for any reason you wish. Even if the reason is considered vanity by some, who cares what they think. Yoga gurus and websites do indeed make us feel bad for wanting to do yoga just for physical reasons but why is this considered wrong? You do yoga for any reason you wish. Be brave and say that you are not interested in anything other than the stretching branch of yoga if that is how you feel. No one can say anything to you because they cannot disregard the truth. Krishnamurti once said, "It is truth that liberates, not your effort to be free". I would much rather have an honest student who just wishes for a firmer backside, or someone who only wants more flexible hamstrings, so it is easier for them to tie their shoe laces than someone who says they are doing yoga to be "one with the divine". Maybe it is me, but I think those chasing enlightenment are frankly deluded souls. The student who loves life and wants new hamstrings is much more likely to reach his goal and not just because it is a more accessible goal, but simply because his goal is genuine and true to their nature.

The teacher, student or website that says true yoga is more than asana and to be respectful to the tradition, we should do more than just asana are often just saying what they feel needs to be heard to create the awe of authority and wisdom. It is like saying you cannot listen to one genre of music. It is usually the self-proclaimed music geeks who say so and never just a casual lover of music. You must listen to different genres, they say, because the expressions of music cannot be put into words, and if you limit your mind to only one genre, then you are limiting your possibilities. But what if you only like a single genre?

"Music is a refuge where you can lose yourself in your daydreams," says my wife "But you won't experience this by just listening to LL Cool J (and NWA) all the time". (She says with tongue in cheek - of course). My reply? "Momma said knock you out". But I see her point. I should probably move on from 80s-90s rap music. But at the same time, why should I? It could be argued that without deviation, progress is not possible. But is that really true? What if total immersion and absolute involvement in one genre is enough to set your soul free? Who says that listening to all genres will give you all the answers? And who says you have to look for answers anyway? Can you not just keep on listening to 80s rap if that is what puts a genuine smile your face? Is it wrong to listen to just one genre because that is what you like? I would say no, because it is that which fills your heart and sets your soul on fire (I know this is a cliché, but I couldn't think of anything else).

Kahlil Gibran said, "Work is love made visible. And if you cannot work with love, but only with distaste, it is better that you should leave your work and sit at the gate of the temple and take alms from those who work with joy. For if you bake bread with indifference, you bake a bitter bread that feeds but half our hunger"[15].

Make asana your work as I and so many other yoga teachers have done before you. A perfect example is the great B. K. S Iyengar. Your total involvement in your asana is what will create the melodies within your soul and not the feeling that you are doing something wrong by "just doing the poses".

Asana produces the kind of comfort that my human nature cannot possibly do without. Asana invigorates my bones and cultivates my cells. It hardens my nerves and reinforces my will. It nourishes my brain and sustains my resolve. It enhances my love and brings harmony to my soul. Based on this argument, who has the right to tell me that I should be doing more than asana?

*"I am what I am. Are you what you are?"* - Alanis Morissette

# Science

This answer will involve some science.

Your nervous, muscular and skeletal systems are collectively known as your kinetic chain[16] ("kinetic" meaning something that is concerned with movement). Your kinetic chain seeks to maintain a state of physiological balance, also known as homeostasis. To do this, your body must be capable of adapting to the physical stresses placed on it. This ability to adapt to "stress" is known as the general adaption syndrome. This general pattern of adaption was brought forth by Hans Seyle who showed that the kinetic chain responds and then adapts to the stresses placed on it. To respond, however, the body must be confronted with a stressor that warrants a response. In yoga, the body will respond initially to a new pose with caution and then over time, the body will adapt to this pose. It will then continue to adapt if the body is pushed further in the pose.

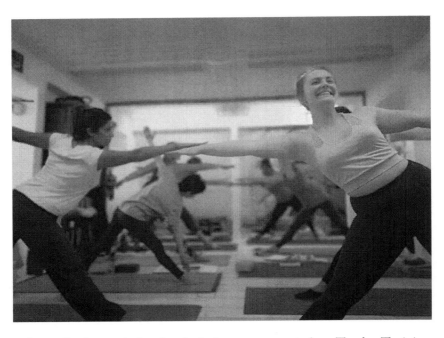

*above - Students enjoying the physical asanas as part of our Teacher Training programme.*

The body responds, at first, in what is known as an "alarm reaction". The yoga poses stress the body, increasing oxygen and blood supply to the necessary areas of the body. There is no real change at this stage. The body is just trying to understand what you are attempting to do. After a period of time that is unique to an individual, the body then goes into the "resistance development" stage. This is the part where the body is adapting to the pose. It is during this second stage that the individual perhaps notices their body changing and going further into the pose. Once adapted, the body will require increased stress to produce a new response. In other words, the individual will need to continue to push themselves to notice more of a change.

The early stages of yoga are undoubtably the most frustrating. We need to not expect too much too soon. When we first adopt a pose, the body has to understand the stress being placed on it before it can adapt. The neural network will eventually adapt to the new pattern. The science is that the more we engage in a particular movement pattern or patterns, the stronger and more efficient our neural network becomes. If we expect an increase in flexibility after just a few classes, we will no doubt be left frustrated and disheartened.

*Disciple - How long do we stay in the first "alarm reaction" stage?*

There is no way anyone can correctly answer that. Everyone is different. An individual's exercise history, work patterns and injuries will all play a key role in determining when the body is ready for stage two. The key is to be patient and persevere. The famous footballer Pele once said, "Success is no accident. It is hard work, perseverance, learning, studying, sacrifice and most of all, love of what you are doing or learning to do".

*Disciple – Culturally speaking, how long will it take to adapt and progress in yoga?*

It is said that a disciple went to the holy sage Narada with tears in his eyes. He said that he had spent his whole life seeking, so he wanted his master Narada to please tell him how to become a Buddha. How to become a Shiva? How to find my enlightenment. How can I awaken? It is said that the sage Narada just slapped the taste out of his disciple's mouth. "What are you doing?" screamed the disciple. The wise Narada explained; "Stop this nonsense. You are a buddha. You have always been. But your questions and seeking will take you further and further away. How can you become something that you already are?"

How does this relate to yoga and the asanas? Well, if you come to me with tears rolling down your cheeks asking me how long it will take you to progress and become more flexible, I will follow the example of the sage Narada and pimp slap you. I will explain, "Stop this nonsense. You are flexible. You have always been. But your seeking is taking you further away".

Allow me to elaborate. Our muscles are flexible. There is nothing wrong with our muscles. They are not too tight. Theoretically there is no such thing as a tight muscle. When we have movement restrictions, what is the actual cause of this restriction - the muscles or is it our nervous system? (the brains and its corresponding nerves). If we think the front of our hips are tight, for argument's sake, this is because we have created such a pattern of movement in our everyday lives that the front of our hips (psoas, rec fem muscles and so on) stay in a position more suited to the demand being constantly placed on them every day. So, if you sit down a lot, the front of your hips are "tighter" than you would like because your brain and nervous system are actually readying you to sit again. The nervous system becomes accustomed to this pattern of movement. You have created a neural pathway that has become like second nature. Remember there is no such thing as general, overall flexibility. Flexibility as we know it is specific to joints and joint action[17].

When you come to yoga class and ask your front hips to do something that is the exact opposite of what you do all day long (lunge stretch for example), the brain and nervous system are confused. So, they send a message to your hips telling them to tighten - the exact opposite of what you wish to do. This is a defence mechanism. The very efficiency of our nervous system is the reason we can feel the tightness. So at least something positive comes from such tightness. At least we know our nervous system is working! What we have to do is be patient and keep repeating the action of the hip stretch over and over again until the brain and nervous system allow the hip muscles to relax, which it will. Then, you can go further. Essentially, this just brings about your dormant flexibility. Thus, the restriction is not in the muscles. It is your brain and nervous system.

Remember Patanjali calls this "*abhyasa*" - constant inner practice. It is the repetition of something over and over again that will move that pattern from the conscious brain into the unconscious brain. This is when we feel we have become more flexible and we rejoice. What has actually happened is our brain and nervous system have simply adapted. So, if we are patient and persevere, we will understand the sage Narada's theory. We have always been flexible. It will just take time for us to come to this realisation.

*Disciple: Will yoga poses make me stronger?*

Yes and no. The answer is not as straightforward as you may think. Plenty of students have commented over the years that yoga has made them stronger. Plenty of yoga teachers promote classes to build strength. But technically, you cannot build strength from yoga.

Before the shock makes you choke on your Avocado, allow me to explain. When someone arrives to do yoga for the first time, they perhaps do so having been out of action for a while or having not exercised for some time. They arrive and are not in, what I consider, peak physical condition. Their muscles are "tight", and some muscles are weaker than they should be. You could say that such a person is 'deconditioned'. Let us take the 'core' as an example. Your core could be lazy, weak or inefficient. After weeks or months of yoga, a student comes back and is thankful because yoga has now made their core stronger than it has felt in years. I nod along and share their enthusiasm (I don't want to bust their groove), but the reality is that they have not got stronger, they have just returned to what they should have been like before they stopped exercising. They are no longer deconditioned but have returned to their optimum baseline. Essentially, the muscles have regained their efficiency. The student will argue and say, "No. My core is so much stronger now". And I will say yes, it is "stronger" than before because before you returned to yoga, you had become weak. Your muscles had switched off. All you have done is switch on your muscles again and restore the muscles' potential to generate force. You have awakened dormant muscles. You are now as efficient as you should have been before you arrived to yoga.

You know this to be true if you think about it. A sportsperson who has a solid foundation of fitness would never say, "I am going to yoga to get stronger". It would never happen because they know subconsciously that in order to get stronger than you are, you are required to work with an external resistance (weights) that yoga does not provide. Using my friend, Sheree, who teaches at the studio, as an example. She was a professional Muay Thai boxer for many years. If she felt she needed to get stronger, would her instincts send her to yoga, or would they send her to the gym? If you are in rehab and you need to work certain muscles again after surgery to make them stronger, the physical therapist doesn't say "Go do yoga". They tell you to go to the gym.

I once saw a sign that said, "Build strength in yoga". If I went to that class, would that class make ME stronger?

It would make me stronger only if my muscles were weak (deconditioned) in the first place. Once you restore your muscles efficiency, the only way to get stronger is to work with external resistance.

So, what actually happens as a result of yoga?

What you can do is build endurance, which is your body's capacity to endure physical stress. Take the warrior 2 pose for example. If I get you to hold warrior 2 for five minutes, will this make you stronger or will it improve your body's ability to tolerate physical stress (endurance)? The answer is obvious. Unless you have my niece crawling all over you while you are in warrior 2 there is no external resistance so you cannot build strength. Holding a pose, be it the warrior, downward dog or headstand, does not make you stronger. All it does is improve the muscles' efficiency to tolerate that particular stress. This is called endurance. Again, Endurance is your bodies ability to maintain its efficiency under the influence of gravity.

Holding a headstand for five minutes does not require strength. Strength is your muscles' capacity to generate force, to oppose or withstand an external resistance and to lift a significant weight. Endurance is your muscles' capacity to tolerate physical stress. So, holding headstand for five minutes is more to do with the endurance capacity of your muscles (as it overcomes gravity) than it has to do with strength. Holding a headstand for five minutes will not make you stronger. It will make your muscles more efficient at supporting your skeleton while in a headstand.

Yoga essentially helps you build endurance and maintain your strength levels only if you do not shy away from the more advanced poses.

So, although yoga teachers promote yoga to build strength, technically speaking, this is not accurate and, in my opinion, is very misleading. The accurate term would be "to restore your dormant strength" - all this does is make you feel stronger (psychologically) and create the feeling of toned muscle. All you have really done is restore your base levels of strength. Hence, the answer to the question is a "yes and no". It depends in how you have come to understand strength.

Some so-called yoga experts say that yoga can 'build muscle'. The logic being that by lifting your own body weight (handstand for example) can stimulate the muscles to grow in size. In the gym world this is referred to as hypertrophy. Some yoga experts and websites even go as far as to claim that yoga poses can replace and be just as effective in building muscle as going to the gym. Does this really satisfy your logical mind? For me this is the most misleading yogic claim of all (a close second is the cleansing of chakras). Yoga experts even make such ludicrous claims such as 'chair pose' can build muscle. Chair pose? Really?

You build muscles via progressive overload. Which means increasing the load over a period of time. So how can a static chair pose increase muscles size and volume when the stimulus on the muscles remains the same throughout?

'Yoga can BUILD muscles' is just another in the long line of preposterous yoga claim made my people who may be yoga teachers but, are not health and fitness professionals. This is the ludicrous world of yoga.

Mika Janhunen is a chiropractor and the author of "Survival Guide to Your Home". His clinic is based in Shepperton, Surrey. Mika, on the question of whether yoga makes you stronger, said "It depends! It depends on how you define strength and improving strength". He also said that often we can gain emotional strength from returning to yoga. This means that we can gain more confidence in our ability to do things in yoga, which is why we feel stronger. Mika continues, "The central governor (the brain) needs to be reminded of the capabilities of the body through the myriad proprioceptive stimuli and the physiological challenges that yoga poses, and flows place upon the brain. When coming back from a hiatus (de-conditioning), the brain has to first connect with the body and establish adequate functioning of all relevant systems, which leads to a huge barrage of stimulation (that in itself feels absolutely wonderful and euphoric) arising in all different nerve endings in the body - very much akin to an ice cold plunge, but sustained, and not freezing". This stage, Mika says, is where we feel we have become stronger and are ready to put our new-found strength to the test. Essentially, you have now re-opened old neural pathways. This means that the electric signal from one room to another was "lost" simply as a result of inactivity, but by visiting that room and switching everything back on again, you literally re-awakened the neural pathway.

Mika continues, "As the person attends yoga classes and practices at home, his brain is able to relearn that he is able to move safely through a broader range of motion and intensity, which results in convincing the brain to allow them to return to improved performance. With diligent yoga practice, I am sure, the person would be able to improve his movement efficiency to such a degree that it would manifest in real strength gains as well. Take handstands for example. A person who learns to balance his body in an inverted position will gain strength in the core muscles and the upper body in that direction. Most of us are pathetically weak in inversion, but by learning to do it, we become stronger and more skilled at the same time. Will that result in bulging biceps? Don't know and don't care, but I feel that there would be a quantifiable difference from the beginning to the end of the programme".

Essentially, Mika is saying we can get stronger, but I sort of disagree, we are just more efficient! But I shouldn't argue with Mika, he could school me on knowledge all day long! The disparity is simply down to how we have learnt through our lives to understand and interpret the word "strength". In order to answer the question for yourself, just think to yourself, can warrior 2 make me stronger or will doing warrior 2 for 5 minutes make my legs more efficient at holding warrior 2?

But do you regard your capacity to hold warrior 2 as strength or endurance? Look up the word's "strength" and "endurance" and ultimately, draw your own conclusion.

I appreciate that these are just words, and you could question whether it even matters how we interpret 'strength' and 'endurance'? I see your point. In many respects, it does not matter but in some respects, it does. Socrates, I believe, once said, "The beginning of wisdom is the definition of terms." This is why the yoga world is full of nonsensical claims, because yoga people do not appear to be taking the time to understand and define such terms.

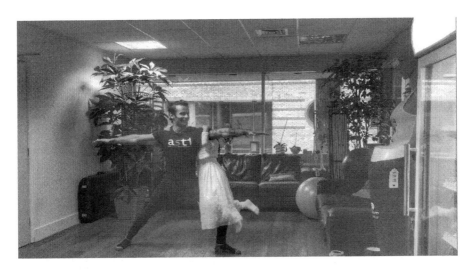

*above - My niece attempts to climb around me whilst I hold the Warrior 2 pose. The additional weight of her body is a new challenge. So the muscles in my legs must work much harder than they would without her. They are fighting an external resistance thus they get "stronger".*

# Ego

*Disciple: My teacher told me that advanced yoga poses are for show offs and all about the ego.*

*"There are some who never try, get left behind, forever dying. they just sit it by the sidelines while they criticise, hide and scrutinise; but then there are others who are tough enough, who stand to risk their wrongs, flying high, as they rise up in this life and thus, fight right through the lies."[18] - Chris Jammies*

I once went to a yoga class in London many years ago, and after class, I asked the teacher if any of the teachers taught headstands/handstands and the like. Her reply was a resounding "No". She said it was because headstands are not really yoga but just things people do for their ego. "We don't do ego here," she said. I thought that was admirable. But you know what else I thought? This teacher doesn't think headstands should be taught because she can't do a headstand for herself. It's that simple. We don't do that which we fear for ourselves. Rather than admit we can't do something, is it not easier to dismiss it altogether? Interestingly, the teacher was dressed head to toe in what I consider the more fashionable of modern-day yoga attire. Is that not of the ego? The teacher's hair was immaculate - Not one strand had been disturbed in class. It was a miracle.

Why do we dress and wear our hair a certain way? It is for our own self esteem for sure, but we also dress for others. We want people to notice how we look. Anyone who denies this is deluded. This is our human nature. Is this not the work of the ego? When we do a headstand or handstand, we do it for ourselves and not for anyone else. This is about how we want to feel for ourselves. We want to be the best version of ourselves. So, the handstand is all about ourselves while our clothes and appearance are about us as well as how we want to be identified by others. So, which is more egotistical?

Some of the poses I teach can appear advanced at first, and I can see why people are a little put off. But to avoid the more advanced poses all together is missing the point of what a yoga pose is. A yoga pose is not just a stretch, a yoga pose also tries to help us deal with the conflict we are in with our minds. If this is not understood, then I can see why teachers tell their students to avoid "advanced poses". My response to the above statement that advanced poses are all for show offs and are about the ego is to say that will all due respect, I don't think the teacher saying this really understands yoga.

Nietzsche once said, "The higher we soar the smaller we appear to those who cannot fly". Teachers who say advanced poses are for show offs want to remain within the conflicts of their own minds, essentially enslaving themselves and their students too.

Remember yoga is psychological as well as physical. Teachers sometimes feel insecure in not wanting their students to advance beyond their own level, so they prevent their students from even trying more advanced poses. This is not just done in yoga. This is a common problem with anything that is taught. The teacher, whatever the subject, must be the authority. When that authority is threatened, a deep fear arises, and our insecurity creates a trap for the student to ensure we remain credible and remain the teacher. They say the inmates cannot run the asylum. Thus, teachers overrun by their own fears and insecurities cannot help their students advance. This is a psychological problem that is a very human problem. This is why I have put such an emphasis on yoga being psychological. Through the immersion in yoga comes the realisation when the mind is creating worry, anxiety and insecurity. We should be proud to see our students develop and encourage them to move on to more advanced poses if their minds are ready. It is here the student really unlocks their potential. If you prevent students from unlocking this potential, you are keeping them prisoners in their own minds. Teachers must thus allow their students to fly. I once read that one repays a teacher badly if one always remains nothing but a student.

Then again, upon further analysis, maybe this teacher has a point. Let's call her Wendy - Wendy, the 200-hour yoga alliance teacher. Wendy thinks advanced poses are about the ego. Let's use the handstand as an example of an advanced pose to give you context. Wendy says that the handstand is about the ego. And is she right but wrong at the same time. It's like she on to something, but she is seeing it upside down. A handstand is about the ego, but it's more about taming or killing the ego, not adding fuel to it. See in my opinion, remember this is just my opinion, Wendy fears failure. She fears falling and or failing in her headstand. Her mind is behind this insecurity. Her mind has her convinced that she cannot do that pose. So the mind convinces Wendy that the handstand pose is not really yoga and for show offs only. She wants to stay within the compulsions of her mind as here, life is safer and more secure. For Wendy, remaining within the confines of her comfort zone is her reality. However, deep down, she realises that she only fears failure. You see her ego does not want to fail. The ego is more bruised when you fall in a handstand. For anyone who has fallen, it does not hurt as much as you think it will. Often when I ask the question, "Are you okay?", students jokingly reply, "Yes, but my pride is shattered". So they pick up the pieces of their shattered ego and try again

Nietzsche once said, "There are no beautiful surfaces without a terrible depth". Thus, with each attempt, the ego is tamed. The mind convinces you to revert back to your restorative approach to yoga. And there is nothing wrong with this, I guess, but you end up missing out on so much.

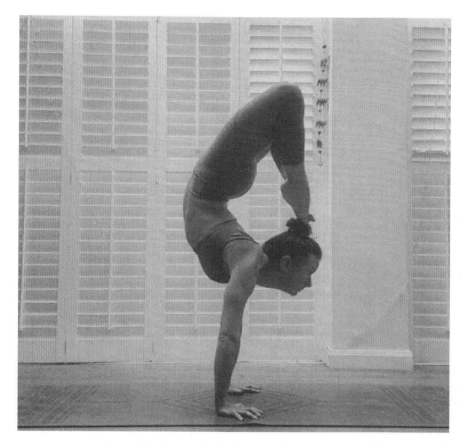

*above - Laura in the "advanced" scorpion posture.*

When my Laura teaches poses that some consider advanced, is she teaching them because she is egotistical? Is she teaching others to be egotistical? Or does Laura just inspire? Based on the attendance of her classes, you would say she inspires.

I too teach "advanced poses", and the response I get when students realise they can do the pose reminds me of why I teach yoga for a living. I often joke that I feel like a proud father after class. In one class, I had twenty-one women (of all shapes and sizes) try and almost succeed at *Ashtavakrasna* (arm balance). The look on their faces when I demoed the pose was a look of pure horror. I told them the biggest barrier is not physical. "I am convinced you all have the physical capacity for the pose. The pose is about finding your centre of gravity and then fighting your mind to create the expression of the pose."

The first thing to do is to pause for a second and see the beauty within the pose. See the artistic expression of what you are trying to create. This is the first step in defeating your mind. If you think the pose requires the gain of something external first, you will never do the pose. If you think the *Ashtavakrasana* arm balance requires you to get stronger or you are not strong enough, then you can never achieve this pose. Your mind has convinced you that something external is required, so you cannot do it. There is no way for you to do the pose if you are always running away from it. Once there is this realisation, once you stop listening to your mind, you realise that all that is required to do the pose exists inside of you in your will and the mind's greatest enemy, your heart. All that is required is in your heart. And your heart is what defeats the mind. You put aside any notion that you are not strong enough for the pose and you use "heart" to try and ultimately succeed.

When I taught the arm balance pose, some failed to complete the pose physically, but I felt that they achieved the objective psychologically. This is yoga - the battle with the conflicted mind. You cannot say that these poses are for show offs until you have taught them and seen the response from the students once they understand that what is required of them is heart. You can call this a mini moment of enlightenment as well. Yoga students show many of these mini moments the more you teach them. There is nothing more satisfying as a yoga teacher when you see people show genuine heart in trying yoga poses they assumed were too advanced for them.

There is an Urdu word *"himmat"* that translates to mean "heart/courage". But that word is more beautiful and poetic than courage. Courage is a very direct whereas *himmat* is more charming as a word. It almost implies divine spirit or strength, something so dormant that when it manifests, it overwhelms. It refers to that innate boldness that helps you to do battle in times of grief and the real you that only expresses itself as the rest of you is falling apart.

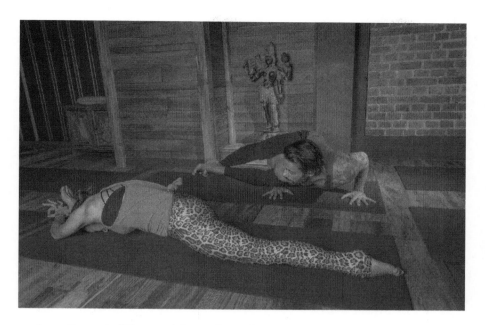

*above - Laura in 'Hanuman' front splits and myself in the 'Ashtavakra' arm balance.*

When I was younger, my mum would say to me, "Whatever you do, however small a task, *dill laga ke kaam karo*", which means put your heart into everything you do. My mum was essentially saying, "show heart" or "show your resolve". Along the same lines, Nietzsche says "live life like existence is a work of art". Both require courage. Art is only an expression of love. My mum would also add in the word "*himmat*" where necessary. But it is not an overused word like courage, which loses its vitality as we become so immune to its meaning. "*Himmat karo*" means "show strength" or "show courage" but not "be strong", which implies that strength or courage could be external or something that can be gained. "Show courage" says that all is already within us.

I have remembered my mum's mantra my whole life. At the various times in my life when I have felt disheartened, as we all do, I have tried to recall my mum's wise words. She wasn't well read or educated and is actually illiterate. She didn't finish school as so many other young women did not in Kashmir in the 60s. But it doesn't take education and knowledge to understand that if you trust in your heart, you can overcome many obstacles in life. She was actually wise despite her lack of education. I don't quite remember who said somewhere that life is not beautiful because you are perfect. Life is perfect because you put your heart into everything you do. Put your heart into the asanas, defeat your mind and you are well on your way to truly understanding yoga.

In "Om Shanti Om" (a Bollywood movie), Shah Rukh Khan's character says, "If you want something with all your heart, the entire universe conspires to bring it to you". What a great scene!

It happened.

Once the great Indian monk, Swami Vivekananda was walking on a lonely road in Banaras (India). Suddenly, a few red-faced monkeys started to follow him. Vivekananda was scared and started running to save himself from these monkeys. However, the monkeys continued to chase him. The faster he ran, the faster the monkeys came after him. Just then, Vivekananda heard a stern voice, "Don't run! Face them!" On hearing these words, Vivekananda stopped running, turned and stood bravely in front of the monkeys. And what a surprise! All the monkeys stepped back and ran away. From this experience, Vivekananda said, "This is the lesson for all life – face the brutes, face the terrible, face it boldly. Like the monkeys, the hardships of life fall back when we cease to flee from them"[19]

So the yoga teacher who says that certain poses are just for ego gratification doesn't understand yoga. The very poses the yoga teachers says are egotistical are in B. K. S Iyengar's "Light on Yoga". Anyone who says that advancing in any capacity is ego driven has a very immature or a naive understanding of the mind. When we learn more about how our mind works, we realise it is this very ego we blame that does not want us to explore and conquer the mind.

The reality is those who say advanced poses are for shows off have never had the courage to try. As a consequence, they have simply lost heart.

Muhammad Ali said, "Often it isn't the mountains ahead that wear you out, it's the little pebble in your shoe".

*Disciple: So, what of the ego? I hear much about the ego in discussions on yoga. What is it exactly?*

In its most simplistic explanation, ego is the part of the mind that creates an identity. If you look up the word, a quick search helps us makes sense of what it means. It is defined as "the fact of being who or what a person or thing is". All the major religions and cultures of the world appear to agree on only one concept - the necessary demise of the ego. Our egos are veils that obscure our reality.

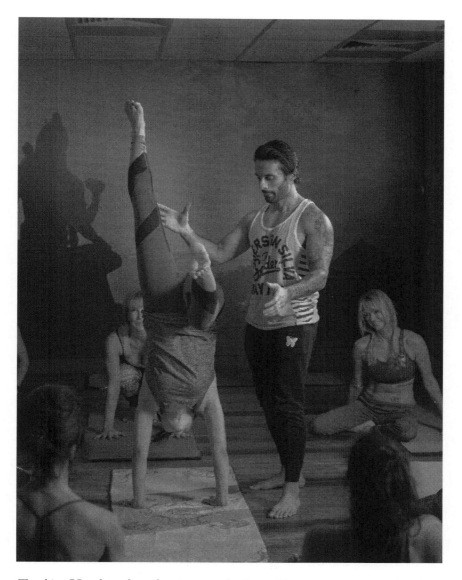

*Teaching Handstands and seeing a student's confidence grow as a result has been one of my greatest joys as a yoga teacher.*

I always viewed "ego" as another word for my self-esteem. So, I found it odd when religions and yoga spoke so negatively about it. Just like all aspects of the mind (as the ego is), the ego can be used for good and bad. I remember John Lennon saying that if people want to call him egotistical for believing in himself then they should go ahead. He didn't think there was anything wrong with that. Most people would agree. This Eastern idea that ego is the root of all destruction just isn't correct. Ego can create desire, dreams, aspirations, ambition and hope. If all of this creates security, income, a sense of achievement and a better sense of self and who you are (self-esteem) then why is that wrong? It would only be wrong if that ego, that sense of identity, then mutates and you become an ego-maniac like Donald Trump, for example. There is no better example of an ego-maniac than Mr. Trump.

So, for the sake of understanding the ego, I think we have to look at two different types of ego or even two different levels of the ego. There is a good ego that is in all of us. As long as we have neurons inside our brains, as long as we can think and have a terrestrial human consciousness, we will also have an ego. So, the ego cannot be destroyed or let go off or killed. It will always exist. This is like our shadows that will always follow us around. There is no point in fighting this. We cannot win. This permanent sidekick of ours, the ego, is actually our acquaintance and does want the best for us. It is this identity of self that will make us feel better and good about ourselves. We cannot allow religions and yoga philosophy (generally just the opinion of robed men remember) to make us feel bad for having an ego. Our ego, when managed, is the link between man and god as Rumi once said. The idea is to not let our ego morph into something or someone in whom love, and compassion is replaced with pride and prejudice.

I have heard many yoga experts and teachers talk so negatively about the ego like they don't have one, which is nonsense. We cannot survive without an identification of self. This is how the human species has supposedly thrived and is now the most advanced species on the planet. We are at the peak of our evolution. People who reject the ego do so because it's easier to reject what they do not understand.

Ego is our friend until we create an attachment to this identity of self. A problem arises when our identity starts override our personality, and we think our identity is correct or better than someone else's identity. We can become a personality hitherto undreamt of.

*"Did you seriously just say hitherto undreamt of?" - Iron Man*
*(Avengers – Infinity War).*

Think of the root cause of suffering in the world. I used to say it was religion. How much blood has been shed since the dawn of man in the name of religion? But it is not religion as I have learnt to understand over time. It is man's identification with that religion and the attachment to that identity. My mum is deeply religious. But you would never know. On the surface, she just wants happiness for her children and eventual oneness with her god. Islam (her religion) is her identity. So, she is an example of having an ego, an identity, but not being attached to that identity. It causes no real threat or destruction as she does not believe her faith is right and yours is wrong. She is only concerned with her own submission to god (as is the genuine non-fundamentalist Islamic way). Then consider the religious extremists - the Christian extremist in the states, ISIS, the raging holy man in India who won't allow women into temples - and away from religion, the KKK. These men (not always men but generally) have an identity and a complete sense of attachment to this identity. They believe in who they are and what they are and their belief (which is their identity) is correct, and those who do not share the same belief are wrong. This is an example of an ego maniac. This is what all true religions are actually against.

The ego-maniac is not just born from being attached to one's identity, it also flourishes when we lust for more than we have, when we are no longer satisfied with our current identity, when our appetite for more and more overrides our logical mind, our ego starts to become out of control. Our ego becomes the Donald Trump of your own world. We have a distorted and grander identification of self. Do you think there is enough money in the world to soothe the bruised ego of a Trump? The divine light is present in us all but our larger than life ego, our superior sense of who we are (or want to be) and how proud we are of who we have become crates such a shadow that we lose any real sense of what or who we truly are. The ego-maniac is the root cause of suffering in the world - not the ego itself. The human species needs ego for survival and evolution but does not need egomania. Look at the legacy of man. Look at history. Do you think Einstein, Darwin, Hawkins, Nietzsche, Newton, da Vinci, Aristotle, Socrates as well as athletes like Muhammed Ali and Michael Jordan were without ego? How about Marie Curie, Helen Keller and Nur Jahan. Were they without ego? It is their ego that has left such a lasting and inspiring legacy. Those who have left destruction, war, blood and hate after they have died were egomaniacs like Alexander and Hitler. And maybe even one day, Donald Trump. So, there is a fine line between ego and egomaniac but on reflection, this is a very clear line. Ego can be used as a mechanism and as a tool to create, inspire and lead or it can be used to cause destruction of both us and those around us. The idea in a philosophical sense as Ice Cube once said is to check yourself before you wreck yourself.

If ego helps drive us forward in our yoga poses, if we want the very best for ourselves, why is that bad/wrong/not yogic? Why should we allow yoga teachers to tell us that being ego driven is not yogic? If ego drives you to have an identity of self, one that is not weak, miserable and suffering, and if ego helps your self-esteem and makes you a happier and a more content version of yourself then how can it be such a bad thing? If we develop into an ego-maniac and act like a terrible person then yes, this is bad. We have lost our self and have morphed into something that not everyone will enjoy being around.

Most people use the ego as a device to help them achieve their handstands and arm balances so they can be the best version of who they are. They can then share this and inspire others. Yoga teachers who shy away and say certain poses are just ego driven don't understand yoga or the subject of ego.

The ego is not against us, and we shouldn't be against the ego. The idea that you are better than someone else is the work of the ego-maniac. We should be against this idea. But the regular ego itself just wants the best for us and is not interested in others and what somebody else might be doing. When we create a superior identity, this is our work. We create the ego-maniac. We should stop blaming the regular ego because we have created the monster for ourselves.

If you have an identity, you have an ego. If you think you are a Hindu, a Muslim or even a yogi, you have an ego. Because again, the ego creates the sense of personal identity. So, if you are religious, are you then egotistical? (some would say yes) If you call yourself a yogi, are you also egotistical?

The ego is your shadow. Nietzsche said that whenever we walk, we are followed by a dog called ego. Your ego is our friend. If we keep our feet on the ground so to speak, our ego will follow us or lead us into all the yoga poses we ever aspired to do. If our yoga poses make us think we are better than those who cannot do the poses, then this is the work of the ego-maniac. In all my experiences till date, I have not met a single yoga teacher/student capable of advanced poses who thinks they are better than somebody else. Practitioners, such as my Laura, Claire Berghorst, Mr. Tenconi, and countless others just have an idea of what they are worth. Their *dharma* and their responsibility unto themselves is to be the best version of who they are. Why should they settle for anything less? Why should they stop advancing because a few insecure yoga teachers think they are showing off? Such yoga teachers with an 'advanced' practice, along with many others do not think they are better than anyone else. They wish for nothing more than to share their journey and inspire others.

In "Light on Life", B. K. S Iyengar admits that he is fanatical with himself when practicing yoga. He goes on to say, "You should be fanatical with yourself but not with others. My guru was fanatical with everyone including me. He applied his standards to everyone. I try to know my students' abilities and to help them to reach their highest potential, not mine"[20].

So, don't let your yoga teacher tell you that ego is behind anything or that it is the root of all problems. Instead, try to understand your ego better. Use your ego constructively to rise to your potential. Ultimately, the reason a yoga teacher will say certain poses are all about the ego is because that particular pose is beyond the ability of that teacher. You won't hear my Laura, or a Claire Berghorst say; "Handstands are all about the ego".

Swami Vivekananda said, "Throw away all weakness. Tell your body that it is strong, tell your mind that it is strong, and have unbounded faith and hope in yourself"[21].

With the above statement is the great Vivekananda asking us to be egotistical? Or is he asking us to embrace the divinity within? Do we need an identity of ourselves to achieve this realisation? The answer is yes.

A yoga teacher will tell us to drop our egos like yesterday's newspaper. We must kill the ego and be done with it. They will say that the handstand and the third series of ashtanga are all just the work of the ego. But are they really? The teacher who says such things, do they own a car? If yes, what car do they drive? Do they live in a nice house? Do they wear fashionable leggings? Do they look after their bodies? Is this not ego? Without a personal identity. Without a value of self. Is it ego to want a nicer car for yourself or to apply for a promotion or to have dreams and aspirations?

So, according to the logic of such yoga teachers it is okay to have an ego if it earns you money and allows you to earn a living, but that same sense of worth and identity, the ego, is not allowed to push us into an advanced pose? So now we can be even more selective about what our ego is. Essentially, ego is whatever the religious man, the yogi or the yoga teacher wants it to be. Their idea of the ego thus suits their agendas and insecurities at that given time.

On a final note, yogis often say we must surrender. They mean that we must surrender our ego. But unless we know our egos, what is there to surrender? Yoga asks that we surrender our identification with oneself by surrendering the "I am". But unless you know who you are, there is no surrender. Yoga says let go of desire and surrender the ego. But unless both have been experienced, you are lost because you do not know what it is you are giving up. Some beautiful paths cannot be discovered without first getting lost. We cannot surrender that which we are not acquainted with. We must make friends with our ego - do not walk in front of it or behind it but rather walk side by side with it where it can cause no harm.

# Danger in Yoga Poses

*Disciple: You have said before that nothing is dangerous in a yoga class, yet when you are teaching, you are very specific about what you want people to do and how. Is this not to prevent students from hurting themselves?*

When I ask a student to adopt a certain position or to create an alignment or correct their posture, this is NOT because of safety. I ask them to follow my specific cues as well as they can because I want them to get the maximum benefit out of the pose. I am demanding due to the rewards I know are available from doing the pose with good positioning and awareness. But not listening to me or not being able to apply what I say does not make the pose dangerous.

So yes, I am demanding, but that is because doing the pose in a specific way can totally transform your body and mind. Doing it with arches collapsed in your feet, knees falling out and a rounded back almost blocks any benefits potentially gained from the pose. But it is not dangerous. All this means is that you are unnecessarily making the body work harder than it needs to. By doing a pose in a certain way, you can encourage the right muscles to work and other muscles to switch off. This creates energy efficiency that allows you to sustain the pose and get the maximum benefits.

I have heard lots of teachers say, "Never do this or never do that. This is dangerous or that is dangerous". The reality is hardly anything is dangerous. If it is, a student will instinctively stop. Most yoga teachers love to talk about what is dangerous because it makes them feel authoritative and educated when the truth is this is a theory they have read and are now sharing with others without any real research or investigation of their own. A student once asked me, "I was told a headstand after shoulderstand is dangerous and should never be done" (it may be the other way around - it was a long time ago). Out of respect, this student didn't ask the teacher why it was dangerous, so she asked me. My reaction was to question as to how it is dangerous? What is the logical argument? This comment was made to the whole class. By saying such a statement, the teacher didn't consider any ability or experience levels in the class. She made an absolute statement that a headstand after shoulderstand or vice versa is dangerous. What if my wife Laura who reads and sleeps on her head or I am in your class? Is it dangerous for us? You could also have Mary the first timer to yoga who has done a little Pilates before. You also have a gymnast in your class as well as a large burly builder. You also have a keen yoga teacher trainee in your class. Does this caution of not doing headstand after shoulderstand (or vice versa) apply to everyone in this class? My Laura defies the laws of physics at times. Is she to NEVER do these poses in that sequence because it is dangerous? What logic is this rule based on let alone any science?

The basic laws of health and fitness say that when you are writing an exercise programme for a client, the exercises selected should be suitable for that client's ability levels. This is common sense. So, nothing is dangerous if the client or student has been built up for the more complicated exercises. In a yoga class, nothing is dangerous if the student has the capacity to tolerate the stress. So, saying one should never do this or do that is absolutely incorrect. The teacher just wants to be perceived by the class as authoritative and knowledgeable and I sympathise. In the modern and very competitive yoga teacher market, what teacher wants to tell their students that everything is fine? If I say to students, "Yeah, just do whatever as long as it doesn't make you cry" and another teacher says, "You should never lock the knee", which teacher appears knowledgeable to the new student? It certainly is not me.

Yoga teachers put too much stock in what some senior teacher said or what they hear. Very little of what they say is based on actual evidence. It was the Buddha who urged us all to find and seek for ourselves. We should also apply these wise words to our teaching. The Buddha taught us to know for ourselves what is hurtful or divisive. The emphasis is always on seeing and knowing, not on calculating and believing as seeing creates wisdom. Knowledge that has been imposed on us or borrowed from someone else is not wisdom. We must be convinced of our own logic before we tell our students what they should or shouldn't do.

The more one studies the human body, the more you question what you read. The more you read about the intricacies of the human body, the more you realise how little you know and is actually known about the body. Everything we know is theoretical anyway. So, we must stop telling people that they can hurt themselves in a yoga class. We must encourage them to be free and move more freely. We must encourage students (as hard as it may be) to listen to their bodies. And we as yoga teachers must be more observant of the different body shapes and ability levels in class and consider this before we make absolute statements.

*Disciple: I am always told the knee should NEVER travel over the toe. Many yoga teachers swear by this fundamental anatomical "rule".*

This type of a teaching point that many yoga teachers have as part of their verbal repertoire (the NEVER part) is regarded as an absolute truth. This is something that is believed to be true at all times. It is something that is always true no matter what the circumstances. It is a fact that cannot be changed. Have you heard the wise old saying that anytime somebody is absolutely certain about something, they are almost always absolutely wrong?

What we have to understand is the concept of "athletic capacity". What does that mean? It is the stress your body can tolerate when you create movement. If you run after your kids, you move athletically. If you do Zumba in your lounge, you are moving athletically. Thus, the physical stress your body can endure is your athletic capacity.

So, what is your athletic capacity? What stress can your body/joints endure? Being specific to this question, what stress can your knee tolerate? From my years of teaching and observation, it is more than most yoga teachers understand.

The next time you are in class, take a look at the various students. Look at the variable sizes, shapes, genders, abilities, experiences and the types of bodies - including those who are athletic, muscular or ex-dancers. The types of bodies and people you get in a yoga class are vast. Each body is unique in what it can and cannot do and the how much stress/load it can tolerate. So, is the absolute statement of saying "the knee should NEVER travel over the toe" applicable to each and every one of these students/bodies? Does a statement like this account for the different bodies and abilities in the class? Does this absolute teaching point leave room for variation?

Coming from a gym/personal trainer and biomechanics background, I have come to understand that it is perfectly safe for the knee to travel over the line of the toe. It all depends on what is happening as it relates to gravity at that time for it to be considered dangerous and even how far the knee travels over the toe. Are we talking millimeters or inches? Where do we draw the line?

The question should be, can the knee travel over the line of the toe? The answer is a resounding yes as this is the design of the knee. Mother nature has designed the human knee to act as a hinge.

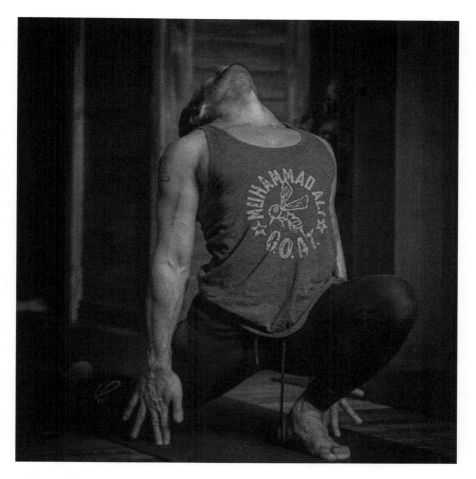

*above - My front knee is over my toe. So is my back knee. How is this unsafe if I have the physical capacity to tolerate this 'stress'?*

The second question is how far can it go? The answer to that depends on the time spent in that position, the load, the purpose for doing so, a person's individual capacity to tolerate such a load (which will differ from one person to another) as well as the sizes of the bones in the lower limbs relative to each other. What if the individual has very small feet relative to their thigh and shin bones?

So, the knee can indeed travel over the toe as this is a biomechanical function of the knee, a student should be encouraged to allow their knee to travel as far forward as is comfortable.

On the subject of this nonsensical yoga teaching point, I asked the following question to Dr. Jacob Harden, (Doctor of Chiropractic degree from the Palmer College of Chiropractic in Port Orange, FL, US): "What is your theory on the knee never travelling over the toes? (as it relates to yoga).

Dr Harden's response was "There is no basis to it (the statement). Yes, moving the knee forward increases the load on the knee but without some sort of measure as to what the knee can tolerate, that information is useless. Load is what makes us adapt so rather than saying it shouldn't go forward, we should be asking if it is an adequate stressor or an excessive stressor. And a lot of that comes down to how does it feel to you."

I asked the same question to my tutors at the National Endurance Sports Trainers Association with whom I studied biomechanics. One of the tutors, who was always vague with his answers, was mainly concerned about the amount of force going through the knee. Is there an external resistance? In our yoga poses, the answer is no. It is just our body weight.

In the Warrior 2 pose, if the knee travels over the toe, the quadricep muscles of the front leg works harder than it needs to. We know this because we can feel it. If we just adjust our weight distribution slightly and the front knee is stacked over the ankle, it makes the pose more stable. This means that we can hold it for longer. It is not because all of a sudden, the pose is safer. This has to be understood. And every now and again, why not challenge students and ask them to take their knee further forward than usual? What could happen? Again, to reiterate, the quadricep muscles of the front leg appears to be working harder while the knee itself is fine when it travels past the toe. When a student says, "It hurts my knee", most of the time I ask, "Really or is it your muscles?" Nearly every time, the student touches their thigh and says, "I feel it here!" I then say, "That isn't your knee!". And even if it was the knee, our understanding of biomechanics suggests that under this new stress, the knee will, in fact, adapt and get stronger with time because, as I keep saying, our knee is designed to do this. It is nature! But a yoga teacher with a 200-hour qualification, where sometimes 10 hours of that is spent on anatomy, apparently knows more about the knee than a doctor and a chiropractor and thinks that mother nature made a mistake in the way our knee was designed.

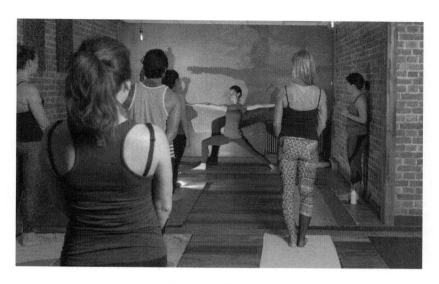

*above - Emma in Warrior 2*

*"There is more wisdom in your body than in your deepest philosophy." — Nietzsche*

*Disciple: Where did this almost universal teaching point even come from?*

I heard way back in my gym instructor days that this idea of the knees not travelling over the toes first gained notoriety in the 70s as the sports science departments of universities tried to establish the safest and most effective way to squat (with an external resistance on your back) without creating shear forces within the knee.

They did, in fact, conclude that when the knee travelled over the toe, the knee was subjected to a greater increase in stress and load; this does sound obvious. Thus, they categorically and authoritatively said, "The knee shall never travel over the toe".

Many years later and after many more experiments and studies, sports scientists have drawn the conclusion that if we don't allow the knee to travel forward as far as is comfortable in a squat, we overload the hip joints. The bending of the knee and the natural way in which it travels forward takes some of the load off the hip and makes the movement less stressful on that part of the body. Essentially, this allows for the weight to be evenly distributed throughout the body. So, restricting the knee from moving forward as it would naturally move in a squat puts excessive load on the hips and lower back.

The problem in group classes at a gym is that the instruction of "don't let your knees go over your toes" had been long established. It had been an effective general rule when trying to teach an exercise to a room full of people with different skill levels, ability levels and tolerance levels. With the change in mindset that many people can allow their knees to travel forward without injury, it became very difficult to apply that to a class full of varied ability and tolerance levels. What if the length of someone's shin and thigh bones meant the knee had to travel forward?

In a class that has a large number of participants, it is difficult to help each individual participant with their specific range of movement. How do you know who may find it stressful? Even if there is a small chance it may create discomfort, what can be done? So, providing a general "don't let your knees go past your toes" instruction has become an effective way of erring on the side of caution for the class exercise instructor. As yoga began to be taught in gyms by teachers, many of whom were not level 2 gym qualified teachers (for a time, the minimum qualification required to work in a gym), they started to copy and recite many of the dialogues being used in the other more gym-based classes.

Today, I can squat with a very heavy load on my back and allow my knees to travel naturally over the toe, but god forbid I allow my knee to travel over my toe in my yoga lunge where there is no resistance. Do you see where my disregard for such a teaching point comes from?

The yoga anatomist David Kiel was asked the question on his website if it was safe for the knee to travel over the ankle in warrior[2].

"This is something that comes up a lot in yoga classes. I've been asked this question many times before about knees as I tell people often to take their knee past their ankle. My position on it has always been there is nothing inherently wrong with your knee moving past your ankle joint. Really far forward is going to add more stress and strain to the knee joint itself, but it's not like we're loading loads of weight onto our back while doing it, which would of course increase the forces going into the knee."[22]

David concludes, "So, in summary, if your knee goes past your ankle a little bit, it shouldn't be a problem. That's normal, natural movement. We should be able to sustain that without any trouble. If it's tilting in, that's more problematic. And remember, if the pressure's coming out of the knee, it's going into somewhere else, which you can also use to your advantage".

Mika Janhunen (the Chiropractor mentioned earlier) visited the studio recently to speak on anatomy and the human body to help graduate teachers better understand the sometimes complex but often uncomplicated subject. On the question of the knee travelling over the toe, Mika was very casual in his explanation that he does not see a problem with it because "to bend" is the functional design of the knee. He then demonstrated from a standing position how the knee travels over the toe and also demonstrated his deep squat position where his knee clearly travels over the line of his toes. In both instances, he said he experienced zero pain! It is the same as walking up and down the stairs. The pain can be experienced sometimes because we are looking for it! It comes down to conditioning.

*Disciple: So, who do I listen to? You or my teacher who I assume will still stick to her guns regardless of what you and your friends say!*

Listen to your instincts and your own body. If it feels okay, then it is okay. If it hurts then it is only you who can decide if this is something you need or something you wish to avoid. But try and listen to instincts and not your conditioning. Most of the time when we think for ourselves, the first few dozen thoughts are actually not our own. They are conditioned thoughts handed down to us from other people. I once heard, "It is what it is because you let it be so". We have to go beyond this to try to find our own reasoning and intellect.

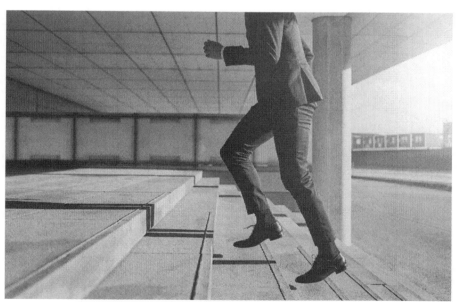

*A businessman runs up the stairs as we all do, day in day out. The knee always travels over the toe.*

We walk up and down the stairs all day long with a tremendous amount of weight on our knees. When the knee bends, the knee travels over the toe and this leg then takes all your weight and pushes you up the stairs. And somehow miraculously, your knee survives. This is because you have not been conditioned to think this is unsafe. So, your body just does what is perfectly natural. Try walking up and down the stairs and be conscious of NOT letting your knee travel over the toe. You can see for yourself how unnatural it is.

*"One believes things because one has been conditioned to believe them." –*
*Aldous Huxley, Brave New World*

*Disciple: My yoga teacher says you should never lock the knee?*

(Before I delve into this topic, I would like to point out that when I refer to locking the knee, I am talking about straightening the leg to its full range of motion. I am not referring to the more medical term where the knees locks and then cannot bend because they are stuck).

*"By some need to appear intellectual, non-thinkers will instantly and without question subscribe to the opinions of those they feel other people think are educated"[23] - Chris Jami, Healology*

I will first explain some of the science behind this without over complicating things as again, I wish to keep this book as simple as I can. Your knee is a hinge joint in that it opens and closes like a hinge joint on a door (it can also rotate a little but again, I wish to keep my explanations simple). The knee can what is called knee flexion (bending the knee) and then straighten in what is called knee extension. Interestingly, despite what Wendy the yoga teacher may say, the knee can actually hyperextend. (Gasp!) This means that it can go beyond the straight line. For most of us, this is completely normal. Normal can also be up to 8-10 degrees of what some people refer to as hyperextension. This is not dangerous; this is your anatomy.

As an exercise, sit down on your posterior and extend your legs out in front of you so they are straight. This is knee extension. Now squeeze your thighs as much as you can. Do your heels come off the ground? If the answer is yes, you can easily hyperextend your knees. This does not mean you are hypermobile. This just means that when you stand up with straight legs, chances are your legs are not in a straight line or don't look straight to the naked eye. They may not look straight to the average yoga teacher, but your legs are perfectly straight

218

I have been told before that I should bend my knees ever so slightly while in the mountain pose. "Soft knees" is the command in an even softer yoga voice. In a basic standing upright position, I am told to soften the knee. For what purpose? I have asked this question before. Why should I soften the knee when I am just being a human and standing up? With no external resistance on my body when I am just standing, I am being told to keep my knees slightly bent? Is this to protect my knee? The teacher will say, "Yes, to protect the knee". Upon further enquiry, on my part of course, they will tell me that this is just what their teacher told them or that they read it on a reputed yoga website.

*"But what good is the popular opinion, if the lot of us just process like minions?"*[24]
*- Chris Jami, Healology*

So, let me get this straight . . . How exactly will softening my knees in a standing pose protect my knee?" Should I, as a new student, ask my teacher to explain why softening my knees is safer? Should I walk around in everyday life and making sure I never lock my knee? Try it. Try walking without locking the knee (fully straightening). When we walk, our legs straighten fully. This is done to preserve energy. When our legs fully straighten, this takes the load or pressure off the muscles around the knee. The load or force of your body is now on the bones or the knee joint. So, if the muscles are not working, they are preserving energy. This allows you to walk for long periods of time. Try walking with micro bent knees. First, you will just feel weird. Second, you will not be able to maintain it for the same duration as you would with fully straight legs because you are wasting energy. Additionally, when you walk normally with straight legs, the bones that make up the knee joint are receiving constant stimulus, which is what the bones require to stay healthy. Bones need good stress to remain healthy too.

I was standing waiting for a train yesterday and I was standing upright with my legs perfectly straight and my knees locked. Everyone else waiting (who were also standing) were standing with their knees locked. I could just picture a yoga teacher or fitness instructor running around concerned for the knee health of these commuters. "Please you must soften your knees! It's true. My teacher told me!" So why was everyone standing up and waiting for the train with locked knees? Two reasons. Reason one is because they can! This causes no risk whatsoever. There were many who were also in what some people would call "hyperextension". The commuter would not be standing like this if it was not comfortable. This is because we have an inbuilt system that detects faulty movement. The second reason we were all waiting with locked knees is because this is energy efficient. When my knees are locked, my surrounding muscles switch off, so my body is more relaxed. Next time you are waiting for something, unlock your knees and stand like you are ready to accelerate. Feel the difference in your legs. The muscles are working to support you. Then lock your knees and literally feel them switch off. Now you can wait for longer without tiring.

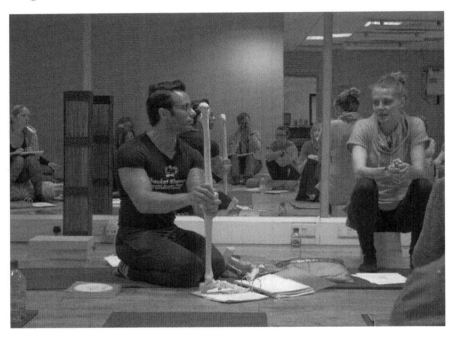

*above - Teaching 'anatomy of the knee' as part of our Teacher Training programme with my friend and fellow yoga teacher, Dr Laurie Ramsay.*

Think of a squat at the gym. If you have squatted with a bar before, you can picture this well. You have more than your bodyweight on your back. If you weigh 70 kg, it is perfectly normal for you to have 100 kg on the bar. So, you place the bar as you would on your shoulders, you think about your core and then you sit back into a squat. You then ascend from the squat back to a standing position with locked knees or fully straightened legs. This is because the body instinctively wishes to recover between repetitions and with the knees bent, this cannot happen. The muscles have to switch off in order to recover. If you kept them bent to "protect your knees", you would soon buckle and fall. The stress would be too much. So, a gym goer, a heavy squatter and even a power lifter must lock or fully straighten the knees when at the top of their movements, but we cannot straighten our legs in a yoga class where there is no external resistance? Where is the common sense in that?

I had a client recently who tore his hamstring away from his sit bones - a very painful injury. I had a similar injury but not as severe, so I was sympathetic towards his pain. Once he was off using crutches and back to walking, he was told by his physiotherapists that he must learn to fully straighten his leg. This gets the muscles to remember what their full range of motion is. Thus, our legs are designed to be full straightened. We even have a muscle named the Popliteus that has the specific job of 'screwing' the knee into position and 'unlocking' the knee when walking. If the knee was not designed to 'lock' then why do we have this muscle?

Let's look at the Warrior 3 - a "balancing" pose, whereby once I am in the full expression of the pose, my body resembles a "T" shape. A lot of teachers and fitness instructors, through the years, have said that we should NEVER lock the standing leg in this position as this can damage the knee. This very commanding instruction will be blurted in class in front of other students to create an illusion of authority and education. Ironically, this could not be further from the truth

If you look at B. K. S Iyengar's standing leg in all his balancing/standing poses in the images available in "Light on Yoga" (page 50), there is no softening of the knee. Iyengar's knee is actually in a position that to the average eye looks like hyperextension. Most modern teachers would be gasping in horror. Does Mr. Iyengar not know about knee safety? Has he not read the article on the knee written by someone random on an even more random website? You see, although Iyengar is a pioneer who revolutionised physical yoga and is perhaps the reason I can write this book and why you are all interested in yoga, most modern yoga teachers appear to know better. This is the problem we have in the West. We take any sort of system from the East, and we think we know better. This has been going on for centuries and is not likely to change. This reminds me of a quote from the Lebanese poet Kahlil Gibran: "Trees are poems the earth writes upon the sky. We cut them down and turn them into paper. Then we record our emptiness".

*Disciple: So why do so many fitness instructors and yoga teachers say locking the knee is dangerous?*

Einstein once said, "Wisdom is not a product of schooling but of the lifelong attempt to acquire it".

Most instructors and yoga teachers, in my experience, just assume they have all the answers after their teacher training. If they have been told something categoric, then that is just the way it is now. However, what they forget is we should continue to develop and refine ourselves and our understanding of the body. One of my favourite footballers as a child, Roberto Baggio, once said, "Kids today don't play using their instincts, but only do what they've been taught. So, their personality, in footballing terms, doesn't come through completely". This is the same as the regimented conveyor belt of yoga teachers being mass produced. No one has any individuality. The yoga teacher upon completion of the course needs to further their studies and understanding of the human body out of concern for their future students. This is not achieved by reading articles on the internet. It is attained through further education and contact with real people from the real world.

I have spent years questioning doctors, physiotherapists, chiropractors and yoga anatomists. I am never satisfied with the answers, and I still have more questions than answers. You should be satisfied only when you have no more questions. I sincerely feel like all yoga teachers should have the same level of inquiry. I say to students at my yoga teacher training that I wish for them to leave thinking their inquisitive nature has been awakened from its slumber. Teacher training only opens the door for them, and the rest of the journey is their own. I want them to leave the teacher training with more questions than answers. The Buddha once said, "Be the light unto yourselves". The more you learn about anatomy and physiology, the more ignorant you will know you are. We know so little fact, all of this just theory.

2,400 years ago, a wise oracle in Athens was asked, "Is anyone wiser than Socrates?" The answer from the oracle was "No". When Socrates was told about this, he laughed. He said, "How can this be? I know so little?" The reality was that Socrates became the patron saint of philosophy because he questioned everything. Life, he declared, is only worth living if you think about what you are doing. An unexamined existence is all right for cattle but not for human beings.

Take life with a pinch of salt. Take this book, philosophy, understanding, wisdom, yogis and teachers with a pinch of salt.

Remember a pinch of salt is all you need to add flavour to a dish. There are supposedly two different types of people in the world: those who want to know, and those who want to believe. Don't join the flock and believe in everything.

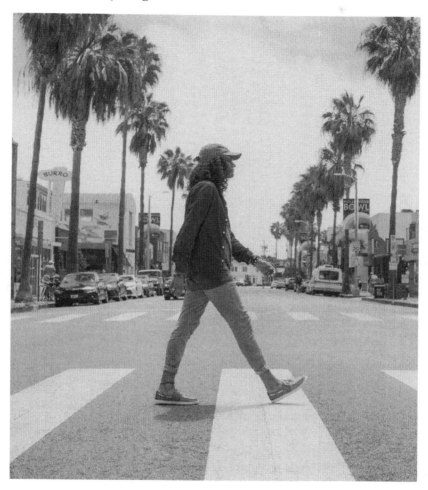

*When you walk, do you fully straighten / lock your knees?*

In a world of suppressed insecure minions, be more like Socrates.

The Buddha has said, "Don't go by reports, by legends, by traditions, by scripture, by logical conjecture, by inference, by analogies, by agreement through pondering views, by probability, or by the thought, 'This contemplative is our teacher'. When you know for yourselves that, 'These qualities are skillful; these qualities are blameless; these qualities are praised by the wise; these qualities, when adopted & carried out, lead to welfare & to happiness' — then you should enter and remain in them"[25]

The above quote from the Buddha is a really important read for all yoga teachers and students as we continue our asana journey. I have often heard yoga teachers say that they do certain things because that is what their teacher has told or taught them. What they forget or perhaps have not realised is the teacher who has taught them is teaching what they have come to understand over years of personal inquiry. Chances are that teacher has added or changed what it was that they were taught by their own teacher or guru to make yoga more accessible to their audience.

As an example, B. K. S Iyengar modified his teachings from his guru because the modified form of yoga he was teaching was better suited to his students in Pune. Iyengar said that he modified the yoga taught by his guru, and this was okay. He fully expected someone to one day modify what he taught. This is how we evolve. In 2019, science is the dominant mode of discovering reality. We have to adapt our teaching the more science opens our eyes about the complexities of human movement.

The Buddha himself asked his followers not to accept his authority as set down in the scriptures simply out of respect for him. He also told them to test the truth of what he said. Further, the Dalai Lama said, "If science discovers that a belief of Buddhism is wrong, that it violates an indisputable truth of science, then Buddhism must abandon that view of scriptural teaching. Even if it prevailed for a millennia"[26].

To say once should NEVER lock the knee just does not bear fruit. Speak to anyone who has had a knee operation or problems with their knees, and they are encouraged to regain the full range of movement, even if to the eyes of the yoga teacher this looks like hyperextension.

Warrior 3 done with a straight leg is not going to damage your knee. The two bones that make up your knee has a padding in between called the meniscus. This meniscus cushions weight so the bones do not rub against each other. The bones and the meniscus are actually designed to sit on each other perfectly. This padding is actually a very clever design. This placing of the bones on top of each other in the way they are designed to sit has a name - joint congruency.

The meniscus is designed to take the load of the bone from both sides and will not be affected if the load is even. If you had a meniscus in your hand and were able to apply even pressure through the meniscus on both sides (trying to squash it), you would probably hurt your hands through the pressure of pushing before you even come close to creating any damage to the meniscus.

Both my menisci are torn and or damaged. This is a result of my pre-yoga life as a boy who played football. I straighten my legs fully in all postures (where required), and there is not a hint of discomfort in either damaged knee. This is because the load applied on the meniscus is even. Ironically, there is mild discomfort when I micro bend the knee. This is because the load through the meniscus is now uneven. Most of the pressure is now on the front part of the meniscus. The meniscus requires the challenge of a straight leg so it can maintain its integrity. In the same way bones need stress too. No stress on the bones weakens them overtime. We thus have to stop wrapping ourselves in cotton wool.

I appreciate that this is an over simplification. But yoga teachers in teacher training need to ask more questions and not blindly believe what they are being told or what they read online. Yoga teacher trainees need to be more inquisitive and more challenging. They also need to ask what science or research something is based on if it does not agree with their logic. The first time I was told to never lock my knee, I questioned it. But guess what, I never got a straightforward answer. I was told it was bad for my knees and that is all. I politely challenged the teacher after class to explain her logic. She said it was bad for my cartilage. I replied, "No, it isn't". And immediately, she said "Well, that is what my teacher told me". The yoga alliance and their quality control (or lack of) had struck again.

The reality is that telling your students to not lock their knees in class because it is dangerous makes you feel credible and educated. You want to appear knowledgeable in front of your students - how ironic!

Terry Pratchett once said, "It would seem that you have no useful skill or talent whatsoever. Have you thought of going into teaching?"

The following happened. These are all true stories, I didn't just make them up.

When Shiva's loyal vehicle Nandi was preaching at a temple, the demi god Indra, was jealous of his large audience and wanted to debate with him. Indra himself wanted to speak to the audience. He wanted this large audience to know that he was much wiser than Nandi.

Nandi was in the midst of speaking when Indra appeared. Indra made such a disturbance that Nandi stopped his discourse and asked about the noise.

"I am Indra and I can perform miracles. I can hold a brush in my hand on the banks of the river Ganga, my attendant can hold up a piece of paper on the other bank, and I can write the holy name of Shiva through the air onto this paper. Can you do such a wonderful thing?"

Nandi replied lightly, "Perhaps you can perform that trick, but that is not the manner of yoga. My miracle is that when I feel hungry, I eat, and when I feel thirsty, I drink".

The moral of the story is that many people want to be extraordinary - so many, in fact, that what is actually extraordinary is wanting to just be ordinary. Nandi had large audiences because he had no gimmicks and was just himself - his own dialogue, his own discourse and his own words. Nothing was borrowed from "how to teach yoga" websites. His teachings were inspired by his teacher Shiva, but his delivery and his tone were all his own. Indra believed that talking nonsense and giving absolute statements would give him authority and a larger crowd. But it did not. People soon learn to see past this kind of nonsense.

Getting back to the question whether locking the knee is dangerous, the answer is no. Unless, for whatever reason, locking the knee hurts. If it hurts, you must learn to straighten your legs using quadricep contraction - squeezing your thighs. If you squeeze your thighs and one muscle in particular (the vastus medialis - the quad muscle more on the inside of the front thigh), the knee will not go to a place that creates pain.

So as a summary, most people will NOT hurt or injure their knees by locking the knees in the various standing and balancing poses. If there is any pain, the person in pain needs to be educated to use the quadriceps to straighten the legs. If there is still pain, find any point within that pose that eliminates the pain.

Another reason for knee pain is the sudden straightening of legs without much care and control. You can straighten the leg slowly with conscious control and feel zero discomfort or you can snap the joint back in a heartbeat. The snap back generally feels awful. So, the speed at which the knee straightens is also an issue. You are thus encouraged to go into a straight leg pose with grace rather than force.

*Disciple: Is there any truth to yoga teachers saying we can release negative emotions from our hips by partaking in hip-openers?*

In many ways, this is similar to an earlier question. Does courage really reside inside the heart? The heart is a muscular organ that pumps blood around the body to keep you alive. As I mentioned earlier, it is a very nice romantic notion that your heart has emotions and can speak to you and encourage you or release courage into your body as it pumps blood around your body at the same time. Anatomically, this is not the case. Courage is a part of the mind. So, courage, along with all other emotions, are all part of our conscious mental world.

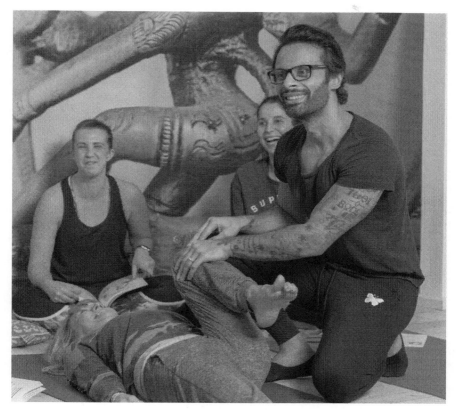

*Above is my initial reaction to the question.*

Every day, we are placed in innumerable situations that elicit emotional responses including fear, anger, sadness, joy, disgust, surprise, courage and the like. These emotional responses occur inside our heads, in our brains. We thus have a neurological response to emotional states. This response is born in the emotional core of our brain - the limbic system. And in particular, the part of the brain that my niece and I have a lot of fun pronouncing, the "amygdala" (the sort of gateway to the limbic system). There are two amygdalae per person with one on each side of the brain. They are responsible for emotions, survival instincts and memory.

As discussed, emotions are born from within the brain. But can our hips store emotions as so often claimed by yoga 'professionals'? If our bodies/cells do store emotions, can we release these emotions in a yoga class as is so often claimed? I personally am not convinced of the latter. Before you get too emotional, here are some questions to ponder.

What emotions are we talking about - the negative ones or the positive ones too? I once heard from a yoga teacher that the hips store negative emotions. So where do the positive ones go? Can our body really store, and house separate positive and negative emotions?

If our hips (or more specifically, our psoas muscles) really holds emotions, does everyone who has a tight psoas muscle repress their emotions until they partake in "juicy hip openers" as part of a yoga class?

Do cyclists and other athletes who dominantly use their front hip muscles need a hug as well as a yoga 'lizard stretch'?

What about all the amazing back bending students in a class? Is it safe to say that their hips/psoas muscles do not hold onto emotions? Was their childhood different? Were the students with amazing backbends always emotionally expressive as children and never made to feel that they had to hold in their emotions?

Have these back-benders just not suffered any emotional trauma? Are those who enjoy back-bending more emotionally stable that someone with tight hips?

With someone who has tight hips, are emotions the main restriction ahead of even the nervous system, or do we only say that people who cry in class hold emotions in their hips? On the flip side, has anyone ever had their tears of joy rain down like a monsoon after having stretched their hips or again, are these just negative emotions that can be 'released'?

These are the kind of questions I have to ask myself when I hear or read something 'yogic' from someone or something online. It needs to satisfy my logical way of thinking, and in all honesty, this idea that you can release negative emotions from a hip stretch does not.

Some 'experts' will say that you can store emotions in your body. There is no distinction, you see, between mind and body. It used to be common thought that mind and body were both very separate. This was the thinking of René Descartes, the French philosopher, mathematician and scientist, some 400 years ago. But today, we view things rather differently. The body is the gross part of the mind, and the mind is the subtle part of the body. If you believe they are not separate, then there is every possibility that your body can express, experience and store your emotions. Dr. Candace Pert the author of "Molecules of Emotion: The Science Behind Mind-Body Medicine" says, "A feeling sparked in our mind or body will translate as a peptide

228

being released somewhere. (Organs, tissues, skin, muscle and endocrine glands), they all have peptide receptors on them and can access and store emotional information. This means the emotional memory is stored in many places in the body, not just or even primarily, in the brain. You can access emotional memory anywhere in the peptide/receptor network, in any number of ways. I think unexpressed emotions are literally lodged in the body. The real true emotions that need to be expressed are in the body, trying to move up and be expressed and thereby integrated, made whole, and healed"[27].

So, there is abundant "information" easily available that supports the idea that we can store emotions in our bodies. Here is another example with regards to the idea that our inner thighs store our fear of vulnerability.

"Are you nervous and untrusting around other people? If you struggle with social anxiety, you might also have inner thigh pain. Because our legs are biologically programmed to run when we first spot danger, fear towards others is often stored here."[28]

After reading the above for the first time, my instinctive response was to hit my head with my palm in the way my niece and I do anytime we hear or read something that ludicrous.

According to some 'experts' and yoga teachers, parts of our bodies store emotions. This, I guess, would include every yoga teacher's favourite muscle - the psoas. Our psoas area is generally restricted due to sports and occupations, and it is believed that by stretching this muscle in a yoga class, it can make the person very emotional. In some cases, students begin to bawl their eyes out. They are then left confused and shook up as to the sudden outbreak of tears. They are then comforted by "yogis" who explain that this is perfectly normal. This happens all the time. "We hold emotions in our hips and sometimes when the muscles releases, so do our emotions". The yogi then hugs the student who has now experienced a moment of spirituality. There is little to no actual scientific data that illuminates our understanding of the relationship between emotions and our hips[28a], but who am I to argue with a yoga teacher?

Has the above experience of a student crying after hip stretching ever happened to me? Err . . . No - not as a student and not as a teacher. As a student, my hips have been worked on for years. But has a lunge backbend ever made me cry a river? "Birds of Paradise" has made me cry in the past but that is because it is the most ridiculous yoga pose ever (anything we can't do properly is always ridiculous). But I personally have never got emotional while stretching my muscles in a yoga class. Am I suppressing my emotions or is my body just not storing them? No student has ever told me that the wheel pose has made them cry. Is that because the student could not express their feelings to a male teacher? Once they left the studio, did they run to the changing rooms and cry like I just stole their lunch money or do the students who come to me just not have suppressed emotions?

Modern scientific research is still trying to figure out the impact of emotions on the body. Some science says that our emotions are all just responses by our brains. Others say that our body stores these emotional memories, and they need to be released by some means such as meditation, yoga, exercise and so on. Research has proven that within the first few seconds of experiencing a negative emotion, people automatically tense the muscles in their jaw and around their eyes and mouth.

In my opinion, many people believe they can release stored emotions from their hips almost through conditioning. Yoga professionals chant this so regularly as part of a rehearsed dialogue that students often believe it to be true. If you cry in a yoga class, I believe it is because you have an emotional nature, and maybe the environments you are regularly in are not allowing you to express these emotions. This emotional nature can be exacerbated by poor posture, lack of sleep, unhealthy eating and other such negative habits. Your colleagues at work and your family at home all expect you to be more in control of your emotions, but this can be a struggle and there is only so much we can take. Then you visit a yoga class that opposed to a gym slows down your entire system, your body and most importantly, your breathing. Your body is slowed down at such an alarming rate that it creates a realisation of just how hectic and manic your life is. Your brain, at this stage, senses signs of distress as you, mid pose, start to ponder the hectic nature of your life. The amygdala portion of the brain triggers the limbic fear response and starts to fire neural signals making your breathing shallow, your pulse quickens, and your forehead sweat. Your reaction to this is overwhelming, so you begin to cry. And remember, the act of crying is generally an expression of anxiety, pain or distress. Then, towards the end of the class, you come to realise just how much you needed just to get out of the house today. You realise that making time for yourself was the best decision you have made in a long time. You remind yourself that looking after yourself should now be your number one priority. This starts to elicit more of an emotional response from you. You start to cry again and don't really understand why.

The truth is you just needed to cry because life has been taking its toll on you, and you have not been making time to take care of your health. But the teacher tells you it is because of the hip openers you just did in class. "This is the power of the pigeon," they will say. They have that authoritative look about them so really, who are we to argue? The reality is you could have felt the same in a body balance class or a mindfulness meditation - essentially, any activity or environment that asks you to just slow everything down. You didn't cry through the power of hip-openers, you cried because you were emotionally overwhelmed and in an environment that perhaps encourage you to let it all out.

Modern yogis say that the mind, body and spirit are all one and the same, and what happens to the mind effects your body, which it does. But does a yoga pose release stored emotions from your body? Again, I don't think so. Many yogis will swear adamantly that inner tension is stored in your body and a "juicy" hip stretch is all you need. I would say spending time by yourself in an empty room reflecting on life is likely to do the same thing. So, to answer your question, can we release emotions from our hips? The modern yoga teacher would say yes. They would say, "As we move through asanas, we literally twist and bend the stagnant emotions out from our bodies. Because the body stores emotions, moving and breathing creates space and helps us process these feelings on an energetic level"[29]. In my opinion that is all extremely untrue (that is me putting it nicely – trust me). But then again, I am a man and way too macho to admit to my emotions, right? Maybe we do store emotions, I can possibly come around to believing that idea, but can a yoga pose release these emotions? It is this that I am not convinced of. Like I said, someone crying in class is not sufficient evidence that a hip stretch can elicit an emotional outbreak. All this means is that person is having a difficult time in their life, and it just so happened to be in a yoga class that things caught up with them. It is not due to the power of yoga despite what yoga teachers would have you believe.

The easy thing for me to do with answering the aforementioned question is to say "Yes, we do store emotions in the hips and yes, we can release these emotions via hip openers" because this is what all yoga teachers say. But I am not a puppet, and this just doesn't agree with my logical mind or as yoga teachers love to say, this does not "resonate with me".

When I hear a yoga teacher say, "the feelings of fear, anxiety and sadness are stored in the hips and we can remove them in camel (pose)", I cannot help but shake my head in disbelief. This shaking of the head is the unconscious response by the brain when it finds something so stupid, no words can do it justice. Again, my question is "Where are all the other emotions stored?" There is a positive to every negative. So, if a hip stretch can make you cry, why does a forward fold (potentially the opposite movement) not make me break out into uncontrollable laughter or joy?

Dr Paul Ekman and American psychologist has identified six basic human emotions: anger, disgust, fear, happiness, sadness, and surprise. We do go through these varied emotions in a class but are they a result of a specific body part? Is a stretch for a specific muscle likely to release the same emotion from every student in the class? Will a cradle stretch release disgust in everyone? Will the pigeon pose release fear in mankind? The whole idea is utterly ridiculous. We are not supposed to blindly agree with everything that is said or understood within yoga. We need to take the information available and apply our own experiences and common sense to it. Until this supposed "logic" convinces me, maybe through my own experiences, I should remain a sceptic as should you about any subject in yoga that does not reach out to you. I have looked for evidence and asked professionals, such as doctors and chiropractors for any science-based evidence on such claims, and there is none. All of these are just theories as is everything.

The subject of storing 'emotions in your hips' is very much like other wild and ignorant yogic claims such as yoga poses "stimulating digestion" or certain poses "wringing out toxins". You can throw in moronic claims that yoga poses can balance your chakras in there too.

I read in an article an answer from a scientist who was looking into the so-called benefits of yoga. The response was; "[Teachers are] basing it on personal experience, on anecdote, on the lineage of practice that's been handed down," he said. "They are probably not basing it on Western-style analytic techniques that followed a control trial design"[30].

A philosopher, having made an appointment to dispute the philosophy and views of Mullah Nasreddin, called and found him away from home. Infuriated, the philosopher picked up a piece of chalk and wrote "Stupid Oaf" on Nasiruddin's front door.

As soon as the Mulla got home and saw this message, the Mulla rushed to the philosopher's house. "I had forgotten," he said, "I had such a busy day at work, and I sincerely apologise for having not been at home when you called. Of course, I remembered the appointment as soon as I saw that you had left your name on my front door."

One man's philosopher is thus another man's fool. For me, a fool is someone who blindly believes everything they hear or read. I am not trying to convince you that we cannot release stored emotions from our hips, I personally just don't buy it. You as a student/teacher have to reach a conclusion for yourself and not just blindly agree with what is considered the vogue thing to say.

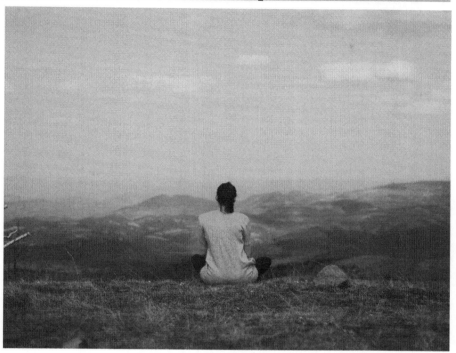

Meditation in the yoga tradition is not something you do. You cannot suddenly decide now is the time to sit down and meditate. This is not how yogic meditation works.

One falls into a state of meditation. Mediation in the yoga tradition is a destination. What we do when we close our eyes and say we are meditating is just the limited Western interpretation. You can call this silent reflection, but it is not "mediation" in the purest yogic sense of the word. An argument could be made that this silent reflection can be a precursor to meditation.

Let us consider the two types of "meditation". We will begin by examining the modern understanding and practice of meditation - what it is we do as a practice to bring about a sense of calmness and wellbeing. Subsequently, we shall consider meditation in the purest yogic sense. You will soon see why I often say that we do not and cannot meditate. Often, people get very flustered and defensive when I say this. I am not mocking modern meditation or our modern therapeutic type of meditation at all. I am just trying to explain so you can understand the difference between yogic mediation and our more modern version of meditation. Ultimately my aim is to help you understand that what we do in the West under the title of "meditation", could be considered something that you might actually do to arrive to meditation.

*Disciple: Okay, I heard that. This is kind of like how we call the poses "yoga" when in reality, it is not yoga but "asana". Essentially "asana" helps us reach "yoga" (union)? Is that right?*

You are a wise one, my young apprentice.

*Disciple: Okay, so before we break it down, what does mediation even mean?*

The English word "meditation" is derived from the Latin word "meditatio" from the verb "meditari" meaning "to think, contemplate, devise and ponder". The modern understanding of the word refers to contemplating or even fantasising or daydreaming. Often, when an important decision is to be made, modern yogis say, "Let me meditate on it". Implying that once they are alone and away from the chaos and confusion of everyday life, they can better hear and understand their "instincts". Silent reflection and contemplation apparently helps us make better decisions. In silent reflection, our decisions are benefited by our intellect rather than our emotions. In theory anyway.

Other forms of modern-day meditation involve just silence - just sitting alone with the eyes closed with a focus on breathing (or anything else) and nothing more. This is why many people like to begin yoga class by sitting or lying down in silence. In this silence, we attempt to become a witness to our thoughts. We simply observe passing mental events like clouds in the sky. We do not evaluate them or waste time on them. We let them pass. Unlike words and mantras, silence has no barriers or obstacles. This type of meditation, as we will see later in the chapter, is exercise for our brains. Neuroscience tells us that this type of silent meditation (when done long-term) has been shown to thicken our brains. A thicker brain does not mean a smarter brain but a healthier one.

*Disciple: So, meditation as it is understood separate from yogic tradition, simply means being silent and/or reflection and contemplation?*

Correct.

*Disciple: So, what does "meditation" mean in the yoga tradition?*

The word meditation in yoga circles is used to translate the Sanskrit word, *'Dhyana'*. Dhyana does not translate to meditation directly. It is more of an indirect translation as there is no direct English version of the word. *Dhyana* means "contemplation", "reflection" and "profound, abstract meditation". It could also mean self-directed awareness or even intense and unbroken focus.

In the contemporary sense of the word, *dhyana* refers to a heightened sense of concentration. I was in a taxi in India, and the driver was talking to me while navigating the busy streets. My instinctive choice of words where, "*Bhai saab dhyana se chalao*", which means, "My brother, concentrate as you drive". But I didn't just mean concentrate in this situation. It is a stage above concentration. The word "*dhyana*" is used often in everyday conversation today as a means to express how you should concentrate intensely on something or to contemplate or even when you are in an uninterrupted state of mental concentration. So, although *dhyana* has been translated to mean "meditation", they are actually very different. In many respects, you can say that the modern use of meditation - to think and contemplate - can prepare you for the yogic *dhyana*, which is profound contemplation and reflection. You can say that one precedes the other. This is what I mean when I often say that we do not meditate in the West - closing your eyes is not meditating. But I am merely basing this on my understanding of the yogic form of meditation.

The following is excerpted from Iyengar's "Light on Life" and has formed the foundation of my understanding of meditation[1].

"Contrary to what many teachers try to tell you, meditation is not going to remove stress. Meditation is only possible when one has already achieved a certain 'stress-less' state. To be stress-less, the brain must already be calm and cool. By learning how to relax the brain, one can begin to remove stress. Meditation does not achieve this. You need to achieve all these as a foundation for meditation. However, I am aware that in modern English usage, the word meditation is often used for various forms of stress management and reduction. In this book, I shall be using it in its purest yogic sense as the seventh petal, which can be achieved only when all other physical and mental weaknesses have largely been eliminated. Technically speaking, true meditation in the yogic sense cannot be done by a person who is under stress or who has a weak body, weak lungs, hard muscles, collapsed spine, fluctuating mind, mental agitation or timidity. Often people think that sitting quietly is meditation. This is a misunderstanding. True meditation leads us to wisdom and awareness, and this specifically helps in understanding that we are more than our ego. For this, one needs the preparations of the postures and the breathing, the withdrawal of the senses and concentration. This process of relaxing the brain is achieved through asana. We generally think of mind as being in our head. In asana, our consciousness spreads throughout the body, eventually diffusing in every cell, creating a complete awareness."

Iyengar goes on to say, "Many people have been taught that meditation is a method of stress relief. In yoga, stress must be dealt with before one can truly begin to meditate. True meditation (*dhyana*) is when the knower, the knowledge and the known become one. This is only possible when one is in a stress-less state."[2]

You can clearly see how much of a gulf exists between modern meditation and the yogic *dhyana*. The difference is like day and night. Many Western yoga teachers teach poses for the physical body and then teach meditation to remove stress - but this is not the yogic method. We remove stress and negative emotions in our poses (as explained when looking at handstands and other poses) and then sit peacefully as we arrive at meditation. There is a fundamental reason why so many people struggle to meditate. This is because we carry stress into our meditation. If the monkey mind is super alert when we sit down and close our eyes, this cannot be yogic meditation. The monkey must be put at peace in our asana and only then can we enjoy the peacefulness of our meditation.

*Disciple: Okay, so what I do with Wendy on a Saturday afternoon in her meditation class is a form of meditation, but strictly speaking, it is not "yogic meditation"?*

Correct. From the purest yogic sense, it is not meditation. Again, I am not creating a barrier between the two so as to disparage Wendy's meditation. I am just trying to help you understand the difference.

*Disciple: So, although what we do with Wendy in her meditation class is not yogic meditation, in the purest sense, does it still work as a method, as a means of stress reduction? What we do nowadays, just sit down and close our eyes; does this actually work? You called it silent reflection. I know Iyengar says we should have removed stress first, but Wendy's meditation class does work for me. I do feel leaving de-stressed. Please explain, oh knowledgeable one.*

It definitely works or more appropriately, it can definitely work. Just like the asanas, there is never a guarantee. The meditation of the West, or Wendy's meditation, can help us find some sense of tranquility. This silent reflection can bring about the serenity and happiness we all seek and in doing so, can even help us develop compassion and understanding towards others. Ultimately, this form of meditation, if persevered with (and that is the key) can change a person's life in ways they could not possibly have imagined.

*"It is in your power to withdraw yourself whenever you desire. Perfect tranquillity within consists in the good ordering of the mind, the realm of your own."[3] —* Marcus Aurelius

Thus, I am not implying that silent reflection as a form of mediation does not work. It does, and I will elaborate much more throughout the chapter. I am just trying to help you distinguish between modern and yogic meditation for the sake of your continued investigation into yoga because they are polar opposites. If Patanjali re-wrote the sutras today, chances are he would know how the word meditation is used today and decide on a Sanskrit word that cannot be translated to 'loosely' mean meditation.

Meditation can work but not always. Just like everything else, it depends on the individual. Some people can leave feeling tranquil, others can leave feeling emotional and many just leave feeling confused. Those who are "tranquil" were able to perhaps "switch off" and just follow the rhythmic vibrations of their breathing. The parts of the brain that can overthink and worry (more on that later) go offline, helping the "meditator" feel serene and blissful. However, there are also people who find silent reflection stress-full and aggravating. This can have an adverse effect on the meditator. Perhaps, there are underlying psychological issues that rise to the surface, and they find it difficult to deal with. The arguments made by teachers or others teaching "meditation" is that this pent-up energy or feelings just needs to come out and be dealt with. But is the yoga class or a yoga retreat the right place for this to be brought up? Is the yoga teacher sufficiently qualified to deal with this scenario? I know most teachers think that they are, but the reality is that most are not. If someone suffers psychological trauma as a result of reflecting on something they wished to keep locked away, a yoga teacher and their happy thoughts will not help nor will unintelligent claims of "chakra balance". Thus, there is a risk involved with mediation. Some people find self-reflection arduous and daunting. But there are those that do not and for them, self-reflection and meditation is critical for their self-improvement. Then, there is the third type of "meditator" who is just plain puzzled and baffled by the whole concept of sitting silently. Sometimes, they even question themselves and wonder if there is something wrong! Why can others "meditate" while we can't? So eventually, they start to create stories to "save face". They may say that today's meditation class was wonderful and super spiritual. The truth is they have no idea what was going on or what they were meant to be doing. They just invent a feeling of wellbeing because they do not want to hurt the teacher's delicate feelings.

But let us consider the positive aspects of meditation for now. For the rest of this chapter, we will create what I feel is a very obvious distinction between meditation and yogic meditation. The type of meditation that is done all over the world today, this silent, seated reflective meditation that you can practice with a run-of-the-mill yoga teacher, we will simply call "meditation". The yogic meditation, the meditation BKS Iyengar spoke about earlier, and the meditation of Patanjali, we will refer to simply as *"dhyana"*. I do not believe they are the same thing; so, for the sake of simplicity, let's separate them.

*Disciple: Okay, got it. I think. Let me summarise.*
*If your individual goal is "stillness of mind" and to reach an enlightened state of mind, then you must remove stress before you enter into dhyana. This meditation is a consequence not a practice. You cannot meditate but can only become meditative. So, you cannot do meditation, you can only be in meditation. Correct?*

Yes.

The goal of yoga is stillness or a state of no-mind. This does NOT have to be YOUR goal. Your goal is the same as most who do yoga these days. We are not chasing *Nirvana* or *samadhi*. We just want peace of mind, to be more fluid in our movements, to think more clearly and to be happy. Here, with this goal in mind, our western meditation can work because it makes our goals reachable.

*Disciple: Understood grandmaster.*
*So, modern meditation: What is it again? I'm not talking about the definition, but the practice. How does it work? And does it actually work (from a scientific perspective) or is it just "meditators" sitting around acting the way they wish to be seen by other so-called "yogis"?*

The answer is a bit of both.

To explain, meditation means to "to think, contemplate, devise, ponder". This is often done in a seated position with closed eyes so that we can concentrate and not be distracted by the bright lights or the environment we find ourselves in. So, what happens (theoretically at least) to our brains while we meditate? It is the same thing that happens biologically when we perform our religious prayers (again theoretically).

The frontal lobe (frontal and upper area of the brain) is the most highly evolved part of the brain. It carries out higher mental processes such as thinking, decision-making and planning. During meditation, the frontal cortex tends to go offline - the monkey stops jumping. If you are doing a more focused form of meditation (such as one of Shiva's 112 techniques), you consciously cause more blood to flow to the front lobe of your brain.

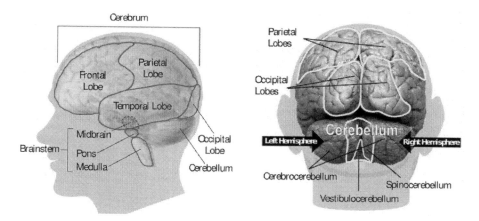

The function of the parietal lobe (upper, back part of the brain) is to processes sensory information that has to do with taste, temperature and touch. This part of the brain processes information about your surroundings and gives you a sense of where you are in time and space. During meditation, activity in the parietal lobe slows down so you start to lose awareness of where you are and your surroundings. This state of "consciousness" creates a sense of freedom from all the stress and anxiety of everyday life.

The thalamus is responsible for relaying information from the sensory receptors to the proper areas of the brain where it can be processed. It is essentially the gatekeeper for the senses. Meditation reduces the flow of incoming information through the brain. Thus, you might not feel a spider crawling on you as you sit like a perfect yogi.

As the brain's sentry, the reticular formation receives incoming stimuli and puts the brain on alert and ready to respond. Meditating dials back the arousal signal of this formation.

So, to reiterate, what has been discussed above is a theoretical biological response to you sitting down and concentrating on your meditation, taking your attention inwards (introspection). Essentially, following one of the 112 techniques Shiva gave us all those many moons ago, we sit silently with our focus inwards. This is what we call "meditation". This, when done for a significant period of time, can have a profound effect on the brain. The parts of the brain that create so much stress and anxiety can theoretically go temporarily offline creating a feeling of bliss or more likely, just a sense of calmness. The argument can be made that meditation is your brain's natural anti-depressant.

I say so because that is all it is. I cannot prove anything. I cannot tell you exactly what meditation will do to your brain just because science has hypothesised what can happen to someone's brain or what they observed to happen in someone's brain. What they have found as a result of their research may not apply to everyone who reads this book. It is the same as when I tell you theoretically what muscles you may stretch in the pigeon pose. The reason this is theory is that although many do feel the stretch in the places where they're supposed to, many do not. So in the world of yoga (and to be fair everywhere else), everything is theoretical. I once heard that an ounce of practice is generally worth more than a ton of theory. So give it a go and see what happens.

*"In theory, there is no difference between theory and practice. But in practice, there is."*

*Disciple - Surely these* THEORETICAL *biological effects do not just happen the moment I sit down and close my eyes. How long does it take for us to feel the benefits of Western meditation? How long before the brain shuts down the parts of the brain that create so much anxiety in us all?*

This is a really good question and one that requires the meditator to ponder on or ironically to meditate on. Research done by intelligent people has shown what the brain goes through during meditation. But what type of meditation are they talking about? How can we measure meditation? Every man and his dog will have a different interpretation of meditation. Does it mean sitting with your eyes closed only? Do you have to focus on your breathing? Will focusing or concentrating on something other than your breathing alter the effects on your brain?

I am not sure how long you have to meditate for or what the parameters are before you elicit the Relaxation Response in which the stressful part of your nervous system shuts down and there is that sense of calmness that rises within you. All we know is that taking the time to meditate can help. I just do not think anyone alive can tell us how long it will take for a positive response. Does it have to be twenty minutes every day? Will it happen after a year? Or does it take a single one-hour meditation session? Our bodies and brains are so unique in how they function that I do not think anyone can answer this.

The same could be said for yoga poses. How long will it take for you to see or feel improvements or progress? How many factors do you think influence this? Putting aside anatomical and physiological elements, what of the practice itself? How regular is it? How much effort is put in? These influence your ability to "advance" in yoga poses (as discussed earlier) in the same way that they affect meditation.

*Disciple: Once we get to a stage where our meditation is more than just sitting with our eyes closed, what else can it do, theoretically anyway?*

This is the same question as "what will happen to my body as a result of my asana practice?" In all honesty, the answer is "I don't know". I cannot say anything for sure because we are all so different. Nevertheless, in the following section, I have discussed what can happen as a consequence of the practice of committed meditation and when one feels that they are going deeper into meditation. However, I cannot guarantee that this will happen to you - it is all theoretical.

When we fall into a "deeper state", meditation can alter the neural processes that affect pain and the ability to feel it. This process gives us more "emotional" control in times of distress. This means that meditation helps us make peace with or deal with something painful. Meditation can also result in increased serotonin (the happy chemical) and dopamine (chemicals that are responsible for transmitting signals between the nerve cells of the brain)[4]. Your act of meditation can also trigger the various circuits within the brain that help fight anxiety and the various stresses of everyday life. Meditation can create a feeling that you can help yourself and that you are not that helpless when dealing with stress.

*Disciple: Okay, I think I followed that. Meditation can work and has innumerable benefits, but we just do not know when it will work for us just like the poses. Correct?*

Yes. We have no idea. We do not know the meditators' trauma. We do not know their minds. We cannot measure their concentration levels. We cannot tell someone when meditation will work for them in the same way that I cannot tell someone how long it will take before they see any benefit from the poses. If you persevere, it will happen all by itself.

*Disciple: How do you actually meditate? I know it is silent reflection, so I imagine sitting down is the first thing; but how can I meditate so as to bring about this theoretical tranquil state of mind?*

At this point, I will introduce you to the "Relaxation Response"[5].

The "Relaxation Response" was coined by Dr. Herbert Benson, a professor, author and cardiologist from the 60s. It was so named because of the physical effects elicited by this response. It is the polar opposite of our "flight or fight" response. As a reminder, our natural human instinct is "fight or flight" when we perceive a situation to be dangerous. This mechanism is essential and evolutionary. It is what allowed our ancestors from Africa to protect themselves from wild beasts and the woolly mammoth. This response allows us today to protect ourselves from impending danger. Nowadays, the response is trigged by our imagination and paranoia rather than actual danger. So, although our ancestors needed this response from our nervous system to fight and survive sabre tooth attacks, this evolution has come at a cost. So efficient and refined is our nervous system that we are now "stressed" at the mere notion of the sabre tooth. In some cases, this flight or fight mode is active while watching a horror movie from the comfort of our sofas.

I was told the following Sufi story when I was 13 years old after creating anxiety from what was apparently nothing.
     Mullah Nasreddin was breathing heavily and hurriedly throwing handfuls of bread crumbs around his house. "What are you doing, you madman?" said his wife. "Keeping the tigers away." "But there are no tigers in these parts." "That's right. Effective, isn't it?"

I was told by the Sufi teacher that our anxiety does not empty tomorrow of its troubles and sorrows. Tomorrow has not even arrived. This anxiety only works in taking away from today's potential fortune and happiness.

When this "flight or fight" response is trigged, our sympathetic nervous system makes our breathing more rapid as well as increases our heart rate and blood pressure. The Relaxation Response does the opposite in that it slows down our heart rate and respiration, stores glucose (for when your body might need it next) and removes waste. Without lowering the formal tone, there is a reason why people who are super relaxed "break wind" in a yoga class.

Dr. Benson describes the "Relaxation Response" as a physical state of deep relaxation. His and other research has shown that the regular use of the Relaxation Response can help with health problems that are caused or exacerbated by chronic stress.
     In fact, you could say the Relaxation Response is another way to describe modern or Western meditation. The response is defined as our ability to encourage our body to release chemicals and brain signals that make our muscles and organs slow down. As a result, blood flow increases to the brain. This, in return, becomes an effective way to

combat "stress" and its related problems. Benson believes that that this method can reduce not only stress itself, but the many illnesses that are exacerbated by chronic stress including insomnia, eating disorders, depression, anxiety and panic attacks, circulatory and heart problems, diabetes and rheumatoid arthritis.

Not forgetting the one thing that gets me more than anything else: mouth ulcers. Are they all completely caused by stress? The answer depends on who you ask. Thus, it is better to meditate than medicate right?

The Technique
1. Sit quietly in a comfortable position.
2. Close your eyes.
3. Deeply relax all your muscles, beginning at your feet and progressing up to your face. Keep them relaxed.
4. Breathe through your nose. Become aware of your breathing. As you breathe out, say the word, "one", silently to yourself. For example, breathe in . . . out, "one", in . . . out, "one", and so on. Breathe easily and naturally.
5. Continue for ten to twenty minutes. You may open your eyes to check the time, but do not use an alarm. When you finish, sit quietly for several minutes, at first with your eyes closed and later with your eyes opened. Do not stand up for a few minutes.
6. Do not worry about whether you are successful in achieving a deep level of relaxation.

Dr. Benson says, "Maintain a passive attitude and permit relaxation to occur at its own pace (this is the key). When distracting thoughts occur, try to ignore them by not dwelling upon them and return to repeating 'one'. With practice, the response should come with little effort. Practice the technique once or twice daily, but not within two hours after any meal, since the digestive processes seem to interfere with the elicitation of the Relaxation Response".

Dr. Benson continues, "You will learn that evoking the Relaxation Response is extremely simple if you follow a very short set of instructions, which incorporate four essential elements: (1) a quiet environment; (2) a mental device such as a word or a phrase which should be repeated in a specific fashion over and over again; (3) the adoption of a passive attitude, which is perhaps the most important of the elements; and (4) a comfortable position. Your appropriate practice of these four elements for ten to twenty minutes once or twice daily should markedly enhance your well-being".

What is the key that unlocks the Relaxation Response?

Benson has said it is "interrupting the train of regular thought". So once this is achieved, the body and mind can benefit.

*Disciple: I had an experience in meditation once. Something "higher" spoke to me. It may have been God. It could have just been Morgan Freeman. I felt really good after. Was all this just my imagination? Please tell me it isn't so.*

Is that really a question? In some cases, the meditator can go beyond just removing stress. The so-called meditator can have "spiritual experiences". But can they be classified as actual experiences? The actual spiritual experience is not something special or mind blowing. It is actually very "normal". Far from making us feel different, elevated and even super spiritual, the yogic spiritual experience makes us feel the same - perfectly normal and ordinary. There is no gift of a third eye from Shiva or an explosion in the heart chakra. The ordinary spiritual experience is just an expansion of mind. The realisation that as you are, you are perfect and happy. We stay with this feeling during our meditation and realise that all that we seek is always a part of us. This is why it is an ordinary experience.

Sometimes (more often than not), our imagination can run amok, and we can think we have had spiritual experiences. But the question is are they real or something your brain has made up based on your innermost desires? (to be more yogic perhaps?) What I mean is that if you wish to talk to god, you can.

In "intense" spiritual meditation, you can decrease the activity in your parietal lobes. This is the part of the brain that helps you find yourself in space and time. When activity in the parietal lobes decreases, we are no longer able to have a sense of where we are. We can feel lost and even immersed into the cosmos. You can literally feel like you are having a conversation with god, and he will be just as you imagined (funnily enough). It may be Morgan Freeman or a burning bush. It will be whatever you mind has imagined to be something or someone "higher". Our mind constructs such images based on our innate theories and beliefs. If you have watched the movie Bruce Almighty, your brain memorises the depiction of Morgan Freeman as God. So, in the future, if you need a divine "pick-me-up", Morgan Freeman will talk to you and make you feel better. This is just a mash-up of memory and imagination. Nothing spiritual has taken place. Nothing has happened here that cannot be explained by science.

Meditation, or intense meditation can play tricks with your brain. Or more accurately, your brain can play tricks on you. This could take place due to DMT, which is a hallucinogenic tryptamine drug that occurs naturally in many plants and animals. It is produced naturally in the body, specifically in the pineal gland in the brain. It is constantly secreted in lower doses during the day, but at night its levels will increase drastically. Thus, when we close our eyes and meditate before we go to sleep, we are meditating under the effects of a psychedelic drug - similar to that of a magic mushroom - in small doses of course. Like everything else in life, this is of course theoretical. When we meditate and have spiritual experiences, it is not because we are experiencing the second coming or that we are enlightened, it means our brain is playing tricks on us again. This experience in meditation, which is a higher state of reality, can be very appealing to the ego. Or more specifically, the part of the ego that competes and thrives on competition. We all have it. It just varies from person to person.

Our brains play tricks on us, and then our super-egos make us play tricks on others as we boast of "amazing meditations". We feel like we are creating a sense of oneness with something that only exists in the imaginative part of our brain. This does not mean that it does not make you feel better. It can and it will. So even if you imagine Morgan Freeman as God talking to you (or Amitabh Bachchan in the Bollywood version), it does not matter as long as it fills you with vitality and strength.

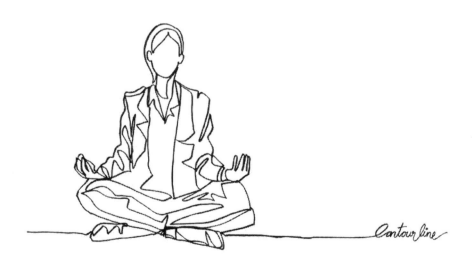

To summarise. the modern form of meditation is simply closing your eyes and slowing down your entire system. You do this. You create this. You send parts of your brain to sleep. This means that the brain begins to respond to our meditation and thus stops processing information as actively as it normally would. This is not religious, spiritual or esoteric. Your experiences in meditation are your own and created by your brain: the organ of your behaviour.

The ability to meditate and receive the many scientifically proven benefits of meditation depends on us and how much we want it to happen. Remember, the brain can change simply based on our thoughts. We can create change by planting a seed of thought and then rewiring the brain with this new action of meditation.

# Depression

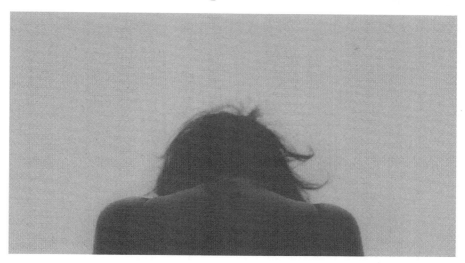

Depression has always been considered something set in stone as a function of the brain about which there is not much that we can do but take medication. Now we know that to be wrong. New findings suggest that changes in the brain can be brought about by pure mental activity such as thinking about something positively or setting intentions. Thinking about things in a certain positive way can restore our mental health. It may appear insubstantial but a thought and/or an intention and the ability to act on that thought can alter the neural connection within our brains and can help us deal with mental illness and improve our overall health. We must first create the thought and wholeheartedly work to get better. This idea that a very thought can alter our brains is, interestingly enough, also a view shared by Buddhism. Since the time of Gautam Buddha, Buddhism has taught us that the mind is an independent force than can be harnessed by will. Francisca Chow (Professor of Buddhist Studies at Georgetown University) says, "By meditative exertion and other mental exercises, you can actively change your feelings, your attitudes and your mind-set"[6].

In order to understand how meditation can help with depression, let us look at how we define depression. There are really two kinds that, today, have been combined to create one mental illness. The first type is when someone is "feeling depressed" with severe despondency and dejection. No human is immune from feeling depressed as it is in our nature. In life, happiness and sorrow are two sides of the same coin. We know they both go hand in hand.

The second type of depression is more of a long-term illness. To be honest the first type of depression (feeling depressed) should not be labelled an illness because it is not. It is simply something we have negotiated with life. Feeling depressed is a sadness. It will pass. The more long-term form of depression, the clinical type of depression, is not just sadness but more of a disease. It has to be treated the same way as a disease with time, patience and potentially medication or other medically supervised intervention.

On the other hand, low self-esteem is not depression. This is something that needs to be understood. Low self-esteem can potentially lead to depression, but it is not depression itself. The problem in modern times is that those with vested interest in our health (pharmaceutical companies) have made us feel like anytime we struggle to get out of bed, we must be depressed. For some reason, we are not considered lazy or hate our jobs or lack ambition or feel down or just feel bad that our last Instagram post did not get 100 likes. The only reason we are down is because we are depressed. Who ultimately profits from labelling us the "depressed generation"? By constantly asking us to talk and admit to our so-called depression, who do you think benefits? Is it us? The depressed? Or the pharmaceutical companies who want us to be drugged up zombies with such little common sense and courage that we go running back with our begging bowls pleading for more pills?

*"Before you heal someone, ask him if he's willing to give up the things that make him sick." - Hippocrates'*

By giving into pharmaceuticals, we are giving up on life too. But in some ways, this is what we want. We want imprisonment. In a twisted way, we want to be in their statistics. We want to be zombies and be experimented on so we can live without awareness. And while we are imprisoned, we feel belonging. It is a deep-rooted psychological problem. By doing this, we are committing the gravest sin. I talk not from a place of authority but a place of experience. The pills destroy our heart and destroy our resolve. We start the year simply feeling down, and we end up with a major depressive disorder. One day, we sit at the edge of our beds with our heads in our hands and our life stripped away from us wondering how it all went wrong?

Life went wrong the moment we decided that we are "depressed". The moment we were given a diagnosis and we stuck the label on our forehead we began to lose the battle with life.

*"You say you're 'depressed' — all I see is resilience. You are allowed to feel messed up and inside out. It doesn't mean you're defective — it just means you're human." - David Mitchell[8]*

Before I continue, I want to be clear that when I talk about 'depression', I am not referring to clinical depression (unless stated). I am talking about man made depression where one convinces themselves they are depressed. The difference between 'depression' and clinical depression are like day and night.

I believe depression is predominantly man-made and manufactured by society. I do not believe it is inherent in us all. When we were children, we laughed. We laughed so much we cried. Some children are born with biochemical defects for sure, and they fall into a different category altogether (clinical depression for example). But those who are not born with "faulty wiring" are born joyful. We only know sadness through experience and life, but our default mode is a joyful and happy one. Our present level of joy or state of mind is determined by millions of mini-experiences throughout our life. Depression does not hit us like a truck. It is like rust that chips away a little every day.

There is nothing more beautiful than a child smiling or laughing. This is because we know it is nature's joy being manifested. It is genuine happiness, and when we see such emotion, we often wish that the child never grows up. We want them to remain the same because we know the moment society gets a hold of them, their smile will slowly wither away. We know that as they grow, to remain part of modern society, a part of them has to be destroyed. You could call it the selling of your soul to the devil. Is this not what is meant by that phrase? The child who was the soul of the household who laughed and brought immeasurable happiness to those around them must one day make the deal with the devil so they can pay their mortgage and spend their 9-5 in a suffocating society where jobs are often uninspiring and even absurd. Does the soulless adult still illuminate the room as they did as a child? Or are they stuck in the shadows with everybody else? Often, the adult becomes as insufferable as the environment they work in. They become the reflection of the life they have made a deal with. The reality of life is that the melancholy of modern life has found a way (through experience) of getting into the minds of modern man. It is such an efficient system that it succeeds almost every time. Yet laughter and life continue to exist in us. We assume laughter has slowly died a death because we cannot see it, but it is inherent in our nature. In our core, our laughing child wishes to celebrate life. What we have is a generation of humans who look back at themselves as children and wonder where their smiles have gone. More often than not, they lost it in stages throughout life. We do not suddenly become depressed - depression grows like a tumour, little by little, through life. As the smile diminishes, the tumour grows.

So, once again to reiterate, there are two types of depression. The clinical kind and the 'man-made kind'. This man-made depression is what people use when they are just having a bad time in their lives. This type of self-diagnosed depression is simply influenced by the demands of life and of society. It seems that this modern-day movement of talking about your mental health is actually creating depression from nothing. To explain, I recently saw a musculoskeletal "specialist" for my chronic back pain who was more interested in my 'mental health' than my back pain. He said; "Let's talk about your mental health". I replied that there was no need. My mental faculties are pretty intact considering my back pain. The doctor just gave me a funny smirk and said; "You know its ok. It's good to talk". I replied and said yes, it is good to talk if you are Bob Hoskins or if you have a genuine issue. But I do not. The doctor none the less continued to try and convince me that I was 'suffering' emotionally because of my back. And I am not! But he was insistent and for the next hour all he did was try to make me feel like I was suffering emotionally. Suffering to the point of medical intervention. Had I met him many years prior he may have even convinced me that I had some form of depression. All he wanted was to give me some pills and stick a slug on the back of my head and send me on my away. This doctor has now created another statistic. This is what talking about depression can do. It can create depression from nothing.

Talking about "mental health" can be helpful for those who need genuine help (the clinically depressed). However, the downside is that people who are just having a bad time in their life are made to feel or are themselves making bold claims of depression and we are all slowly losing our minds as a consequence. We are losing our minds and our hearts. Is it not better to start a new hashtag craze such as "#notme"? I am not depressed. I am just having a terrible day. Welcome to what real life is like.

I do not wish for my niece to grow up. She is now nine. I remember a friend of mine saying that she is one of the happiest children she has ever known. I wish for my niece to stay this way. But I fear the devil will be knocking on her door one day too. I want my niece to love herself and to continue to love who she is. I do not wish for her to one day look in the mirror and feel insecure of how she looks. I want her to be happy. When we can love who we are, our love is vibrant. We find loving ourselves to be the device that allows us to show love to others. This is because we cannot give what we do not have. The problem arises in insecure modern society where if one loves who they are, they are deemed arrogant. I remember being asked once in my younger days if I wished to look like somebody else, another celebrity perhaps or someone else that I may have worked with. I was baffled by the question. I think I responded by saying, "No". I was happy as I was. The consequent response was not a positive one: "You are not that special you know Zahir. You are not all that". I think I was too shocked and disorientated to respond. Upon reflection, I realised that there was no implication that I thought I was special or better than anyone else because I am not. I was just happy and content with who I was and how I looked.

What followed however was the most insecure and bizarre period of my life as for the first time, I began having issues with my self-esteem. I no longer "loved" myself and lost any and all confidence I had. I allowed someone to hold power over how I perceived myself. This lasted some years until I was able to break free from this psychological enslavement I had created for myself. All this began by being made to feel that loving who I was and just being happy with how I looked was somehow wrong. This is the mindset of modern man. If you love who you are, you are arrogant.

How can we expect the next generation of children to not grow into depression if this is the prevailing thought process? How can I expect my niece to grow up feeling like she is just perfect as she is? At some point, she will be made to feel guilty for being happy with the way she looks. Her innocence will be butchered. Here are planted the seeds of depression. And we ignorantly stand around scratching our heads and wonder where it all goes wrong?

In the Prozac Nation, Liz Wurtzel said, "That's the thing about depression: A human being can survive almost anything, as long as she sees the end in sight. But depression is so insidious, and it compounds daily, that it is impossible to ever see the end."[9]

The difference between feeling depressed and actual clinical depression is so great that I will not trivialize the subject by using a metaphor. You can look into the eyes of someone who feels depressed, but you somehow see all the way through someone who is really depressed. Their eyes show no life and no dreams. They are drowning in their anguish. The depressed often find it difficult to see the light at the end of the tunnel. On so many occasions, it feels easier to take their own lives than is to endure it. If it was not for fear of the unknown, then perhaps it would be easier. Or do we not take our own lives for a different reason? Do we decide that life is worth enduring for the sake of somebody else?

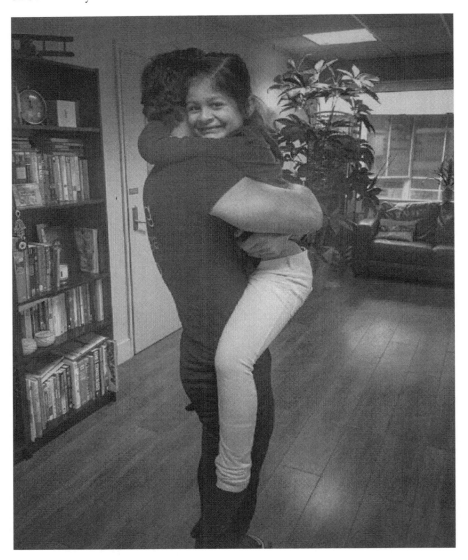

*above - With my niece 'kalegi ka tukra' at the old studio. I was overwhelmed by love when she first came dancing into my life.*

Whatever the reasons are, here we are. We rejoice life. We have the heart to continue the fight for our sanity. The problem today is that we have become trained to somehow think that saying we are "depressed" is normal. In modern times, it has become fashionable to say you have mental distress. I feel sorry for those who genuinely suffer from mental health problems, however, many just say they have mental health illness when they do not. It becomes almost impossible to see the difference. Unlike physical ailments, mental health problems cannot be measured by taking blood pressure and conducting other such tests. It can only be measured by our "state of mind". Rather than being made to feel brave (as is the yogic way), we are told that depression is perfectly normal. This mindset can create actual mental problems. We can literally create something out of nothing.

The Buddha said that our every thought will become reality. If we say we are depressed, then depression will follow. If we think something may make us anxious, then it probably will. Tantra says the same thing. It is us who is creating the world around us. Whatsoever we think, creates our existence. Tantra says that misery is our creation. So, if misery is man-made, so is bliss and so is happiness. Depression is not like a mythological Hindu god that follows you around with a hammer and hits you on the head when you least expect. it These myths, just like our depression, are man-made and created in our own heads by us and us alone. Tantra says we can become "enlightened" and experience real life the moment the realisation dawns on us that the world we are living in is created by us.

The world will go on and the chaos will continue but it is how we respond to the madness of the world around us that creates our madness or our "meditation".

*"On an incredibly simplistic level, you can think of depression as occurring when your cortex thinks an abstract thought and manages to convince the rest of the brain that this is as real as a physical stressor." -*
*Robert M. Sapolsky, Zebras Don't Get Ulcers*

# Restoring Mental Health via Meditation

Often, it is the ignorance about our true nature that keeps us trapped in this cycle of depression. If we do not meditate (or just call it mental training), we can take this "down feeling" with us into old age where it becomes almost impossible to come back from. As we get older and get lesser and lesser brain stimuli, our chances of improving our mental health decreases. It could just be our second nature to think that mental health problems are normal. The other problem is that Western thought and medicine makes us feel like our goal is merely the absence of mental illness. We have been conditioned to think that being happy is too much of a leap. It is too far for us to reach. This is why we feel depression is normal. We have to make our goal in life not simply being free from mental illness but striving for optimum mental health. The goal of yoga is not to be free from mental illness but to create such a way of thinking that you cannot possibly feel depressed again. We achieve this via our meditation. I will not provide statistics or evidence to explain the benefits of meditation mainly because they cannot convince someone feeling depressed that meditation can help them feel better.

When I was younger and would fast, before it was time to eat after a long grueling day of starvation, my mum would say, "Eat very little. Your stomach has shrunk so don't eat like an animal. Eat a little". Do you think I listened? After a long day of fasting, all logic goes out of the window. We want immediate gratification. This is a human condition. We are so addicted to instant gratification that we have no concern, at times, for the long-term impacts. If I asked someone who is depressed to meditate, try to picture his or her reaction? When we are at our lowest point, our instant gratification is to medicate. We have no regard for the long-term effects. We want to feel better now. We always give long-term health less importance over a pill that promises immediate relief. I read that we are officially the "instant civilisation"[10]. Everything is now. We want an instant cure, instant dinner, instant weight loss, instant spirituality, instant movies, instant delivery (Amazon prime), and instant dates (dating apps). Where does it stop? We have lost our understanding of the basic principle of patience. This is made even worse when one has money. We have become a society so obsessed that we will willingly turn a blind eye to anything that we know may help us, if in return, it asks for a long-term investment. Not only are we obsessed with instant gratification, we are also dangerously drawn to liars and charlatans. The chakra cleansers? The spiritual sadhus? What do they promise you? What can they give us? We are drawn to sadhus and holy men because we believe they can save us from ourselves. We as the instant civilisation are lazy and impatient zombies who want someone to give us something now, today.

Thus, I cannot convince anyone to try meditation. It has to come through their own journey and struggle. When the pain medication no longer works, when we become closer to mad men than the Buddha, we will turn to meditation ourselves. That is the hope anyway.

As stated previously, we are all zombies and thus we will soon become all too predictable. Many zombies do not fear death. They have no fear of death because they have no concept of life. Many people in the world fighting with the various metal illnesses do not fear death either because deep inside, they already feel dead. Zombies perhaps do not even realise that they are dead and devoid of life. What is the difference between them and us who roam around aimlessly through the desolate wastelands of life with no purpose and seemingly no cure? We, like our brain-eating friends, sleepwalk through the valleys of depression and anxiety with no one to listen to our thoughts, let alone hold our hands. We accept our brokenness and our lifeless states. Zombies do have one thing right though: they are more interested in our brains that our bodies.

The difference between us and zombies is that their minds are total and the real person inside is lost. We have lost our minds too, but the real person inside of us is screaming to come out. We are zombies because, simply put, our machinery is faulty. Our brains are either running too fast or too slow. This nature of suffering is also hardwired into our brains, and we have come to accept this as being okay.

The Buddhists have often said, "Birth is *dukkha* (suffering), ageing is *dukkha*, death is *dukkha*". Life is suffering.

But is life suffering? Should we just accept it for what it is?

Zombies say that our minds are a terrible thing to waste. A zombie is a person who appears apathetic or completely unresponsive to their surroundings. They are essentially lifeless. We, however, deep inside still have our humanity intact. We still have a life worth salvaging. We have just created the appearance of zombies. The more we accept suffering as our nature, the more we lose hope and the less human we become.

I have always believed that the only inevitability in life is suffering and it is how we react to this suffering that will determine the quality of our life. This is the mantra that has been embedded deep into my subconscious throughout my life. But can we erase suffering? Or can we minimise suffering? Why should we accept suffering as such an inevitability? Have those who are "depressed" - and I don't mean those people who join in the movement to get more Instagram likes - I mean those with actual clinical depression, been advised to try meditation? Will the person suffering with depression have the patience for meditation? They should because it will work. It is just not a quick fix. Meditation, which is self-understanding and self-healing, is a lifetime endeavour and one that society has shown it does not have the patience for. This is why we chose to medicate. We simply lack the patience for meditation. And when we do meditate, we often stop after a short time saying it does not work, or our pride fabricates all sorts of nonsense on the power of meditation. As with our asanas, we operate in extremes.

We have come to understand that there is something fundamentally wrong with us when we are down or feeling depressed. I am not talking of clinical depression but the feeling of being depressed. Most of the time, there simply isn't anything wrong and if there is, do not worry, it will pass. Maybe the neurons in our brain are misfiring or not running as we would like them to but that can all be corrected. So let us first throw out the idea that something is wrong with us when life gets us down. We are not depressed. We have faulty wiring, which science has shown can be corrected via positive thinking and meditation, NOT medication. It is not okay to think of this type of depression as being okay. If we do, what is the difference between us and lifeless zombies? Meditation can help us to understand that what we perceive in our minds that troubles us and creates so much anxiety is nothing more than a thought. It is not real. Once we start to understand that we are giving too much emphasis to a thought, we start to become more aware of what anxiety actually is. Then we can start the process of rewiring of our brains, which involves learning to let go of passing thoughts and emotions. The new wiring does not allow the brain to create such anxiety when a thought of what might happen tomorrow pops into our head.

The amygdala portion of the brain is closely linked to emotions such as fear and anxiety and its activity can be reduced via long-term meditation (of course it is not a quick fix). So to reiterate, the parts of the brain that create anxiety and fear can be overcome through meditation.

When I was struggling with my back a few years ago, I had to seek medical help because nerve pain is something that meditation could not help me with. So I was given drugs that had the side effects of "depression". These drugs can make us feel so low about life, how can we possible recover? At the time, the side effects of these drugs I was on was so powerful that it began affecting my memory, mood and most important of all, my self-esteem. How can we recover from this?

Is it the power of the pharmaceutical companies who don't want us to get better, or is it the underpaid and overworked doctor who just wants us out of their office? Who has the time now to work closely with patients? The easiest thing to do today is feed our impatience and give us drugs. We might walk into a doctor's office looking human but more often than not, we will leave like zombies after a few visits. Our mental faculties are barely intact, so the outside world is not going to help us. We must have the heart to take care of ourselves. The misuse of medication is not a disease, it is a decision as Phillip Dick (American writer 1928-1982) has said.

But there has to be an end in sight. We cannot be without hope. Then what is the purpose of living? We can fight depression and mental illness, and the process begins by understanding that we can change the circuitry of the brain. The end is in sight. It has to be. Globally, 350 million people of all ages suffer from depression. This is a statistic taken from the Brain & Behaviour Research Foundation website (www.bbrfoundation.org), which I believe to be incorrect as I think it is higher. The most alarming is that two out of 100 young children have depression as do eight out of ten teenagers. With the Instagram and social media boom, this is likely to get worse. So, is there really an end in sight? According to Aristotle, we have a "telos" as humans, which is our goal or purpose to fulfil. The telos of human life according to Aristotle is happiness.

*"Happiness is the meaning and the purpose of life, the whole aim and end of human existence."- Aristotle[11]*

This thought process has been challenged by many thinkers and philosophers since the time of Aristotle. But think of how life would be if our parents, schools, churches and temples taught us this basic fundamental teaching rather than making us feel like who we are is not good enough and that we are sinners and to fight sin is our purpose in life. We would have grown up to become happy and peaceful adults.

# Meditation for Depression

I appreciate that there are many ways to treat depression. Antidepressants and psychotherapy are definitely the usual first-line treatments for sure, but ongoing research has suggested that regular meditation can assist by changing how the brain responds to stress and anxiety. Today, we have brain-scanning technologies like fMRI (functional magnetic resonance imaging) that have shown that meditation produces discernible changes in brain activity[12]. If modern day Western meditation is all created in our brains, this means we have the power to change. Before this understanding, we could easily close our eyes and hope for the best (which many people do). They usually then say that meditation does not work. However, we can make ourselves feel better with the level of meditation we are capable of practicing. We can elicit the Relaxation Response and improve the quality of our life. All the power of mediation is ours. This is why I believe it should be practiced alone.

The experience of our meditation - whatever it is we may see and experience - is all created and imagined within our brains. This is not spiritual. This may sound disheartening to the spiritual Western seekers but what we gather from this is that our mental health can be made better and improved by us alone and not a spiritual teacher or by seeking spirituality. Mental health is created in our own brains and can be destroyed by our own brains alone. If we put our hopes in spiritual teachers and medicine, we are fighting an uphill battle (there is definitely a place, however, for medicine in our world). Ultimately our health, both physical and mental, is in our own hands. And by that, I mean brains! We are the causes of our own suffering. We are the poison and we are the antidote.

The Dalai Lama once said that the most powerful influence on the mind comes from within our own mind[13]. Happiness or whatever our goal is can be cultivated through meditating. Buddhism teaches that meditation mutes the negative and destructive feelings within the brain. If you are feeling depressed or enduring the worst time of your life, the only way from here is to ascend. We owe this to life. If we think of life as a tree, we can understand that the deeper the roots the higher the branches. The roots represent our depression - our sadness and sorrow. The branches represent our joy - our happiness. The roots and branches both go hand in hand. So, if we open our eyes, we come to the realisation that life is a balance. Our happiness has its roots in sadness. We must experience the depths to one day reach for the sky. There is a saying that life begins where fear ends. Once you reach the heights, you leave fear behind, but this is only possible due to our roots in sadness. We can only understand the whole of life and its meaning when we understand the dynamic interplay of life. This is why we must look up and lift our heads. Then, we fully understand that depression and happiness are two ends of the spectrum. They come to life hand in hand.

In Cat's Cradle, the author Kurt Vonnegut has said; "In the beginning, God created the earth, and he looked upon it in His cosmic loneliness. And God said, 'Let Us make living creatures out of mud, so the mud can see what We have done'. And God created every living creature that now moveth, and one was man. Mud as man alone could speak. God leaned close to mud as man sat up, looked around and spoke. Man blinked. 'What is the purpose of all this?' he asked politely. 'Everything must have a purpose?' asked God. 'Certainly', said man. 'Then I leave it to you to think of one for all this', said God. And He went away."[14]

Yoga teaches us that each soul arrives at life with a specific destiny. He or she has somewhere to reach or something to fulfil. Perhaps, some words are to be spoken or a message to be delivered. Maybe, there is someone who awaits your inspiration or love or kindness. Our destiny is to complete this task, which includes adding love to another soul. We are not here as an error of nature. Our birth is no accident. We are here because our life has meaning. We have meaning. We all have a purpose. A soul is waiting to be touched by us. A life is waiting to be influenced by us.

Nietzsche once said, "He who has a why to live for can bear almost any how"[15]. Maybe our purpose is not just to be happy but also to make one other person on this earth happy. We must fight our depression and believe in our hearts, our will, meditation, yoga and science. Vivekananda said, "Be brave! Be strong! Be fearless! Once you have taken up the spiritual life, fight as long as there is any life in you."[16] We must believe that we are meant for a life where we are loved, and we will share love. Our life has purpose and many miracles will happen. The truth is that the universe or god or the cosmos or nature or whatever it is that we individually believe in wants us to be happy. Life does not want us to be depressed because depression is a disease that can spread. On the other hand, our happiness is contagious. Our happiness flowers, and its fragrance can penetrate even the bitterest of souls. Happiness can travel afar with the wind and touches the core of every living organism around. There is nothing more contagious than the sounds and effects of happiness and laughter.

In The Reengineers, author Indu Muralidharan has said; "Become aware of yourself. Everything will come to you, when you are in that most wonderful place on earth, the centre of your being. If you learn just one thing, let it be that once you are aware of yourself, depression cannot hold you back any more than a tiger can be trapped in a spider's web."[17]

The first battle when you encounter depression is to remember that in life, there is a purpose. It may not be clear in that moment but that does not mean we do not have one. In the 80s tv show, "Monkey", the lead character says, "If clouds obscure the sun, does the sun hurry past them? Clouds will pass. The storm will pass. Every day the sun rises again". We have to find our purpose and then give our whole heart and soul to it. We can find this purpose via meditation through turning inwards. The deeper we look in, the smaller and increasingly insignificant our troubles appear.

Buddha has said that once we understand that we are lost, we have no choice but to find our own way. There is no help coming. When we understand this, we become responsible. We start to look after ourselves. We save ourselves from ourselves. Meditation can help us fight our depression and restore our faith in life. Meditation gives us all the tools needed - everything we can think of. Meditation gives us wings to fly as well as the roots to stand tall. It gives us the confidence to smile and the patience to love. It is a skill just like learning to play an instrument. We can, with time, ultimately master this skill.

It is just like our asanas. Our asanas are not magic. Our asanas and our mastery of asanas come from a willingness to improve, and science then takes care of the rest. Our meditation and mental health are the same. If we have a willingness and the patience to sit still, over time, science will take care of the rest. It took the Buddha six years of "soul searching" to find his true nature. And this was a twenty-four hour immersion. How long will it take before we can benefit? It could perhaps take a lifetime and that is okay. We just need to make sure we are not deluded by what we see or experience on our journey. We must also remember that nothing is permanent. The monkey mind is not permanent. Whatever arises in the mind will cease. If the will is there, the potential is immense. When we meditate, the experience that is created by the hundred billion or so neurons should be kept and remembered as a unique personal experience. The minute we share this with others, we realise we are "meditating" for all the wrong reasons. We should meditate to simply maintain, improve and/or restore our mental health.

## Meditation: Summary

Ultimately, if we wish to know mediation and understand it, we should meditate until we know. To fully realise meditation and to acquire the many benefits, one has to dedicate many years to training the mind. The process of rewiring the brain, where we slowly erase or replace old faulty and dangerous wiring with new ones, can take many years of commitment and observance.

*"Hard work it is to train the mind, which goes where it likes and does what it wants, but a trained mind brings health and happiness" - The Dhammapada[18]*

Meditation is not a quick fix. Going to a monastery does not automatically make us "Zen". Going to a yoga class or doing "the yoga" does not make us yogis. Meditating with others does not mean we know meditation or are, in fact, even meditating. All we are is a witness or a clueless observer of someone else looking just as hopeless as ourselves. The reason most people say they struggle to meditate is because they are doing so in groups. The best practice is done alone. We should not be spectators of meditation but become the meditation ourselves. For this, we do not need a workshop or a teacher or an app. We need a small space, silence and willingness. This can be difficult as for many people, being alone with their thoughts is a source of anxiety in itself. Self-doubt, guilt and paranoia all kick into overdrive as they sit silently and witness as the monkey mind use the opportunity to ironically make a real show of himself. The untrained mind is a playing field for our simian friend. The monkey thrives as he swings from one thought and emotion to another. The monkey mind wishes to expand itself and achieves this goal when we fear being alone with it. But this monkey inside our heads cannot and does not swing forever. It will rest. With patience, the monkey can be trained. This stage, the early stage of controlling the monkey mind, is by far the hardest.

In the earlier mentioned Japanese television show "Monkey", the title character says. "The trouble with the illusion of magic is that mere belief in it creates more demons". The same is with our monkey minds. The fact that we give it so much attention is what makes it go so crazy. So we should sit still and let him play. Simply witness and let the thoughts pass. The monkey will rest. He has to.

*Disciple: Apart from Dr. Benson's technique, is there another type of "meditation" one can practice to find peace of mind?*

There is no ready-made path for us when it comes to meditation. We create our own path by walking it for ourselves. We just close our eyes and listen to our unconscious breaths. That is all. Nothing more is needed. We close our eyes and first observe the silence. This is the single most important part of meditation: observing the silence. We have to use the mind to observe. Only by using the mind, we move beyond the mind. We stay observing until the silence is a natural phenomenon. It becomes a spontaneous silence. We cannot fake this part. This is why so many people fail in their meditation too. It is because we do not have the capacity (just yet) to allow the silence to arrive naturally. We force it. So we use the mind to create silence and the mind "stops" and just the silence remains. We have tamed the monkey mind. Within this silence, we observe and feel as oxygen comes in through the nose. The important part is to feel the life force of oxygen as it enters and touches the core of the body. We then hold the breath and observe the pause. In the Tantra, Shiva says that at this point (between breaths), we are beyond the world. So fixed observance is required at the point that we hold our breaths. It may just be for a moment. Then we exhale (at length) and empty the stomach. There is no pause between the exhale and the next inhale. We keep this pattern going until the day arrives that we understand meditation for ourselves. If this moment does not arrive then what does this mean? Could it be that we have not meditated enough? It is the same when someone says they still cannot do certain yoga poses. I ask how long they have been practicing. They say, "A few months". Mastery can take a lifetime.

*Disciple: Is there a secret to meditation?*

Patience is the most common answer to that question. But I kind of disagree.

*Disciple: Of course you do!*

Let us consider the concept of "patience". Have you heard the saying that "trees that are slow to grow bear the best fruit"? Philosophy, culture and religion are all full of quotes and anecdotes all reminding us of the benefits of patience. It is a virtue after all. But what is patience? It is the ability or capacity to tolerate delays, stress and even suffering. It could be thought of as your mental endurance. How long can we endure the stress before the weight of the world crashes on our shoulders and pins us to the ground?

Patience only works as a device in meditation if we are aware of what awaits us. If I say to my niece; "Be patient while the iPad charges, it will charge in its own time". She will smile and just get on with another task. Her exercise in patience is determined by the outcome. She knows what she will get as a reward for her supposed "hardship".

She knows the iPad will charge, so the concept of patience will work for her. If I ask someone who is feeling depressed to meditate and be patient with their task, they will look at me like I am a fool. This is because they cannot see the reward their patience will bring them. So patience only works and is the key to meditation if we believe in the eventual outcome. But who does? Meditation seldom works because we do not know what we are doing and what we can hope to achieve. If your reply is that a blissful mind awaits, I will still be confused. So for me, patience is not the secret to meditation.

Remember, patience is endurance; it is not waiting and hoping - this is what you can end up doing in meditation if you do not know anything about the end goal. You are simply waiting for something to happen. Telling someone to be patient in meditation is a hard thing to do when they feel like all they are doing is waiting and hoping for something to happen.

Patanjali, in the Yoga Sutras, I believe is telling us to learn things and to do things little by little. Nothing that means anything happens quickly even though that is what we want and that is what it may seem like from the outside. The action of drawing back a bow and sending the arrow straight into the target takes only a split second, but it can take a lifetime to master. Many people talk of their accomplishments (generally via Instagram), and we are often amazed at them but what we do not see is the whole cycle of becoming. The small pieces and fragments that collectively create this "whole" have taken many years of discipline and perhaps even taken a lifetime to piece together. What we should do is not be concerned with the whole but focus our attention on the small pieces. We should look at achieving our goal of meditation bit by bit. Today, we should just rejoice in our ability to sit down. This in itself may be the biggest obstacle of all. We should not worry about meditation but concern ourselves with just sitting. When this goal has been achieved, we can then work towards the next: breathing. However, if too much is added too soon, we lose sight and eventually lose heart. You could think of it as travelling to a destination with a map. Without a map, the journey may not go according to plan. Yet a map allows us to make short-term stops that will allow us to arrive to our eventual destination. This is what "mindfulness" helps people to focus on. We should have one goal at a time. It helps us to be more relaxed and patient as well as develop a sense of understanding towards the eventual goal. Once we learn to sit, we learn to be grateful simply for what we already have; the argument being that what makes you think you would be happy with more if you are not happy with the now. In the same way, people say you cannot love others until you truly love who you are. Thus, we need to cultivate the experience of being happy with our short-term goals in meditation.

We learn to sit first and everything that we are deserving of will follow. So to answer the question what do I feel is the key to meditation? The answer is learning to sit and then being happy with achieving this goal. Everything else follows.

However, perhaps in the purest yogic sense, all the above is not in agreement with yogic lore. One cannot have a goal. One cannot desire meditation. If the desire for meditation is there, then the mind is always in the future. You then cannot arrive at meditation because your physical body is always chasing the goal that has been set and created by the mind. The mind is in the future with the goal and the body is here. Remember meditation in the yogic sense is stillness of the mind. When this happens, you can be in or do meditation. In yoga, we are not here to attain anything. We are here to come to a realisation that we cannot find meditation. What makes this yogic meditation so difficult is that even saying in our heads, "I must not desire meditation" is a desire in itself. It is a paradox. Your mind wants meditation and your mind is convincing you at the same time that you do not really want it. But we do! In many ways, we simply cannot win. This is why in the purest yogic sense. we cannot do meditation. For us Westerners, it is too arduous a task.

So as a summary before we talk about *dhyana*, the yogic form of meditation, Western yoga meditation can be described as sitting with the eyes closed and trying to elicit the Relaxation Response. We are trying to send the parts of our brain that create stress, worry and anxiety offline so that we can attain a level of peacefulness and fill our hearts with quiet joy. This type of meditation has many benefits and we should all, in an ideal world, meditate as often as we can. In my opinion, this should however be a personal practice and not done in groups.

*Disciple: When is the best time in our lives to meditate?*

Now is the best time because most people come to meditation when they are in anguish. Then it can be too late. Meditation at that stage is one of the hardest things you will ever do. This is why medication is so popular because in such a crisis, meditation seldom works. The best thing to do is to start meditation when life is good so that there is a better chance of training the brain, so it does not create too much stress and anxiety. Of course, when you are happy the last thing you want to do is meditate! Why should you? Life is sweet. You should thus meditate so as to not reach a state of crisis.

*Disciple: What is your experience with meditating? How did it, or how does it make you feel?*

I once had minor "success" in meditating, I felt like I was daydreaming. I was on the verge of sleep but somehow, the part of my brain that was not resting, kept me awake. The rest of the brain that is responsible for my understanding of where I am in space and time was resting as was the proverbial monkey. My frontal cortex had gone temporarily offline or it was convalescing. The part of my brain that was still alert was firing electrical currents around my brain, creating a dazzling array of lights inside my head. Similar to the firework display at my wedding (maybe the parts of my brain that are responsible for memory were still online - possibly the amygdala, the hippocampus, the cerebellum and the prefrontal cortex). I was experiencing a heightened sense of self in that I was experiencing space and the vast emptiness of my mind. All the while, I could see the constant firework display of my neurons all firing away in the distant part of my brain. After fifteen minutes or so, everything began to die down. What transpired (which was obviously just memory and visualisation and not anything esoteric) was now in the past. I could just see the emptiness of space as I slowly started to absorb myself into it. I then started to feel like I was falling asleep again. I was living in a body of death that was no longer my own. The awareness of my body was slowly going offline. I then saw a light in front of me that was so powerful, it felt like someone had just switched on the lights inside my head. This was the deathless part of me. Was it my consciousness? I stayed with this light until its essence slowly dawned on me. This was my soul. I was creating oneness or union with my soul. I was being a simple witness of my thought processes as they slowly started disappearing and de-cluttering my mind. I experienced the calmness and pure harmony of my being for the first time. I could even hear the divine sound of a stringed instrument in the background.

Then Laura switched on the lights and came into the room. "What are you doing you weirdo?" she asked. "Just meditating". She looked stunned and proud of me at the same time. "I knew you had it in you. How was it?" I replied that it was the usual. The whole time I was in "meditation", my imagination was running wild. I explained to my adoring wife that for me, right now, there is no escape from the monkey mind. The saying is that the ocean can calm itself and so can we. But the ocean can also unpredictably explode and so do we. On this occasion, my mind exploded with imagination. I realised that forcing myself to meditate is not the answer.

*Disciple: So is it hard to shut down the part of your brain that creates imagination in meditation? And rather than admit that your imagination is overactive, do most people believe that they had a genuine spiritual experience?*

Yes. If my aforementioned "imaginative" experience happened in a meditation class (as opposed to the bedroom), it would have been easy for me to wax lyrical on what a spiritual experience it was. You see the environment you are in will also dictate how special or spiritual you feel your actual experience was.

This is not an attack on any one individual as it is our innate human nature. We want spirituality (especially keen yogis) and our desire for more and to evolve into spiritual beings makes us create something from nothing. Deep down, we know the experience we just had was all our imagination, but we somehow convince ourselves it was so much more. This is just the way we are. It is the evolution of us humans. We are, by nature, hungry for more and never satisfied. This is how we evolved. We cannot just sit and be still. We must first sit and then we absolutely must tell others what wonderful meditators we are and share our experiences even though we know it was all made up by our imaginations. We will exaggerate and even create our own personal reality using nothing more than the gift of our inventiveness and then poetically describe these fabricated experiences to others.

Essentially what I am saying is if someone tells you of their experiences in meditation, the "reality" they describe is limited by their vocabulary. Can they find the words to match their imagination? If they can, they are philosophers or yogis or both. We will then foolishly call them our gurus because we need an authority - someone to show us the way. Again, this is down to how our species has evolved. If the meditator cannot find the words, then perhaps they are the real meditators. The meditator sees the world for what it really is in all its glory stripped bare of any illusion. The feeling of meditation and the loss of self within the brain is so unique and serene that history tells us we should be lost for words and experience a feeling of blissful loss. Real meditation I believe can only be practiced alone. Gautam Buddha once said, "Be Lamps onto yourselves. Rely on yourselves, do not rely on external help. Hold fast to the truth as a lamp. See salvation alone in the truth".

Real meditation works once the monkey mind is understood. The monkey will create an alternate reality in our brains as we close our eyes. The idea here is that we should just be a witness. Let the monkey roam. Let him be free. Soon, he will tire. Your brain will slowly start to shut down the parts it no longer needs to sustain you in your seated posture. Here, you will find that feeling of calmness we all crave so dearly. From my own experience explained above, I could easily tell people of how spiritual it was and how "connected" I was to the cosmos. The reality is that nothing spiritual happened to me at all. It was a similar experience to daydreaming. The difference was I was just more aware in my "meditation". My imagination and my memories created a reality, and my eyes showed this to me in a strange way that was hard for me to grasp. The mind was recalling memories (of my wedding to create the lights) and my mind was recalling a previous guided visualised meditation (the oneness of space) to produce this glittering show reel in my brain. Blood supply and oxygen to my eyes were also probably depleted leaving me with retinal ischemia, which caused the bright tunnel of light that I foolishly thought was my soul. It felt like had had an "out of body" experience, and I was not wrong - it was out of body. It was ALL manufactured in my mesmerising overactive brain. It all occurred in the fascinating 3lbs of matter that is inside my head.

*Disciple: So if someone tells me they had a spiritual experience in my meditation class, they are simply full of hot air?*

This is correct. In my opinion of course.

# Dhyana – The Meditation of Yoga

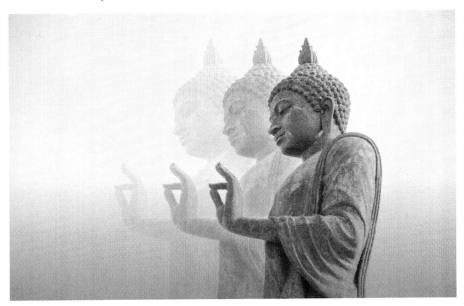

At this point, let us discuss *dhyana* - the purest sense of yogic meditation. In the Sutras of Patanjali, *dhyana* is referred to as an unbroken stream of consciousness. *Dhyana* is not a practice but a destination. When we think of "meditation" in a general sense, we often think of the Buddha. We imagine him seated with his eyes closed and lost in another dimension of life. What we need to understand about this imagery is that technically speaking, Buddha is "meditative", which allows him to be in or do meditation.

Before the Buddha was "Buddha" (meaning awakened /enlightened), he was just Siddhartha Gautama. Siddhartha felt that he was on the verge of death having spent years searching for enlightenment. It was a bright full moon night. He relaxed under the Bodhi tree and could barely hold himself up. The sounds of the birds and the river flowing that had kept him sane for six years was now beginning to sound distant. Siddhartha was tired, pale and bloodless. He remained with life long enough to simply focus on his breathing and nothing more. The outside world was slowly dying to him. He remembered a breathing technique he was taught on his travels. Yoga tradition says that this breathing technique (perhaps unknowingly) was technique one of the 112 that Shiva taught his wife all those years earlier.

With regards to the technique, Shiva says to Parvati, "Radiant one, this experience may dawn between two breaths. After breath comes in (down) and just before turning up (out) - the beneficence."[19]

Thus, the experience or beneficence or Nirvana may manifest between two breaths. The gap or pause between breathes is very short, but keen sincere observation, Shiva has said, will make us "feel" and penetrate this gap. Because the Buddha used this technique for his enlightenment, it has been called *Anapanasati* Yoga (meaning mindful breathing).

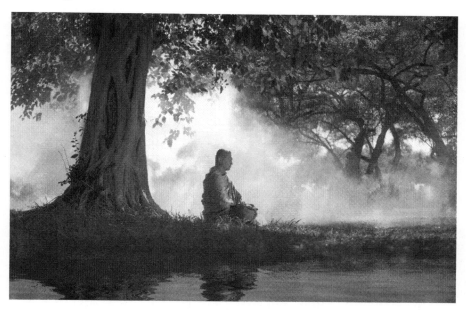

So, going back to the story, Siddhartha had given up on the desire to be "awakened". He was just breathing and being one with nature. Suddenly Siddhartha's body started to feel cold. He felt like a corpse. Then all of a sudden, he felt his mind disappear, like when water evaporates. Siddhartha was close to his death and at this point, he became attuned to his inner flame. Suddenly, a new energy came upon him because of his relaxation. His eyes remained closed, but a new vitality came to him. He fell into a state of meditation. He was now a Buddha. He was a Buddha and would remain eternally awakened. This is the moment where the Buddha came to the realisation that hell is a state of mind and heaven is the harmony when one goes beyond the mind. This was the great realisation of meditation. Siddhartha had thus left or died, and the Buddha had arrived. This was a re-birth. This is why the great yogi Goraknath has said; "Die o yogi die". Because meditation is a rebirth. The past has to die for one to become open to the future. The Sufi's have also said; "Die as you are so that you can become that which you really are".

Siddharth had gone and the Buddha had arrived. Buddha had arrived to meditation. And blessed are those to whom it comes. But how to describe this destination of meditation? There was no way to express this or communicate it. What was this experience that could not be expressed? This was Nirvana or the cessation of self. So Gautam Buddha did not meditate. He arrived at a state of meditation that Patanjali calls "*dhyana*".

*Dhyana* is the doorway to the "ultimate". This experience of the "ultimate" or the "highest state of our consciousness" is actually not an experience in itself in that the one having the experience is now lost. The knowledge is present, but the knower is not. The drop of water (which is us) merges with the ocean of divinity (the highest consciousness). If the drop is dissolved into the divine, then what can the drop say of this experience? It cannot say anything. This is why the Buddha has said nothing about his experience of *dhyana*. The whole of the Buddha and the whole of Shiva has become one with *dhyana*. They know that words will not help so silence is all that seekers can listen to. The cosmos, enlightenment and *dhyana* are all silent. It is just the "yogis" who are so full of noise.

Upon the Buddha's enlightenment, many men gathered together including many kings and many men from the far reaches of the world. They all wanted to hear what the Buddha had to say. He was so unique that people were convinced he was enlightened just by being in his presence such was his charisma. A man like the Buddha did not need to convince anyone of his "realisation". Thus, many men gathered and waited patiently to receive the divine wisdom of the awakened one. However, the Buddha was troubled as he had no way to express his thoughts on this realisation and meditative state. He thus preferred to stay silent. After seven days, the kings gathered before him and touched his feet. They begged the Buddha to not remain silent. They asked him not to be like an eagle that soars through the sky without leaving a trace or a footprint in the sand that is soon washed away. They begged the Buddha to share the secrets of life. Then, the Buddha finally spoke, "For seven days, I have been thinking of all the pros and cons. I do not see the point of speaking. People are deaf, people are blind. They can hear, but they cannot listen".

Nevertheless, the followers pleaded and begged to know what the Buddha had achieved from his quest. Buddha said, "I can only say I have lost something - the ego, the mind - I have not achieved anything at all. Now, I know that all that I have was always there. I was blind.

So, I have lost my blindness; I have not achieved anything, I have lost something". Thus, to teach the method, Buddha now turned to silence. Many people including seekers, kings and emperors had gathered before him They wanted to know how he had achieved his enlightenment. They wished to experience it. But the Buddha remained silent.

I heard a story once that a question was asked to a Zen master: "What do you think of all of us crazy Zen students?" He replied, "I think you're all deeply enlightened . . . Until you open your mouths".

*Dhyana* was not communicated because the Buddha understood the futility of words. Words were irresponsible, lifeless, dead and meaningless to the Buddha. Rumi once said, "Words are a pretext. It is the inner bond that draws one person to another, not words". We can fear words and distort them. We can also misinterpret words and twist them into any shape. As I mentioned earlier, words can create barriers but with silence, there are no obstacles. Words can destroy because the very meaning of these words can be interpreted so incorrectly. The silence of *dhyana* and Patanjali are a source of life. This silence itself has a unique sound. In this silence, we are blessed, and in this silence, we will understand. In "The Prophet", Kahlil Gibran says, "Your hearts know in silence the secrets of the days and the nights"[20]

"*Dhyana*" is the same as "Zen": both are above Western meditation (that is the meditation of modern times). One is required "to do" in meditation, but there is no doing in *dhyana*. In the West, we can say "Meditate on the thought . . . " or "Meditate on a feeling" . . . We cannot do the same with *dhyana* because it involves non-thinking. When thoughts have vanished, when the mind is still and when the monkey is in a coma, we arrive at *dhyana*. With this arrival, the past, present and future all become a blur. There is no "being present" as there is no longer a concept of time. We arrive at "forever" and can become timeless. This is why Shiva is depicted as beyond space and time. He is immersed in this reality, and he invites us to join him through the methods of *dhyana*. Here, in this endless ocean of bliss, love and harmony, there is no beginning and no end. Shiva is sometimes depicted as this column of fire that travels forever in both directions. It does not travel to eternity as it is eternity itself. We become blissfully lost in this never-ending space.

However, maybe, there is no state of *dhyana*. There is no state of no-mind. Maybe, this is all the product of man's imagination. This soma induced hopeful existence has been carved up by those with all the time in the world to concoct such a hopeful reality. Can we ever reach the yogic *dhyana*? Is it even possible for a place that is in a perpetual state of ecstasy where there is no pain, suffering, tears, death, fear, night, depression and anxiety to exist. The very idea is absurd because we do not know any better. It is not for me to convince you that *dhyana* exists and awaits us. We have to find the answers for ourselves. The problem in the West and why I think we are more likely to experience madness than meditation is we try to 'do' yogic meditation. We have a method and hope to reach a conclusion through completing it. And because meditation is so subjective, we have a million yoga teachers all explaining meditation in their own unique way. While this is all reasonable, the yogic meditation of *dhyana*: is not an act of doing. In the East, meditation is the conclusion. We know the conclusion and so the pre-requisites for our meditation are our methods (the Eight step path of Patanjali).

The Buddhist say that there are five hindrances to our meditation: sensual desire, ill will, sleepiness, over excitement or depression and doubt. We must overcome these to "meditate". But in the West, we "meditate" to overcome hindrances. We thus have the whole concept backwards.

Western meditation is always searching for something. When a modern-day student meditates, we are looking for something to happen. We are searching and seeking. However, Eastern meditation says that meditation is in our nature. It exists and only needs to be discovered or in some cases, stumbled upon. But as the Buddha said, we are blind. And we continue to remain blind by closing our eyes and searching for *dhyana* with Wendy in the church hall.

I know *dhyana* has been translated to mean "meditation". And this is because it is perhaps the closest English word. But the word is still far from describing the essence of *dhyana*. *Dhyana* as a concept for us Westerners is a foreign one. We can speculate and discuss it all day long, but we may never truly understand it. This is why it remains such a fascinating subject.

Shiva implied that keen sincere observation is required to create this expansion of consciousness. For a time, we need to disappear from the world. No one or no-thing can penetrate our thoughts. We appear lost yet we may never be more alive. While a teacher may guide us into the right posture and provide instructions on how best to observe and follow our breathing, no yoga teacher can teach us anything of *dhyana*/meditation. This expansion of our consciousness comes through practice and patience. All of the knowledge contained within the cosmos will be downloaded by us when we can go beyond the mind. Thus, we must begin our meditation by using our mind. We should listen, sit, breathe and prepare - all of which is required by the mind. We should use the mind and then effort should be made to go beyond the mind. Where your mind ends, meditation begins. However, whatever is achieved is only achieved through the mind. So yoga is not against the mind. Yoga tries to get us to understand that the mind is the nemesis but is still required for our evolution. The Italian poet Dante once said, "The path to paradise begins in hell". The path to no-mind/meditation begins with the mind. Remember, the mind must become the slave. All it takes, as Vivekananda said, is patience, purity and perseverance.

# 8 Limbs of Yoga

To better understand *dhyana*, let us go back to many thousands of years ago to the time of Patanjali, who was as unique as the Buddha himself. Patanjali has given us a really simple yet intelligent system to experience this state of no-mind or higher reality. Patanjali refers to this higher reality as *samadhi*. You can look at this as the great homecoming where man experiences ultimate reality - the same as the *Nirvana* of Buddha. This is beyond *dhyana* but for the sake of simplicity, you could say that *dhyana*/meditation, *samadhi* and a state of no-mind are all the same thing.

1 & 2) *Yam and Niyama*: These are your moral and ethical codes
3) *Asana*: Poses
4) *Pranayama*: Expansion of breath
5) *Pratyahara*: Withdrawal of senses
6) *Dharana:* Concentration
7) *Dhyana*: Meditation
8) *Samadhi*: Enlightenment

*Disciple - Before you explain the eight steps in a little more detail, could you please explain the concept of "non-attachment" that Patanjali also talks about? It is incredibly confusing.*

Earlier in the Yoga Sutras, 1.15, Patanjali also introduces us to the famous 'non-attachment' or '*vairagya*'.

Second only to *dhyana*, I would say the word "*vairagya*" is the most misunderstood in all of yogic lore. *Vairagya* translates loosely to 'non-attachment' or 'detachment' The idea is to free the mind of that which it is attached to: repulsion, fear, attraction, pain, pleasure and the like. It does not mean that we must create an environment of "non-attachment" as suggested by many people. But then again, this is open for interpretation. The idea of Patanjali's non-attachment is very misunderstood in yoga circles.

Most yoga people have little idea of what *vairagya* means, how to apply this concept to their lives, or even whether they should apply this to their lives. Yoga teachers just speak of non-attachment because like most yoga terms, repeating them over and over again in front of naive Western students will make them all look like yoga gurus. They pretend to be this yoga character and feed this projected image with Sanskrit words that they seldom understand. As long as this deception is not discovered or exposed by others, the social character (not the real character) keeps on going from strength to strength. At some point in time, the so-called yogi can no longer tell the difference between themselves and the character they so shamefully portray. The reason for such fabrication is that deep down, we all suffer from an inferiority complex. Deep down, we fear we are a nobody. So, we go through life finding ways to hide this insecurity from others. We create many illusions all trying to prove to others (not ourselves) that we are somebody special. We are not ordinary but yogis. If we do not keep up this appearance, then maybe someday someone will recognise that we are simply ordinary. So the next time you hear someone speak about "non-attachment" in a yoga class, roll your eyes and ask for a refund.

Non-attachment could also mean that we should try and not be dependable on certain things as a source of our happiness. If we are, there is a possibility that we could become attached to the source. However, this is a warning and not a religious commandment. If non-attachment is to be understood directly and as a commandment, is being attached to my wife wrong? Patanjali would say this is only true if it is an unhealthy attachment that can create suffering. He would ask if we are both independent and can we survive without each other? The answer is yes. Somehow, we survived life before we met so we can survive without (although not ideal!). Love is not an attachment. If your happiness is dependent on the other, you become dangerously attached. This will become a possible source of your suffering. Further, this is not true love anyway as attachment is not love, it is possession.

In 1923 the Lebanese poet Kahlil Gibran, in his celebrated work, "The Prophet" said, "Let there be spaces in your togetherness, and let the winds of the heavens dance between you. Love one another but make not a bond of love: Let it rather be a moving sea between the shores of your souls. Fill each other's cup but drink not from one cup. Give one another of your bread but eat not from the same loaf. Sing and dance together and be joyous, but let each one of you be alone, Even, as the strings of a lute are alone though they quiver with the same music. Give your hearts, but not into each other's keeping. For only the hand of Life can contain your hearts. And stand together, yet not too near together: For the pillars of the temple stand apart, and the oak tree and the cypress grow not in each other's shadow"[21].

I personally consider "The Prophet" to be one of the most beautiful books ever written and have been reading it to my wife's pregnant belly over the past few nights.

The concept of non-attachment does not mean a literal non-attachment. If I am attached to certain people and certain things, this does not mean that I am against Patanjali's yoga. Patanjali is not against us enjoying life, he is simply recommending that we do not make our life and happiness dependent on anything. This is not an immediate action but a lifelong process. Patanjali implies that the reason man is unhappy, disillusioned, sick and highly stressed is because of an unhealthy attachment to things and people. We rely on these "things" for our sanity. We have created an unhealthy attachment to certain emotions. Gorakhnath famously said, "Die o yogi die". If you are afraid of death, then you will desperately hold on to life and various attachments. If we let go of the attachments that have become our sources of happiness, we lose the fear of dying. Gorakhnath also said, "Die as a drop and become the ocean. The art of dying is the art of attaining to absolute life". We in the West cannot be expected to let go of all attachments immediately. But yoga is a sadhana - a lifelong dedicated practice after all.

So *vairagya* or non-attachment can be summarised as follows: Attachment may or may not lead to suffering. The Buddha supposedly said that attachment is the source of all suffering. This is something we should think about and understand. It is not a commandment: "Thou shall not be attached". This has to be understood because we may misunderstand and assume that Patanjali is against life. He just warns us of the pitfalls, but we are in charge of our own lives. Religion appears to create obstacles and drills what we should not do into our minds. However, Patanjali does not do this. He just makes us aware of the potential danger. This is another reason why raja yoga, the yoga of Patanjali, is not a religion - it is moral guidance that is accessible to all.

Let us now go back to the eight steps.

The eight steps outlined by the genius Patanjali are very logical and straightforward. These steps are essentially a map or a guide that takes you from where you are to your ultimate destination. It follows a very logical and methodical sequence: One step after another.

Steps 1 & 2: *Yam* and *Niyama*

The first two steps, *yam* and *niyama*, could be considered as your moral, social or ethical code. An entire book could be devoted to the first two steps so my apologies for my simplification. The idea is that the first thing to be done when embarking on your yoga journey is to ensure you have the read and understood the ethical guidelines: What is expected of you? How should you behave?

They are broken down into two sections:

The *yamas* are often translated to mean "restraint". These include the following:

* *Ahimsa* (non-harming or non-violence in thought, word and deed);

*Ahimsa* to mean non-violent is one of the most complicated concepts in all of Patanjali's Sutras. In modern times it has created a vegetarian crase and a one must not harm another life mindset. Which is all fair. But many people miss the point of the overall message from Patanjali. Your act of non-violence has to come from your core and not from your consciousness. By that, I mean your actions of righteousness, towards eating meat etc has to be genuine and true to your nature. If you do not eat meat because you feel that is what is expected of you, that does not mean you are non-violent and adhering to *Ahimsa*. It means you are a puppet and simply conforming to social expectations. If you are raised to not eat meat, then this also does not mean that you are necessarily non-violent. It means you are just acting on your conditioning. You were raised to feel like meat is repugnant. You have made no real moral choice or decision of your own. It is just conditioning. *Ahimsa* has to be something that you grow to understand. You cannot be 'non-violent' (in the yogic sense) because your teacher or your teacher training says you should be. You should be 'non-violent' because this is your understanding. This is now in the core of who you are. If it is not who you are you will always know that deep down, you are being fraudulent. You are just trying to keep up appearances. If one's appetite to be a decent and proper human being is based on greed, it is not decent, but simply greed. What I mean by this is most often, the action of *Ahimsa* is undertaken on the premise that there will be some sort of reward. This could be a social reward where people applaud you for your stand against violence. It could be to gain more Instagram likes. The other type of prize people hope to gain from their *Ahimsa* is a reward from their god. If you abstain from violence, then your god is likely to reward you. This is not real *Ahimsa* but the cunning work of man's overwhelming desire for more. Again, *Ahimsa* has to come from the core of who you are. Similar to prayer and penance.

The Sufi Idries Shah has said; "I will not serve God like a labourer, in expectation of my wages".

The teacher who does not eat meat as an act of *Ahimsa* will still drink a glass of wine. Alcohol and the effects it can have on your body and mind is also against the principle of *Ahimsa*. Alcohol is considered a destruction of one's life hence it is referred to as *Himsa* - something that can cause you harm (the opposite of *Ahimsa*). But 'yogis' have such a limited understanding of *Ahimsa* they only seem to associate it with being non-violent towards animals.

I went to dinner once as I was invited by a friend. I was hesitant as I knew there would be plenty of yoga teachers on the table. I was a few minutes late and everyone else on the table has already ordered. The waitress came over to me and asked if I would like to order. For some reason there was a silence. I replied; "Yes. I will have the Chicken with a side of sweet potato fries". I took a look around the table and there was a look of horror/disgust on most of the faces. One such woman was looking at me like I was pure evil. Then finally one lady said; "Oh I am so glad you are not a vegan! – Can I have the chicken too!". Then another woman laughed and ordered the same thing. They all had a glass of wine too.

Why create a circle of yoga friends when you feel you will be judged for your choices? I am not going to say I don't eat meat because this is expected of me as a yoga teacher. My expectations on myself are more important than how others will perceive me. I eat less meat today than I have done at any stage of my life. And maybe there will be a day where I stop. When I do, it will be an honest, legitimate and wholeheartedly true to who I am and what I have come to understand. Lao Tzu has said that if you constantly act in a way according to the expectations of others, you will always be a slave.

I am not an advocate for meat eaters or saying that anything is right or wrong. What I am trying to say is that whatever decision you reach about your decisions and in regard to *Ahimsa*, should be your own and not something forced. You have to draw the conclusion for yourself and not allow the so-called noble yoga community to make you feel bad for still being on your journey of understanding.

In *Light on Life* - Iyengar has said; "We should not use truth as a club with which to beat other people. Morality is not about looking at other people and finding them inferior to ourselves."[22] This is what *Ahimsa* has become in modern times. A way of showing yogic superiority over others.

I was once asked by a yoga teacher; "Do you eat meat Zahir?" My response was "Yes". She responded; "How can you? That is so un-yogic!". I just laughed at said it wasn't me making the judgement.

Part of *Ahimsa* is compassion and non-judgement. The really interesting things is the less someone understands something or a concept, the more firmly they believe in it. A little knowledge is very dangerous because all this is, is not really knowledge. It's what we think we know. This is the root of ignorance. Gandhi has said; "I cannot teach you violence, as I do not myself believe in it. I can only teach you not to bow your heads before any one even at the cost of your life." And this is what yoga students do and are made to feel like they should do. Bow their heads in shame for being who they are. This is *Himsa*. This is the worse type of violence you can bring onto yourself.

And no, *Ahimsa*/non-violence does not mean you should not push your body in the poses either. Many yoga teachers say this and again it shows such a limited understanding of the concept. If you hurt yourself in a yoga class because you are trying to be the best version of yourself, this does not mean you are being violent with yourself. It means you are adhering to your dharma (your sense of responsibility) and simply trying to do your best so you can be the best version of who you are. You believe in your divinity/ability. You have heart. You are courageous. Your dharma overrides everything.

Martin Luther King has said at the center of non-violence stands the principle of love. So, adhere to your principles through love for what you do. If you wholeheartedly love what you do and love your poses and by doing so inadvertently hurt yourself - this is not *Himsa*. You are doing what you love. So, leave the judgement to the so called 'yogis'. Just keep on going as you are.

Continuing with *Yams*...
* *Satya* (truthfulness);
* *Brahmacharya* (correct use of sexual energy rather than complete suppression);
* *Aparigraha* (non-possessiveness);
* *Asteya* (honesty).

A Zen story I was told on the subject of honesty. An old Indian-Chinese Buddhist tradition holds that someone who makes false statements concerning the dharma, the spiritual way or truth, will lose all their facial hair. So Chan master Cuiyan (9-10th century), at the end of one summer spiritual intensive remarked to all those assembled, "Since the beginning of this summer session, I have talked much. Please see if my eyebrows are still there!"

The following may or may not have happened.

The sage Vasishtha (as in Vasishtha-asana) was one of the seven great sages from India. When he held his yoga "meditation" weekends, pupils from many parts of India were in attendance. During one of these gatherings, a pupil was caught stealing. The matter was reported to Vasishtha with the request that the culprit be expelled. But he ignored the case.

The pupil was later caught in a similar act, and again Vasishtha disregarded the matter. This angered the other pupils who drew up a petition asking for the dismissal of the thief. After he read the petition, Vasishtha called everyone before him. "You are wise brothers," he said, "You know what is right and what is not right. You may go somewhere else to study if you wish, but this poor brother does not even know right from wrong. Who will teach him if I do not? I am going to keep him here even if all the rest of you leave."

Upon analysing this story, we can see how quickly people turn their backs on those who commit crimes such as stealing - just as the pupils did. However, a person who commits a crime is not always a bad person. They could be someone that simply needs to be shown the path, and this is what Patanjali does with the first two steps. He ensures that we understand what is expected of us before we embark on our quest.

The *Niyamas*
* *Saucha* (cleanliness);
* *Santosha* (contentment/cheerfulness);
* *Tapas* (discipline, austerity);
* *Svadhyaya* (self-awareness)
* *Isvara Pranidhana* (surrender to a higher being or the contemplation of a higher power).

If the above, *Isvara Pranidhana* refers to 'god' then this can be looked upon as a religious text. But it does not say A god or thee god. It can be understood to mean your god or an understanding of a 'divine entity'. Be that science or the universe or the cosmos. Something greater than us mortals. The idea is to 'surrender' to this concept, so we don't become overly attached to life.

Assuming that you have been raised with the correct moral code, the basis of the *yamas* and *niyamas* do make sense. The others that sound quite strange to us (restraint of sexual energy and the like) just require more exploration. Interestingly, these other stages eventually make more sense to us once we immerse ourselves into step number three - the *asanas*. Nevertheless, I believe that we Western yoga students will spend the rest of our yoga lives just meandering around within the bottom three stages. And this is perfectly fine.

All the rules or moral guidelines are not easy to apply, but even limited understanding and effort can lead to greater peace of mind.

Step 3: *Asana* (the poses)

Immersion into asanas, the yoga poses, is where most of us commence our yoga journey. We start with the body because that is the outermost layer and the one that is the most accessible to us. This is where we start and, in all honesty, if we are genuinely true to ourselves, this is where our journey ends. I believe that the steps that are above asana are not for the Western yogic practitioner. Not only are they not for us, they are seemingly impossible to attain. This will be discussed in more detail later; for now, let us examine Patanjali's definition.

On *asana*, Patanjali has said, "Steady and comfortable should be the posture". A more contemporary translation of this verse from Mr. Iyengar elaborates on this a little more saying, "*Asana* is perfect firmness of body, steadiness of intelligence and benevolence of spirit". The posture as a summary should be graceful or become graceful. "Graceful" is not fragile, weak, flimsy or frail but is poised and elegant. This elegance of posture is the illumination of the body.

The purpose of an *asana*, according to Patanjali, is to balance the different nerve impulses, feelings of pain and pleasure and all other opposing sensations until the asana becomes steady and comfortable.

Again, Patanjali says the asana when practiced should be steady and comfortable. The meaning of this should be properly understood. In the poses, we work using effort until effort has ceased, therefore making the pose "steady and comfortable". In order for anything to become easy, one must first know hardship. We must experience and then overcome tension in order to know and experience what "steady and comfortable" is. Many yoga teachers will teach their students that each pose when practiced must be steady and comfortable, and this is not an accurate understanding of the sutra. This false understanding of the sutra allows a teacher to remain within their insecure nature. Some teachers fear certain postures, and they use their limited and often naive understanding of "steady and comfortable" to justify their reasons for not advancing in their practice. This is acceptable for them as this is their personal choice. But it is however no longer acceptable when they share this "teaching" to students and limit their potential along with their own. In actuality, the idea is that one must arrive at a stage where the posture is steady and comfortable. But how can one know exactly what is "steady and comfortable"?

How can one know what day is without experiencing night? How can we explain and appreciate the magic of daylight without facing darkness? In order to understand the real meaning of "comfort", we must experience discomfort. You must work through a posture until you arrive at an almost impossible place where all effort has ceased. The *asana* must be so perfectly relaxed that all muscular tension has left the body. There should be no effort or any sign of stress in the pose. There should almost be a loss of awareness of the body. We should no longer think about the body. How can we be comfortable if we are fidgeting or constantly moving? Thus, movement should also cease, and the feeling of the body should be dissolved, and it is then that comfort rises.

Sadhguru Jagi Vasudev said the following on effort: "Logically, somebody who never put effort into anything should be the master of effortlessness. But it is not so. If you want to know effortlessness, you need to know effort. When you reach the peak of effort, you become effortless. Only a person who knows what it is to work understands rest. Paradoxically, those who are always resting know no rest; they only sink into dullness and lethargy. This is the way of life."[23]

On *asana*, Patanjali says the following in the Yoga Sutras, "Perfection is achieved when the effort to perform it becomes effortless and the infinite being within is reached."

This is not an easy achievement. Think of the number of postures you have fought and clawed your way into over the past few years. In how many of these poses have you experienced a cessation of effort? The answer is probably none. Even a simple pose like the mountain pose requires our utmost focus and concentration. It feels like we are constantly up against an iron wall. I am not sure whether we Western students will ever reach a point where we can silently sit down, subdue all effort and then merge into the expanded field of unified consciousness. But is this our goal? Are we trying to merge with the infinite? If not, then we should have no desire to master the practice of *asana.* We should continue to just do the best we can. As I have said earlier, all that is expected of us is our willingness to do the best we can - science will take care of the rest as mentioned in the Asana chapter.

All modern-day yoga practitioners who practice yoga for their health and minds alone without a desire to be one with the universal consciousness or to be with god, should make this step - asana - their goal and destination. As you read on and discover the secrets of the following steps, you will understand why. The remaining steps are not for you and me. They are for the "yogi" who seeks union with the highest form of consciousness with Shiva or *Bhairav* - an experience of Nirvana.

On a final note, without creating confusion, Patanjali could also just be referring only to meditative seated postures and not the modern poses of hatha yoga we are so familiar with today. The practice of physical yoga was perhaps a preparatory practice before one embarked on the yoga journey according to Patanjali. In fact, he begins the Yoga Sutras with, "Now the instruction in yoga . . . " The implication is that one arrives at the *"asana"* rung of Patanjali's ladder having already immersed themselves in the bending and crackling poses of hatha yoga. These hatha yoga poses are an important means in that they make the seated and meditative posture more accessible. Thus, one can argue that Western yoga practitioners, who have accumulated so much stress on their bodies from playing sports, their occupations and injuries caused by simply maintaining their Western lives, will always stay within the realms of hatha yoga - the system that preceded Patanjali's Yoga Sutras. However, this is just a theory believed by some. I have found constant contradiction among translators and commentators on this sutra. Is Patanjali talking about the poses we are so familiar with today? Many commentators say "No" while some say "Yes". Since Mr. Iyengar is one of the few people in the history of yoga teachers who I trust, I will go with his theory that Patanjali is indeed talking about the poses of hatha yoga. Thus, we should continue to work through our poses until all effort has ceased - yes, all of them.

*Student - How is "effortlessness" achieved?*

In the asana chapter, we spoke about the relevance of science in yoga. If you turn up to class and practice with nothing but your willingness to try, science will take care of the rest. Over time, the effort being put in ceases because the body is no longer resisting being distorted into so many shapes. The muscles that you had to train to work now work unconsciously, and the pose is now steady and comfortable.

A Zen master put it so simply when he said, "When walking just walk. When sitting just sit. Above all, do not wobble".

When we first adopt a yoga pose - the headstand is a perfect example - we have to literally switch muscles on to create the integrity of the pose. We have to tell our arms to support us and take the weight, and we have to tell our core muscles to switch on. Why would they switch on automatically? How would they know what to do while you are upside down? We have to consciously switch our muscles on to create the desired pose. After a period of time, the muscles develop memory that is very cleverly called "muscle memory". The muscles now do not wait for you to tell them to switch on, they just switch on unconsciously. This is a little bit like when you walk. You do not need to think about using your hip muscles to walk. They just switch on when you walk. You have trained your muscles to work since you were a child. The same will take place with a headstand. After a period of time, there will be so little energy used to create the pose that it will get steadier and much more comfortable.

The next element to consider is your breathing. If you are holding your breath in the poses, then we have a long way to go. With slow breathing, the body will receive the oxygen it needs, and your mind will stay calm. Why is the mind important? The mind is the voice in your head that first tells you that you cannot do a headstand. It reminds you of how feeble and pathetic you are and convinces you to skip the headstand. This is because there are seeds of doubt in your mind that have been previously planted. These could be from a previous headstand attempt or even your childhood. And by refusing to do the headstand, you water these seeds of doubt and nourish them until they cause the flowering of more doubt. The mind has thus now convinced you that a headstand is not possible for you. But on the flip side, your mind also has seeds of courage and perseverance. You can water these seeds rather than the seeds of doubt. So, the answer exists within your mind. It comes back to the title of the book and the paradox we exist in - the wrong use of the mind is madness, and the correct use of the mind is meditation.

The key for me has been to not overthink a pose by not allowing your mind to pester you. Do not give the mind time to develop a personality. Instead, take courage and try. You should have a willingness to attempt new things. In an old Bollywood movie Kuddah Gawah, I clearly remember Amitabh Bachchan saying, "Don't think so much. If the thoughts become deep, then the decisions become weak" ("Itna mat sooch . . . sooch gehri ho jaaye . . . toh faisle kamzor ho jaate hai").

So once the mind is under your control, once breathing is mastered (in the pose) and once all of the muscles in your body work unconsciously, there is mastery of *asana*. It is as simple as that! You now see why Mr. Iyengar spent his entire life immersed in *asana*. It is an arduous ordeal that is not mastered in just a few years.

People imagine how hard it can be to gain mastery of the poses and find themselves feeling disheartened and disillusioned. It all seems so wonderful at first when the teacher tells you that each pose you do should be steady and comfortable, and no effort is required. But nothing is achieved in life without effort. Nothing in the world is worth having unless they are obtained through effort from the sweat of your own brow. Simply wishing is for fools, but actually doing is for those who thrive. There is no effort that is not beautiful because to exist requires effort. You can easily just float aimlessly and heedlessly through life but to live, to actually live, requires effort.

Step 4: *Pranayama*

So, let's just say you do master asana in this lifetime - stranger things have happened - you move onto rung or step number four: *pranayama*.

*"Breathe in. Breathe out. Breathe in. Breathe out. Forget this and attaining enlightenment will be the least of your problems."*

When broken down, the word *"pranayama"* can be explained as follows: *"prana"* is the subtle life force. It also means breath, respiration, vitality and energy. *"Ayama"* refers to control, restraint or extension – meaning to stretch, regulate, expand or prolong.

The word *"pranayama"* itself simply means the expansion of this subtle life force. It means the prolongation of breath and its restraint. The *sivasamhita* (one of the earliest texts on hatha yoga) calls it *"vayu sadhana"* (*vayu* = breath; *sadhana* = practice, quest).

However, *prana* is not like a gross physical energy - it is a subtle energy. *Prana* or *prana-sakti* is a life principle or life force. This life force expresses itself in each breath. B.K.S Iyengar says, "Prana is usually translated as breath, yet breath is just one of the many manifestations of prana within the human body". Iyengar adds that it is as difficult to explain prana as it is to explain God.

Prana is a subtle biological energy that catches breath and transmits it to the physical body. It is the transportation system that carries oxygen into your body. *Prana* and breath are intertwined. *Prana* is the driving power of the world and can be seen in every manifestation of life.

Tradition says it takes mastery of breathing to experience prana as it takes years to become so sensitive to the subtle sensations of breathing. We must experience the breath in "a touch" - this is the moment the breath is known. Then, we will have known prana - the vitality. It is only experienced upon mastery of the breath. With unconscious control of our breath, we are able to maintain life. This is no small achievement. This is a miracle in itself. Every moment of the day that we function is due to the unconscious management of our breath. Through this, not only are we able to survive, we are also capable of achieving amazing feats: athletically, intellectually and even spiritually.

When we experience first-hand what occurs when we are deprived of oxygen, we start to appreciate why the people of the subcontinent worship this *prana-sakti* as a goddess - Mother Nature is the giver of life.

The science of yoga explores what possibilities lay ahead of us if we are able to control the very *prana* that is responsible for life. If without thinking about our *prana* we as humans can achieve so much, imagine the possibilities if we were able to control, direct and expand our *prana*. Through control and mastery of *prana* via breathing, we are then ready for the next step.

The great Lao Tzu once said, "A perfect man breathes as if he is not breathing at all." Thus, mastery of breathing is life itself.

The *pranayama* of Patanjali is NOT the *pranayama* you may do in a yoga class. These may both have the same name but are very different in actuality. This is similar to how mediation and *Dhyana* are both very different concepts. The *pranayama* done in a yoga class (alternate nostril breathing and the like) are breathing exercises. Patanjali's *pranayama* deals with the retention of breath. The text says, "The asana having been done, *pranayama* is the cessation of the movement of inhalation and exhalation". The cessation of movement is "*kumbhaka*". Retention of breath. The stopping of the breath is *pranayama* according to Patanjali.

Patanjali then says that there are four types of *pranayama*. However, their techniques must be learnt from a guru - an actual realised guru of which there are few on this earth. Thus, *pranayama* can be understood intellectually, but the practice itself has to be guided by a guru and only upon mastery of asana. However, this is almost impossible.

Nevertheless, "teachers" all over the country continue to teach *pranayama* because why not - they are yogis after all.

Or, as most teachers say, "I have done a course".

Step 5: *Pratyahara*

Once there is mastery of breathing control or mastery of the art of breath expansion, the seeker or "yogi" moves effortlessly or glides into step five: *pratyahara*. *Pratyahara* is derived from the Sanskrit roots: *prati* meaning "away" or "against", and *ahara* meaning "nourishment". Therefore, the whole word refers to a withdrawal from that which nourishes the senses.

You could translate this to mean the withdrawal of your senses. This means that if we switch off the input channels to our brains (the senses), there is no way for us to respond to the outside world. We cannot sense the world because the mechanism for the senses has been "switched off". Thus, we desensitise our bodies to the external world. The ultimate law of survival says that we must sense the change in our environments and adapt to the change. These include natural disasters, human interferences or animal interaction. It is actually this law that has made us humans the most advanced species in the world. However, *pratyahara* requires the switching off of these senses - this is essentially sensory deprivation.

You could be sitting silently with your eyes close immersed in your breathing exercise. A spider or two could be crawling on you, but you will not have a reaction. This is because your mind is under your control and is not directed outwards. There is instead an inward turning. There is no reason to flinch and nothing to fear. You cannot fear because your input channels (your sensory nerves) have been told to not respond.

"Just as the tortoise withdraws its limbs, so when a man withdraws his senses from the sense objects, his wisdom becomes steady", explains the Bhagavad Gita. Consciousness becomes far more sensitive when it detaches from the senses. Further, as the senses withdraw, the intuitive mind awakens. It is however impossible for the yogi to explore the inner realms of the mind if one is easily distracted by the external senses.

Next time your yoga teacher is sitting upright with a perfect posture and hands in some sort of mudra teaching "yogic" meditation, go and pinch her arm. If she screams, you can ask why he/she has not withdrawn his/her senses since this is a precursor to meditation and if such a wise teacher is teaching yogic meditation, how did he/she feel that pinch?

Step 6: *Dharana*

"*Dharana*" means the concentration of mind. It is the step before meditation and is concerned with fixing awareness on one object while excluding all others. This is possible because there is no longer external stimuli. Well there actually is, but you have to switch this off. The only stimulus that now exists is the fixed observance of your mind. It could be fixed on breath. You could be so oblivious to the external world that all you experience (internally) is the sensation of breath.

The *dharanas* are what Shiva revealed to Parvati all those years ago when he manifested the existence of 112 concentration techniques. Thus, all Patanjali did is create an order - a list of pre-requisites for Shiva's methods.

Step 7: *Dhyana* or Meditation

This step is an extension of *Dharana*. From *Dharana*, there is a fall into the true reality - this is yogic meditation. The few traces of the mind that remain are collections of thoughts, imaginations and memories that have all been already stored. The external environment has been completely switched off and now all that remains is what is "inside your brain". If these final traces of the mind are switched off too, the mind ceases to exist. This is a state of no-mind, and this is yogic meditation.

The finite is within the mind, but in meditation, the infinite is no-mind.

Step 8: *Samadhi*

"*Samadhi*" is the homecoming. It is self-realisation. It is Nirvana. You are now a Buddha. You are immersed into the universe.

With no-mind, without the monkey mind and without the clouds in the sky, one is able to experience the transcendental state of their consciousness. This is technically not a step but just an extension of *Dhyana*/meditation in the same way that *Dhyana* is not a step above *Dharana* - it is just an extension.

The above is a very simplistic explanation. A more thorough understanding would take many books so my apologies for the simplification.

Let us do a quick review of the steps.

1 & 2) *Yam* and *Niyama*: These are your moral and ethical code

3) *Asana*: Poses

4) *Pranayama*: Expansion of breaths

5) *Pratyahara*: Withdrawal of senses

6) *Dharana*: Concentration

7) *Dhyana*: Meditation

8) *Samadhi*: Enlightenment

The eight steps outlined by Patanjali are very logical and straightforward. These steps are essentially a map or a guide that takes you from where you are to your ultimate destination. It follows a very logical and methodical sequence: One step after another.

*Disciple: I have been "taught" dhyana before in a 'yoga workshop', and if I am honest, I am not sure of what I was doing. I felt like I was not as spiritual as others because I could not "meditate" or get in the zone. Is this why dhyana is so hard - because I have skipped so many proceeding steps?*

Simply put, the answer is "yes". Most teachers nowadays teach the meditation of the West, yet many also believe that they are teaching Patanjali's meditation. Teaching a Western form of meditation is probably harmless but teaching meditation under the yogic umbrella only shows their own ignorance. I mean we are all definitely ignorant in our own ways, but these "meditators" are the most uninformed of us all

My wife once showed me a video of Sadhguru in India talking about why Westerners often fail in meditation. She found this amusing as she knows how I feel about yoga teachers claiming to teach yogic meditation. Just because they did a weekend course with someone who hasn't meditated themselves, they think they are "meditators". It is a case of the blind leading the blind. How can you teach yogic meditation if you have not yourself experienced it? You are simply charging people to sit with their eyes closed. Thus, when Sadhguru was asked why the meditation of Westerners just does not work, he said, "Flowers and fruits will come out of a plant not because you want it, but simply because you created the necessary, conducive atmosphere. Similarly, if you create the necessary atmosphere within yourself, on all the four dimensions of who you are, then meditation will naturally flower within you. It is a certain fragrance that one can enjoy within himself. Meditation is a consequence"[25]

Meditation takes time to blossom. It takes time to develop, grow and mature. By not being patient and not allowing life to follow its natural course, we disturb the natural flow of our sadhana. We know that Rome wasn't built in a day and in the same way, meditation cannot be mastered immediately. In its natural flow, meditation will blossom like the lotus flower from muddy water. By not wanting to work and expecting the fruits, we are inflicting a lot of unnecessary stress onto ourselves. I believe it was the great Lao Tzu who said, "Nature never rushes, yet all is achieved". We must therefore be patient. If we are deserving of meditation, it will arrive at its own time.

*Disciple: Why then are these later stages so misunderstood? Why do some teachers teach the pranayama and dhyana of Patanjali when they are clearly not ready for it, and it is not really for the Western student?*

The answer is perhaps too long for this book. It may require an entire book to be properly explained. A part of the problem is the way in which it is written. These stage and steps are very brief and sometimes cryptic. It is very easy to miss the significance of the verses without a realised guru. Further, because actual gurus are in short supply or have passed away or should not be trusted or are not geographically accessible, we make up our own assumptions and interpretations. I remember reading a commentary some time ago where the author was very clear that the Yoga Sutras are not for academic debate. Thus, they should not be speculated upon but rather practiced - just like Shiva's methods, doing is knowing.

The other perhaps more concrete reason is our image as yoga teachers. Yoga teachers want to be seen as "masters" (definitely not all of them). Our vanity will not allow us to admit to our students that we are still hovering in the bottom three stages of Patanjali's yoga. We thus have to say that we are higher than step three. Because if we say we are on step two or three of eight, we feel this revelation is likely to undermine our image to our students. The truth is the student probably does not care. It is more about the preservation of the image we seek to project onto others. Remember our pride is what we expect for ourselves. Our vanity is how we wish to be perceived by others. If you are a teacher, our vanity says that our position must be infallible. The harsh reality is that when we start teaching much more than asana (and perhaps a few simple breathing exercises), we are showing a complete lack of actual knowledge and a certain amount of self-awareness as well as the inability to be honest about our shortcomings.

A yoga teacher, who I met in London, who said that she does not teach head and handstands because they are not "yogic" will probably mask her shortcomings and insecurities by being more "spiritual". Such teachers will imply that they have now moved on from asana - something which is far from the truth. I know this because as a teacher, I have had my own battles with my inability to do all the poses and the fact that I had become stuck. How can I still be an authority when I am trapped in this spider web of my own inabilities? Should I teach more anatomy? Should I explain more mythology? Will this maintain my position as an authority in my students' eyes? This is just my vanity and remember yoga teachers are not immune from vanity - our vanity is more fragile than you can imagine.

Nietzsche once said, "One sticks to an opinion because he prides himself on having come to it on his own, and another because he has taken great pains to learn it and is proud to have grasped it: and so both do so out of vanity".

On reflection, the main reason is just plain ignorance. You can have a 500-hour qualification and still be ignorant. You can have twenty years of experience, read 1000 books and have a university degree, but none of this makes us immune from man's greatest disease: pure ignorance. Is ego related to ignorance? This could be true. When we are asked a question, rather than admit we do know not, why is it that we try to remember something that we have never even known? Is this ignorance or ego? Every person and every yoga teacher has the right to an opinion for sure. But our lazy minds, our lazy attempts at research (the internet) and our general lazy nature means that rather than gather knowledge and wisdom, we gather nothing but ignorance and stupidity. The wise man speaks to us through a book in one language and rather than study and reflect these words, our nature is to regurgitate that knowledge to suit our own misguided brains.

The root cause of why no one really understands yoga and meditation is because the yoga community who spread the words of yoga have nothing but an accumulation of superficial knowledge. This is the outermost layer of yogic understanding that when viewed by itself has no nucleus, core and essence.

At this juncture, I want to introduce you to something Patanjali talks about in the Yoga Sutras: the concept of "incorrect knowledge".

There are two types of "incorrect knowledge" as per my understanding. One is just pure ignorance. Many a yoga teacher who I have met over the years have a 200-hour alliance certificate and think they are ready to teach the world. They do not leave their teacher training with more questions as they should but leave feeling like they have all the answers. Again, I apologise for being a little harsh, but I am simply talking from my own experience. With regards to this type of ignorance, there is an Arab proverb; "The greatest obstacle to discovery is not ignorance - it is the illusion of knowledge".

The second type of "incorrect knowledge" is the acquiring of knowledge and simply interpreting this to accommodate our desire for immediate enlightenment. Patanjali in his Yoga Sutras warns us of the pit falls in acquiring knowledge we are not ready for. Our mind will interpret this information to suit its needs and desires. We look at Patanjali's eight step system, and we are in such a rush to develop our spirituality that we do not interpret them in the correct way. We simply interpret what we read to accommodate our ego and desires as we are in a rush to be more yogic. Again, because we have no patience, our desire for quick knowledge means we rarely understand the wisdom being bestowed upon us.

*"When disinformation is running rampant, there are two ignorance's that may emerge: the one is actually positive, a sort of pure and intentional emptying of the mind; but the other is of course negative and clogged and polluted."[26] —*
*Criss Jami, Healology*

How is it that today in a time where we have more information at our disposal than ever before we can be so ignorant? Or maybe this overload of information is the reason why? Worrisome are the days in which everyone is an expert.

## Meditation Summary

To summarise this chapter on meditation, any action of the mind cannot be meditation. An act of doing is an action of the mind. So you cannot do meditation. You cannot practice it. The mind cannot contemplate meditation because mind is madness. You have to go beyond the mind to a place of no-mind to know meditation. So the next time you are sitting in lotus with your hands in your favourite mudra, ask yourself, is this action of yours, madness or meditation? The fact that you have to ask yourself says it all.

'Yogic meditation' only begins when the mind ends.

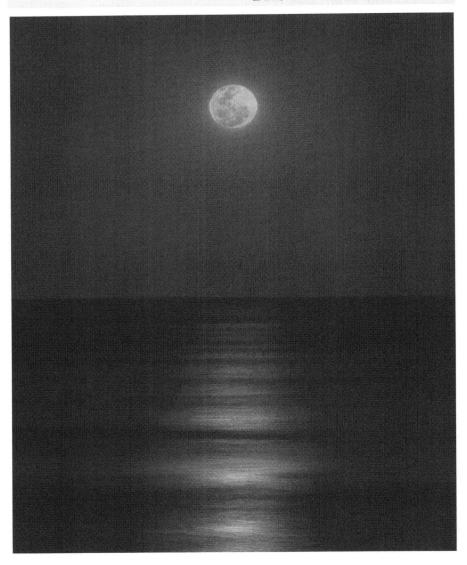

This destination (from *samadhi*, Nirvanai and beyond or 'enlightenment') is also referred to as in the yogic tradition as an "eternal darkness" or an eternal emptiness. In the yogic tradition,

*Mahakala* is the dark emptiness of space (*Mahakala* is also another name/dimension of Shiva). The goddess Kali (another version of Parvati) is also the darkness that pervades existence.

Darkness is eternal. While light comes and goes, darkness is forever. Before there was light, darkness already existed. Light has to travel through darkness. Light has a source, a birth, an origin and an ignition. Darkness is without any birth or conception (this is why Shiva has no family history. He is this darkness described in human form with no origin and no birth). So the reality of *samadhi* is an immersion into the infinite darkness of space and time.

Tradition has it that the dawn of time as we know it is through the eyes of Narayan (one of the three primary Hindu gods – or Vishnu). When he first opened his eyes all he saw was eternal emptiness. Narayan was floating in the vast bliss of total darkness. It is said that for a moment he felt afraid, he was all alone, a speck of dust in the never-ending darkness of infinite possibilities. Narayan was then comforted by this space. Narayan although floating in an empty void was comforted because this void still somehow pulsated with life. Narayan discovered that the darkness that surrounded him was not to be feared, it was to be understood.

*"People will do anything, no matter how absurd, in order to avoid facing their own souls. One does not become enlightened by imagining figures of light, but by making the darkness conscious."* - Carl Jung, Psychology and Alchemy

We students of yoga are blind seekers. We cannot perceive this darkness as our true reality because we have to fight and destroy our evolutionary and hereditary conditioning to not be afraid of the dark. We fear the darkness because we do not know what lies beneath. We have been conditioned to associate darkness with death or misery. How many times have we heard something along the lines of "Fear the darkness inside of you" or "the darkness follows me wherever I go". We all fear or try to be distant from that which is categorised as "darkness". We have been conditioned to think that darkness will always attempt to extinguish light and that light is forever in a battle trying to repress the darkness. However, yogic thinking does not agree with this Western thought. According to the yogic way of thinking Darkness exists as it is. There is no fight. It is all imagined and programmed into us. The light does not fight the darkness but simply allows us moments of clarity.

Man created God as "the light" through evolutionary fear of the dark. And ever since this conception of God as the light, we have feared that which is dark. Thus, we have to destroy this conditioning and we can only do so through the methodical and scientific approach of Patanjali. He has given us a map that leads us to this realisation that reality (or god) is NOT light. The reality is infinite darkness - a dance and harmony between *Kala Bhairava* (another name for Shiva) and *Kali Bhairavi* (Parvati). When the senses have been trained and the negative perspectives of the mind are let go off, how terribly enchanting this darkness will become. It will be bewildering, breath-taking and inexplicably beautiful all at once.

Have you seen images of the great Kali, the "dark mother"?

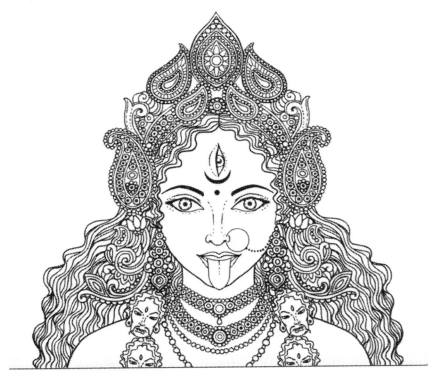

She has been re-imagined so many times that she is barely alive as the symbol she once was. In Sanskrit, time is called "*kala*", and the mother of *kala* is Kali - the "mother of time". This means that time is born out of Kali. She is beyond space and time. She represents creation, preservation and destruction all in one. She is boundless and infinite and remains a mystery. Almost an illusion to the un-awakened souls. Ramakrishna (a 19th-century mystic saint) said, "She is Knowledge Absolute, the Inscrutable Power of Brahman (the supreme reality) and by Her mere will She has given birth to this world. Everything is in Her power to give".

Maybe the birth of the Western God as "light" was a reaction to the Eastern idea that Kali or darkness is the true source of life? Maybe, the Western or Jewish God (as a man) was created by man himself as a macho rebuttal to this idea that what can be described as godliness, the ancient Indians have referred to as the divine mother. Would men not of the Eastern tradition have accepted a female god? And how did the Eastern man feel about this? Were male Hindu gods also created over time as a way to restore man's pride? In perhaps the most unsafe place in the world to be born as a woman[2], would the subcontinent continue to accept divinity as feminine? It is some food for thought.

Here is a riddle that has baffled thinkers for decades.
A man and his son are in a terrible accident and are rushed to the hospital in critical care. Upon arrival, the surgeon takes one look at the boy and exclaims "That's my son!"
How could this be?

The answer is the surgeon is the mother! But our brains and especially that of men cannot grasp that until we are told. In our heads, the surgeon is a man. He must be! Even though life is full of strong brave women, we still think such a job is above women. So how can we expect divinity to be feminine? This is why I believe man elevated Shiva to the status of god and men invented Krishna and Ganesh and so on as manifestation of gods with various masculine qualities. Man cannot fathom that the greatest surgeon of them all is probably wearing a pair of Jimmy Choos.

The real existence in yogic lore is the divine mother - this infinite and eternal darkness. Kali allows light to enter as a guest and witness to her darkness. Light will come and go, but darkness will always remain.
When yogis say, "I have seen the light", they have only seen what their imagination and conditioning has created. Further, when yogi's say, "Love and Light", this is not a yogic term. Yoga is not "light", but it sheds light not on darkness, but our understanding of darkness. This image of Kali may be terrifying and fearful for us in the West but is perhaps dearer than any other to the hearts of Indians.
The only way we can understand and perceive Kali, this dark reality, is if we flow naturally through Patanjali's system. Each step is not really a step or a climb. It is actually an ascension. To climb would imply that whenever we think we are ready, we can step up or climb the ladder. The reality is that we naturally ascend as a consequence of a

lifelong dedicated practice. But we all know the impatience of the modern student of yoga. We cannot jump from steps two and three to seven, which is what so many people attempt. They want to do *dhyana*, the meditation of yoga, and they desperately want others to recognise this.

There are eight steps in Patanjali's yoga. They are steps in the sense that each follows the other. The second cannot come before the first. The fifth cannot come before the third. They are steps with a sequential growth that have to be followed. So if you follow Patanjali's path, you cannot practice *pranayama* and meditation until you have "mastered" posture.

I have heard that patterns cannot be weighed or measured. Patterns must be mapped. You cannot measure success in Patanjali's yoga. You just follow the map.

Interestingly, my wife's dream job would be to do public relations for Kali – such are the misunderstandings that accompany her.

I feel like it is only fair (to my wife) to introduce the mythology that brought the goddess Kali into existence. There are several stories (as always) that tell us of the introduction of Kali into the mythological world. Her first appearance was not her origin but simply her introduction as a human being. Until the point of her dramatic appearance, she existed around humanity just like gravity itself. She is the physical energy that moves the stars and the waves of the sea. She is the source of light and the depth of the darkness that we gaze into at night. She is the vitality in our bodies and the core of our soul. The yogis say that she has been the source of our reality and existence without us even knowing it since the dawn of time – hence, her title of "divine mother" in Indian tradition.

The concept of Kali like all mythological characters is very difficult to fathom, especially for sceptics and logical thinkers who read this book. It can appear bewildering and absurd and in many ways, it is. But also, in many ways, it is just the opposite. Indian mythology is sometimes a fantastic blend of storytelling and artistry. Behind the madness, there is a method that was probably only understood by few at the time of their composition. In the "Power of Myth", Joseph Campbell said, "Mythology is not a lie, mythology is poetry, it is metaphorical. It has been well said that mythology is the penultimate truth – penultimate because the ultimate cannot be put into words. It is beyond words. Beyond images, beyond that bounding rim of the Buddhist Wheel of Becoming. Mythology pitches the mind beyond that rim, to what can be known but not told."

It is said by some regarding the legend of Kali that the entire story of Shiva and Parvati should be rewritten and retold. It was not Parvati who Shiva married after Sati but it was, in fact, Kali. The story goes that Kali was reborn to King Himavat (Parvati's father in the other version) as one of three daughters. Shiva who was mourning the loss of his first wife was offered sanctuary by the King. Shiva not wanting to turn down the benevolence of his devotee stayed at the palace even though it was the absolute opposite of his regular dwelling. Shiva preferred the dusk and obscurity of the burial grounds to the pomp and richness of the king's palace.

One day, as Shiva sat in meditation, his usual concentration was not what it normally was. He kept visualizing art in its finest form. The disturbing part for Shiva was that this art was the body of a woman. This figure was reaching for Shiva and evoking his desire. In order to snap away from these thoughts, Shiva decided to stop his meditation. Upon leaving his room, Shiva was stunned. The very woman he had been seeing each time he closed his eyes was there in the palace courtyard. It was Kali. Shiva immediately began to walk away as history had taught him a severe lesson on love, and he didn't wish to experience it again. He was determined that he would never marry or be with anyone again. But the more Shiva tried the harder it became. In his heart and soul, he knew it was her. It was Sati reborn as the beautiful Kali. No matter what Shiva did, Kali would not leave his thoughts. Kali was soon so imbedded in Shiva's mind that when Shiva's mind wandered, it always went back to her.

One day as Shiva was leaving to return to his abode, he noticed Kali waiting for him at the gates of the palace. Shiva stopped and looked into Kali's brown eyes.

He said; "I have searched throughout the valley of love. I only found your sighs. I wished not to fall in love again, but it was completely beyond my mastery". They held each other consumed by their love as the seasons passed. Kali was the perfect fit for Shiva as her wildness was, on this occasion, tamed by the great yogi.

On one such occasion after marriage, Kali fought the demon, Raktabija. The demon Raktabija had a boon that whenever a drop of his blood fell on the ground, a duplicate Raktabija would be born at that spot. So the more Kali wounded him, the more demons she ended up fighting. In the end, a frustrated Kali stretched her tongue over the earth and licked up each drop of blood pouring from Raktabija's body while the other goddesses wounded him. Kali thus devoured his duplicates into her mouth and eventually annihilated him.

According to the myth, after eating the demon and his entire army, Kali went on a rampage, killing all other creatures as such was her rage. Anyone who got in Kali's way was devoured and destroyed. The news that Kali's anger was out of control feared the gods as there is no force or power in Hindu mythology greater than Kali boiling with rage.

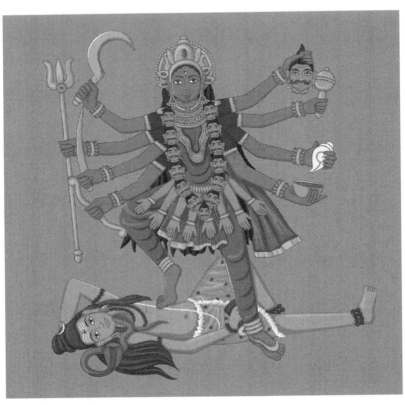

*above - Kali stepping on Shiva's chest has been depicted in many Hindu paintings and portraits.*

Kali's eyes appeared electric, and her weapons were dripping with blood. She carried the heads of demons, and wrath had consumed her core. Narayan (one of the gods) pleaded with Shiva to intervene. Shiva himself was initially at a loss and didn't know what to do. The universe had never experienced Kali's wrath before. But he had to do something, or the world was going to implode with Kali's rage.

Upon seeing Kali approach him, Shiva laid himself down in her way. Kali stepped on Shiva and let out such a huge roar that the continents quivered. Afterwards, when Kali looked down on Shiva's body, she was shaken and ashamed. Anger had consumed her, and she had lost all sense of self. Feeling ashamed at trampling on her beloved,

Kali removed her foot and as she did, she returned back to her less terrifying form.

Kali's other origin stories vary from madness to even more madness. It makes you wonder if these myths carry deep hidden messages as the sages proclaimed or whether it was just escapist fictional writing – the science fiction of its time. It could be that there is no meaning, and one writer wanted his origin story to be superior to the other. However, the same could be argued regarding the stories of Noah, Moses and Jesus. Are they all magical with meaning beyond our intellect or fantasy storytelling to feed our desire for knowledge? The yogis would say, in not so many words, that although we think that their myths are not reality, it is in fact our reality – that is the actual myth.

Interestingly, the design of the famous Rolling Stones logo, the "Tongue and Lip design" was suggested by Mick Jagger, inspired by the goddess Kali[3]. In April 1970, Jon Pasche, a 25-year-old student at the Royal College of Art, was asked by Jagger to create the logo based on a newspaper cutting portraying the goddess that he had seen. Pasche was hesitant at first, but Jagger was insistent. The final image is one of pop culture's most iconic logos

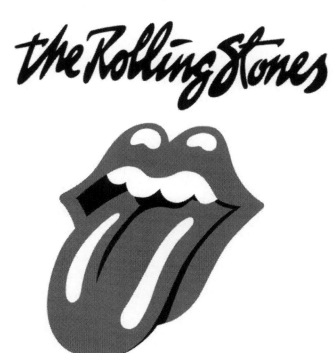

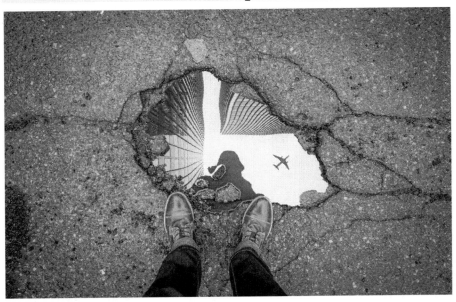

I think it was on my very first date with Laura that my soon-to-be wife told me that I should write a book. Of course, I thought she was trying to flatter me. I also realised that for her to be thinking that, I had obviously gone into one of my many rants about yoga and yogis, so I decided to pipe down and actually let her speak. It's a good thing I did.

The seed, however, was planted. Recently, my teacher training students and new students of the studio inspired me to write a book on yoga that, for once, will not send the reader to sleep. I hope that I have somewhat achieved my goal. I remember someone reading out loud a passage from a well-known book on yoga, and my only thought during the recital was that it was a good thing that I was not operating heavy machinery at the time. So, I decided to put something together with a little more flair. I guess I will know from my all-too-honest students if I have achieved my goal.

    Writing this book, or more like compiling my thoughts, has been a bigger challenge than I could have imagined. As each day passed, my target audience changed. I found myself at odds, wanting to change my thoughts to please the tradition and the next minute I was trying to please the yoga academic. To be truly positive in the eyes of some, you have to risk appearing negative in the eyes of others, so I decided to go down the traditional format where I could expand on my storytelling. Ultimately, I made the students of my studio my audience.

For a time, though, while I was unsure, I had a real battle on my hands. Many students commented on how I looked tired, and the truth is, I was tired. I was stressed and tired of trying to format and articulate my thoughts. So much so that my beautiful wife gifted me a copy of "Why Zebras Don't Get Ulcers".

The biggest challenge was my Bhagavad Gita Chapter in one of my earlier drafts. I had spent longer on this chapter than any other. On reflection, I was trying to be too clever. Reflection has a way of schooling us like that. I wrote almost 40 pages of this chapter, and the overall theme was that, via the discussion I have with my disciple through the book, I as the master would slowly come around to understanding and accepting my own *dharma*. I was very judgemental and overly harsh on the character of Krishna. I started the chapter by dismissing him and his words (more him to be honest) and, by the end of the chapter, through reflection, I came around to Krishna's words in the same way as Arjun does in the Gita. So, the chapter came full circle and so did my view on Krishna and the Gita. Like Arjun, I too am schooled by Krishna.

I structured this chapter and was very proud of what I thought I had accomplished. I sent it off to be proofread by my friend and yoga academic Daniel Simpson. Anyway, he sent it back to me and buried me. He was being polite, but I am sure he wanted to say it was rubbish. He didn't get or appreciate the overall theme I was trying to present because although it sounded like a good idea in my head, it just didn't come across or work within the chapter. Daniel was complimentary on a few parts, but in general my views probably made it sound like Krishna once stole my lunch money and I was trying to get back at him. The structure I had planned failed to work if Daniel didn't get it. It was no reflection on him, but more my inability to articulate my big plan.

Daniel's feedback was deeply disheartening (although I appreciate his honesty) as I had put so much work into that chapter and structured it in a way that made me feel proud, considering that this is my first book. Even writing about yoga can take you to madness or meditation. So, what was I to do? Feel sorry for myself and just drop the whole project? The thought did cross my mind for a moment, as this is a very human reaction. The author of Why Zebras Don't Get Ulcers (Robert M Sapolsky) has said, "It takes surprisingly little in terms of uncontrollable unpleasantness to make humans give up and become helpless in a generalized way"[1]. Rejection is the bitterest pill to swallow. I had followed my heart and gone along with this project, and now the core of my book was in shatters. Just like my self-esteem.

So again, what do I do? The same thing we do when we fail in handstand attempts (or the many other yoga poses). I didn't see it as "failure". I just looked at it as a method that did not work. I tried again. We all encounter moments where we feel like we are being beaten and defeated, but the overall defeat comes from our minds alone. There is a Bollywood song that always plays in my head during times of despair (have I mentioned Amitabh Bachchan in this book yet?). The song loses much of its charm away from its mother tongue – "Today's day will soon be yesterday. Don't look back, keep moving forward…" *Aaj ka ye din kal ban jayega kal… Piche mudke na dekh pyare age chal…* It's a mantra that has played in my head since childhood (who says TV is bad for kids?) and helped me through life in ways I could not possibly explain. Even with my back pain. I was in car accident when I was 18 and the ramifications of that has caught up with my back over the past 10 years. There are days like today when I cannot even tie my shoelaces, and one of the hardest things to do is teach physical yoga when you can barely walk yourself. It's not just physical but emotional pain too, when you strive to inspire but so much of who you are is crumbling under chronic pain. I am in a constant battle with myself for my own sanity. I have found a way, over the years, to hide the pain when I teach (not always though), but my pain remains persistent like a shadow. A mute companion. The pain just doesn't go away. And I have tried everything. More often than not, I leave a yoga class, or the gym feeling worse (more psychologically) than when I went in. But this has been my life. I have failed more in life than I have succeeded. But life is like a river in the law of *Tao*. It keeps moving forward. So what can I do? What can we do? Pain is a by-product of life. It will always exist. Today is a new day and a chance to do something meaningful. Today is a chance to live gloriously. So I can stay at home and feel sorry for myself or I can live like an instrument of nature. What other choice do we have but to live? When I was a child, my mum would tell me to be like a lion. They know nothing of depression and no doctor has stuck it in their heads that there is something wrong with them when they have a bad day. Live gloriously.

So, I had to continue with my book. I don't really know any other way. Staying at home and reading books by other people was not an option. I had to show heart and an iron resolve, so I stopped trying to be so clever, I took Daniel's advice (without compromising on my message) and ended up writing a chapter that was a much better fit in the overall book. I guess you could say I was trying to run before I could walk. But this is how we learn, and this is how we prosper. How many philosophers, parents and teachers have told us that we do not learn from our successes but our failures? There is some wisdom amongst wise men still.

We live, we fail, we learn, we fall, we laugh, and we cry. But through this all, we live. Confucius said, "Studying the past would define the future".

I wanted to write a book that would reach out to you and not give you all the answers, but simply ignite your enquiring minds. There is little fact in this book, going back to what Nietzsche has said at the start of this book. Although I have tried to give you an articulate understanding throughout, the truth is that I do not really know anything. All I have done in this book is give you my theoretical interpretation. Plato once said, "I am the wisest man alive, for I know one thing, and that is that I know nothing". The more I study, the more I research, the more clueless I become. I realise that I cannot cheat time and I cannot buy experience. And that, in essence, is what yoga really is. One man's unique experience over a period of time. What yoga means to you right now won't mean the same thing to you in 10 years' time. This is why it gets harder to tell people what yoga is and what yoga can do for you. The reality is that I just do not know. You must walk the path for yourself, as have I. Then you can come back to me and tell me what yoga is for you. It is a personal expression. A personal revelation. No one can tell you what is waiting for you and no one can lead you. You can only lead and help yourself.

I learnt yoga all on my own. I did a few classes (with Jessica Stretch at BeatBox Gym) and realised that, with my back pain, I would have to practice alone to make yoga fit around my pain. I stumbled across Iyengar's 'Light on Yoga' at a charity shop and pursued my goal of improving the way I moved to relieve some of my physical agony. I am completely self-taught in many respects. I have no guru and had no teacher. I learnt through Iyengar's pictures alone, on my living room floor as my dogs would jump and climb all over me. Hence, I am not a parrot teacher who repeats the same lines their teacher uttered in class. I have learnt with time how to teach yoga and how to do yoga using nothing but the expression of my own personality and the love for my craft. I have arrived at this point in my life where I have never been happier through will and the love for what I do. This is why I say, just do yoga asana. Just do the poses with all you heart and simply observe the natural and generic changes in your life. Put your heart into what you do. Nothing should be forced, and nothing should be fake. Forget about meditation classes and consign chakras and hand mudras into oblivion. None of this is useful to us. It doesn't work. It doesn't do a thing. This is nothing more than the yogic attire that people wear to be noticed by others. There is no spirituality to gain. No chakras to cleanse. This is all an illusion we have come to think of as real. This idea that we can reach for spirituality in a yoga class is all an illusion too, and it derives its power from our deep longing to fit into something. But we were never meant to fit into anything. We are as we are. Just think… There is no esoteric nonsense in yoga. A hand mudra will not unlock your 'spirituality'. There are no energy fields. No third eye. No such concept exists. Stop pressing your fingers on your forehead trying to evoke an imaginary third eye or chakra. Stop believing the nonsense you hear about chakra cleansing. Our desperation for spirituality is only filling the pockets of these charlatans. No chakra has ever opened in a yoga class and no serpent energy has ever exploded in a kundalini class. It has never happened and never will. Your spirituality in many ways is out of your hands. If you are deserving of an 'awakening' it will just happen to you by chance. You also cannot speed up the process by going online and purchasing Chopra's chakra mist spray. Perhaps the biggest load of misleading horse s*** I have ever heard. What a jabroni.

Forget spirituality. Just do your asanas with all your heart. And what transpires as a result of a regular asana practice will not be quantified. It is unique, individual and completely yours. The moment you speak of spirituality, the more deluded you become. When you experience honest and legitimate changes, you won't have the vocabulary. You will say, "Just do the poses as I have done, and you too will transform in ways you could not imagine".

    I have found that people and teachers can act like guides, but no one can show you the way. No one can say, "Just follow me" or "look at me and copy me". That is not the way of the world. We are unique, and uniqueness requires a unique journey. One that is our own and cannot be shared with somebody else. Our transformation from finite to infinite cannot occur if we remain as shadows to those who we aspire to be like. You can have a yoga teacher, a philosophy teacher, a personal trainer, a dietician. But you cannot put your life in their hands. You cannot ask them to lead you to harmony or ask them to show you the way. Most importantly, you cannot try to be somebody you are not. You can admire my Laura. You can respect her drive. Remain gobsmacked at her grace while she hangs upside down. Feel inspired by her arm balances, but you can never be her. You should never try.

    The gravest sin that man can make is to try to be somebody else. Inspiration is one thing and mimicry is another. You were designed and created unique. You may have similar traits as someone, but you will never be like anybody else. Your eyes are unique. You can scour the world and you will never find anyone who has the same eyes as you. No two eyes have exactly the same iris patterns. Each iris has a unique pattern of ridges and folds, specific only to you. Your thumbprint is unique. The surface of our hands and feet form ridges in patterns that are unique to each individual and which do not change over time. Your DNA profile is unique. You are unique. A product of nature made unlike anything else on this planet. How can you sacrilege nature and try to be like somebody else?

In the Avengers Endgame, Thor's mother say's to our valiant hero; "A measure of a person, a hero is how someone succeeds at being who they really are".

Never have wiser words been spoken.

We were never born to be anybody but who we are. Have you noticed how the various characters and gods in Hindu/yoga mythology are all unique? No one deva or god is the same as the next. No one is better. Each is just uniquely different. Each character has a flaw and each character has many traits individual to them. In many ways, they are just like us. Nietzsche has said, "One is fruitful only at the cost of being rich in contradictions". These gods are a blend of contradictions. No god is perfect, because no such concept exists. Perfection does not exist. The stories of these gods would lose their splendour if each god was perfect.

The psychiatrist David D. Burns has said that "Perfection is man's ultimate illusion. It simply doesn't exist in the universe. If you are a perfectionist, you are guaranteed to be a loser in whatever you do"[2]. So we must embark on a journey of self-exploration on our own and for ourselves. To enlighten or illuminate our own understanding of ourselves and life itself. This is not possible if we constantly try to fit into the fake yoga community that, for me, is the most phony and immodest bunch of people of them all. Avoid such company and create a bond with your yoga mat alone.

Anything and everything you are deserving of will come to you in its own time. Joining a yoga community will not speed up your search for spirituality.

I often say to my teacher trainee students that no one should know you do yoga. If you are having lunch with friends and family and they can see that you are a "yogi" and you are "well into" yoga, then you need to slow down. You are starting to lose what is so beautiful about you – you. Yoga should make you a happier version of who you are, not take over who you really are. There is no beauty in trying to be a yogi or trying to fit in to someone's ideal.

I am a fan of LL Cool J's music. I grew up to his music and remember trying to dress like him in the late 80s. In "I'm Bad", LL had on a Kangol hat, no t-shirt, a bare chest and lots of baby oil. This was my go-to outfit, confined to my bedroom of course. I am now a grown man of 40 years. If I dress like LL today, at my age people will think I have lost my mind. Although the bare chest does make an appearance every now and again. Why would I, at my age? I can listen to his music without changing my identity. The yoga community is full of grown men and women dressing themselves up to fit into yoga. A necklace here and some beads there. The uniform is slowly taking shape. You can even do a class with a woman called "Lakshmi Devi" in London.

Her real name is Wendy from Wales, but who wants to do yoga with Wendy when you can supposedly have the real thing and do yoga with 'Lakshmi Devi'?

How genuine can someone be when they have to change their name to fit into a yogic ideal? And this is the person who is going to teach you the 'science of self-realisation'?

This is dressing up to be a yogi. All you do is hide what you feel insecure about, but ironically, it is the most beautiful gift you have been bestowed with. The gift of individuality. Yoga teachers are always looking for a unique selling point. What is going to make them different to the next teacher? Not knowing that their own personality is their unique selling point. The world doesn't need more yoga teachers. There are already far too many. The world needs more individuals who can teach yoga. The difference is like day and night. We don't need to be told to tuck in our tailbones any longer. We don't need these corny dialogues and we don't need these corny outfits.

Yoga is not about dressing yourself up, but sadly, that's what it has become. When we were children, we identified adult uniforms with power, control and authority. As we get older, we create our own uniforms to create our own authority. It's a deep-rooted problem. Our schools want to create an army of children who are all the same and dress the same. If we don't escape this bondage, we spend our whole lives looking for a uniform that will help us fit in. We are just looking to be accepted.

A middle-aged Indian woman had a heart attack and was taken to the hospital. While on the operating table, she has a near-death experience. During that experience she sees Shiva and asks him if this is it. Shiva says, "No. Not yet. This was just a wake-up call". Shiva then explains that the lady still has another 30 years to live. "Treasure it." Upon her recovery, the lady decides to just stay in the hospital and have a nose job, face lift, liposuction, breast augmentation and a tummy tuck.

She wanted to look like her favourite celebrity. She has her hair re-styled and coloured and decides that she will leave her grumpy old husband and start a whole new life. She figured that since she's got another 30 years, she might as well make the most of life. Why waste a gift from god? She wanted to look her best, feel her best and live her life to the fullest. She was not going to waste another day being a householder. She wanted to be like Priyanka Chopra, her favourite Bollywood actress.

She was tired and bored of being a nobody. She walks out of the hospital after the last operation with a newfound zest and swagger. Wolf whistles are blown, and a commotion begins. Dazzled by the locals taking photos of her, the lady attempts to cross the road and is immediately killed by an ambulance speeding by. The despondent woman arrives to the heavenly abode of Shiva and lets out a huge roar and complains, "I thought you said I had another 30 years!"

Shiva, looking shell shocked, replies, "Sorry. I didn't recognise you!"

This is us. We are losing ourselves and our identities slowly each day trying to be like others or trying to look like yogis or our favourite celebrities. At some stage in life, we will look in the mirror and no longer recognise who we are anymore. Clothes and appearances are all superficial. It does nothing but convey our deep insecurities. I prefer the yoga student in her Lululemon outfit who is at least honest of her vanity than the so-called humble yogis in their fake humble outfits as they "do", "live" and practice yoga. The idea to dress humble was once to be humble. Now all it does is create the facade that we are humble. Who is it that we are actually deceiving? The great Chuang Tzu once said, "But a gentleman may embrace a doctrine without necessarily wearing the garb that goes with it, and he may wear the garb without necessarily comprehending the doctrine."[3]

Shiva gave man no philosophy. This is because as we are, we are pure and flawless. Shiva and Tantra say that we can accomplish all that we wish for. All that is required from us to do so, going back to the start of the book is to be "willing". Carl Jung has said that, "Our main task is to discover and fulfil our deep, innate potential". If we participate in yoga and wish for yoga to transform us, first physically and then emotionally, all we are required to have is our Will. Our character, our determination and our heart are all collectively our Will. If we are willing, yoga will lead us to meditation. A destination of physical vitality and emotional tranquility. If we lose or give up our Will to the so called "guru" or to fit into a yogic ideal, then yoga is nothing more than complete madness.

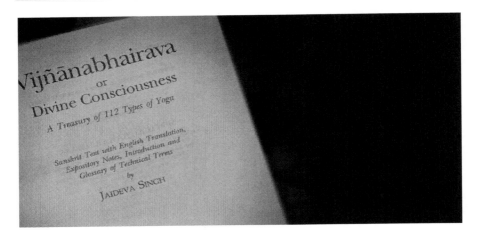

Translated by Paul Reps and Swami Lakshman Joo.

PARVATI SAYS:

O Shiva, what is your reality?
What is this wonder-filled universe?
What constitutes seed?
Who centers the universal wheel?
What is this life beyond form pervading forms?
How may we enter it fully, above space and time, names and
descriptions?
Let my doubts be cleared.

SHIVA REPLIES:

1. Radiant one, this experience may dawn between two breaths. After
breath comes in (down) and just before turning up (out) — the
beneficence.
2. As breath turns down from down to up, and again as breath curves
from up to down — through both these turns, realize.
3. Or, whenever in-breath and out-breath fuse, at this instant touch the
energy-less energy-filled center.

4. Or, when breath is all out (up) and stopped of itself, or all in (down) and stopped – in such universal pause, one's small self, vanishes. This is difficult only for the impure.

5. Consider your essence as light rays rising from center to center up the vertebrae, and so rises livingness in you.

6. Or in the spaces between, feel this as lightning.

7. Devi, imagine the Sanskrit letters in these honey-filled foci of awareness, first as letters, then more subtly as sounds, then as most subtle feeling. Then, leaving them aside, be free.

8. Attention between eyebrows, let mind be before thought. Let form fill with breath-essence to the top of the head and their shower as light.

9. Or, imagine the five-colored circles of the peacock tail to be your five senses in illimitable space. Now let their beauty melt within. Similarly, at any point in space or on a wall — until the point dissolves. Then your wish for another comes true.

10. Eyes closed, see your inner being in detail. Thus, see your true nature.

11. Place your whole attention in the nerve, delicate as the lotus thread, in the center of your spinal column. In such be transformed.

12. Closing the seven openings of the head with your hands, a space between your eyes becomes all-inclusive.

13. Touching eyeballs as a feather, lightness between them opens into heart and there permeates the cosmos.

14. Bathe in the center of sound, as in the continuous sound of a waterfall. Or by putting the fingers in the ears, hear the sound of sounds.

15. Intone a sound, as a-u-m, slowly. As sound enters soundful-ness, so do you.

16. In the beginning and gradual refinement of the sound of any letter, awake.

17. While listening to stringed instruments, hear their composite central sound; thus omnipresence.

18. Intone a sound audibly, then less and less audibly as feeling deepens into this silent harmony.

19. Imagine spirit simultaneously within and around you until the entire universe spiritualizes.

20. Kind Devi, enter etheric presence pervading far above and below your form.

21. Put mind-stuff in such inexpressible fineness above, below and in your heart.

22. Consider any area of your present form as limitlessly spacious.

23. Feel your substance, bones, flesh, blood, saturated with cosmic essence.

24. Suppose your passive form to be an empty room with walls of skin — empty.

25. Blessed one, as senses are absorbed in heart, reach the center of the lotus.

26. Unminding mind, keep in the middle — until.

27. When in worldly activity, keep attentive between the two breaths, and so practicing, in a few days be born anew.

28. Focus on fire rising through your form from the toes up until the body burns to ashes but not you.

29. Meditate on the make-believe world as burning to ashes and become being above human.

30. Feel the fine qualities of creativity permeating your breasts and assuming delicate configurations.

31. With intangible breath in center of forehead, as this reaches heart at the moment of sleep, have direction over dreams and over death itself.

32. As, subjectively, letters flow into words and words into sentences, and as, objectively, circles flow into worlds and worlds into principles, find at last these converging in our being.

33. Gracious one, play the universe is an empty shell wherein your mind frolics infinitely.

34. Look upon a bowl without seeing the sides or the material. In a few moments become aware.

35. Abide in some place endlessly spacious, clear of trees, hills, habitations. Thence comes the end of mind pressures.

36. Sweet-hearted one, meditate on knowing and not knowing, existing and not existing. Then leave both aside that you may be.

37. Look lovingly on some object. Do not go on to another object. Here, in the middle of this object — the blessing.

38. Feel cosmos as translucent ever-living presence.

39. With utmost devotion, center on the two junctions of breath and know the knower.

40. Consider the plenum to be your own body of bliss.

41. While being caressed, sweet princess, enter the caressing as everlasting life.

42. Stop the doors of senses when feeling the creeping of an ant. Then.

43. At the start of sexual union keep attentive on the fire in the beginning, and, so continuing, avoid the embers in the end.

44. When in such embrace your senses are shaken as leaves, enter this shaking.

45. Even remembering union, without the embrace, the transformation.

46. On joyously seeing a long-absent friend, permeate this joy.

47. When eating or drinking, become the taste of the food or drink, and be filled.

48. O lotus-eyed one, sweet of touch, when singing, seeing, tasting, be aware you are and discover the ever-living.

49. Wherever satisfaction is found, in whatever act, actualize this.

50. At the point of sleep when the sleep has not yet come and external wakefulness vanishes, at this point being is revealed.

51. In summer when you see the entire sky endlessly clear, enter such clarity.

52. Lie down as dead. Enraged in wrath, stay so. Or stare without moving an eyelash. Or suck something and become the sucking.

53. Without support for feet or hands, sit only on the buttocks. Suddenly, the centering.

54. In an easy position gradually pervade an area between the armpits into great peace.

55. See as if for the first time a beauteous person or an ordinary object.

56. With mouth slightly open, keep mind in the middle of tongue. Or, as breath comes silently in, feel the sound HH.

57. When on a bed or a seat, let yourself become weightless, beyond mind.

58. In a moving vehicle, by rhythmically swaying, experience. Or in a still vehicle, by letting yourself swing in slowing invisible circles.

59. Simply by looking into the blue sky beyond clouds, the serenity.

60. Shakti, see all space as if already absorbed in your own head in the brilliance.

61. Waking, sleeping, dreaming, knowing you as light.

62. In rain during a black night enter that blackness as the form of forms.

63. When a moonless raining night is not present, close eyes and find blackness before you. Opening eyes, see blackness. So, faults disappear forever.

64. Just as you have the impulse to do something, stop.

65. Center on the sound a-u-m without any a or m.

66. Silently intone a word ending in AH. Then in the HH effortlessly, the spontaneity.

67. Feel yourself as pervading all directions, far, near.

68. Pierce some part of your nectar-filled form with a pin, and gently enter the piercing.

69. Feel: My thought, I-ness, internal organs — me.

70. Illusions deceive. Colors circumscribe. Even divisibles are indivisible.

71. When some desire comes, consider it. Then suddenly, quit it.

72. Before desire and before knowing, how can I say I am? Consider. Dissolve in the beauty.

73. With your entire consciousness in the very start of desire, of knowing, know.

74. O Shakti, each particular perception is limited, disappearing in omnipotence.

75. In truth forms are inseparate. Inseparate are omnipresent being and your own form. Realize each as made of this consciousness.

76. In moods of extreme desire, be undisturbed.

77. This so-called universe appears as a juggling, a picture show. To be happy look upon it so.

78. Oh Beloved, put attention neither on pleasure nor pain but between these.

79. Toss attachment for body aside, realizing I am everywhere. One who is everywhere is joyous.

80. Objects and desires exist in me as in others. So, accepting, let them be translated.

81. The appreciation of objects and subjects is the same for an enlightened as for an unenlightened person. The former has one greatness: he remains in the subjective mood, not lost in things.

82. Feel the consciousness of each person as your own consciousness. So, leaving aside concern for self, become each being.

83. Thinking no thing, will limited-self unlimited.

84. Believe omniscient, omnipotent, pervading.

85. As waves come with water and flames with fire, so the universal waves with us.

86. Roam about until exhausted and then, dropping to the ground, in this dropping be whole.

87. Suppose you are gradually being deprived of strength or of knowledge. At the instant of deprivation, transcend.

88. Listen while the ultimate mystical teaching is imparted: Eyes still, without blinking, at once become absolutely free.

89. Stopping ears by pressing and rectum by contracting, enter the sound of sound.

90. At the edge of a deep well look steadily into its depths until – the wondrousness.

91. Wherever your mind is wandering, internally or externally, at this very place, this.

92. When vividly aware through some particular sense, keep in the awareness.

93. At the start of sneezing, during fright, in anxiety, above a chasm, flying in battle, in extreme curiosity, at the beginning of hunger, at the end of hunger, be uninterruptedly aware.

94. Let attention be at a place where you are seeing some past happening, and even your form, having lost its present characteristics, is transformed.

95. Look upon some object, then slowly withdraw your sight from it, then slowly withdraw you thought from it. Then.

96. Devotion frees.

97. Feel an object before you. Feel the absence of all other objects but this one. Then, leaving aside the object-feeling and the absence-feeling, realize.

98. The purity of other teachings is an impurity to us. In reality, know nothing as pure or impure.

99. This consciousness exists as each being, and nothing else exists.

100. Be the un-same same to friend as to stranger, in honor and dishonor.

101. When a mood against someone or for someone arises, do not place it on the person in question, but remain centered.

102. Suppose you contemplate something beyond perception, beyond grasping, beyond not being, you.

103. Enter space, support-less, eternal, still.

104. Wherever your attention alights, at this very point, experience.

105. Enter the sound of your name and, through this sound, all sounds.

106. I am existing. This is mine. This is this. O beloved, even in such know illimitably.

107. This consciousness is the spirit of guidance of each one. Be this one.

108. Here is a sphere of change, change, change. Through change consume change.

109. As a hen mothers her chicks, mother particular knowing's, particular doings, in reality.

110. Since, in truth, bondage and freedom are relative, these words are only for those terrified with the universe. This universe is a reflection of minds. As you see many suns in water from one sun, so see bondage and liberation.

111. Each thing is perceived through knowing. The self, shines in space through knowing. Perceive one being as knower and known.

112. Beloved, at this moment let mind, knowing, breath, form, be included.

# References -

The stories throughout this book are <u>inspired</u> by the *Puranas*, The Teachings of Sadhguru, The Kumarasambhava of Kalidasa, the works of Osho Rajneesh, Devdutt Pattanaik, Lakshmanjoo, Vanamali, Jaideva Singh, Swami Vivekananda and Ramanaj Prassad as well as many other stories I have read over the years of which I no longer have a reference. I do not agree with everything these writers have spoken about over the years, but they have still inspired me in many ways.

1 - Nietzsche, F., 2017. The Will to Power (Penguin Classics). 3rd ed. England: Penguin Classics; Translation edition (26 Jan. 2017).

2 - Nicholas Ng-A-Fook, K., 2019. Oral History and Education: Theories, Dilemmas, and Practices (Palgrave Studies in Oral History). 1st ed. England: Palgrave Macmillan; Softcover reprint of the original 1st ed. 2017 edition (18 April 2019)

3 - DAN BOX, CRIME REPORTER ( DECEMBER 4, 2014) Yoga guru may have raped seven year old, royal commission told, Available at: https://www.theaustralian.com.au/nation/nation/yoga-guru-may-have-raped-seven-year-old-royal-commission-told/news-story/0b53b8030439d78e69a5c619a3a8b441(Accessed: 2nd September 2018).

4, 5 - Keller, H., 2017. Helen Keller: The Story of My Life and Selected Letters (Classic Thoughts and Thinkers). 2nd ed. U.S, Chartwell Books (4 May 2017).

Chapter 1 - The First Yogi
1 - Paul Reps & Nyogen Senzaki (2000) Zen Flesh, Zen Bones: A Collection of Zen and Pre-Zen Writings, 2nd edn., UK: Penguin.

2 - Friedrich Nietzsche, B., 2016. Friedrich Nietzsche: Quotes & Facts. 1st ed. CreateSpace Independent Publishing Platform; 1 edition (15 Jan. 2016).

3 - Iyengar, B., 2018. Light on Life: The Journey to Wholeness, Inner Peace and Ultimate Freedom. 2nd ed. U.K: Rodale; Reprints edition (2 May 2008) Google Play Online Version.

4 - Vasudev, S., 2017. Adiyogi: The Source of Yoga. 1st ed. India: Harper Collins India (1 Feb. 2017).

5 - booksfact.com/archeology (Unknown) Kalpa Vigraha Oldest Hindu Idol of Lord Siva (26450 BC), Available at: https://www.booksfact.com/archeology/kalpa-vigraha-oldest-hindu-idol-of-lord-siva-26450-bc.html (Accessed: 3rd Jan 2019).
Also - Indian Monk (22 Mar 2018) 26,450 Year Old Hindu Idol of Lord Shiva - Kalpa Vigraha, Available at: https://www.youtube.com/watch?v=qhHQT0HYWq0 (Accessed: 1st Feb 2019).

6 - Sadhguru (2018) Who is Shiva: Man, Myth or Divine?, Available at: https://isha.sadhguru.org/mahashivratri/shiva-adiyogi/who-is-shiva-meaning/ (Accessed: 12 March 2018).

Chapter 2 - Tantra & Love

1 - Singh, J., 2002. Vijnana-bhairava or Divine Consciousness: A Treasury of 112 Types of Yoga. 2nd ed. .: Motilal Banarsidass,; New edition edition (1 Dec. 2002).

2 - Banerjee Divakarun, C., 2019. The Forest of Enchantment. 1st ed. .: HarperCollins India (7 Jan. 2019).

3 - Swami Vivekananda (1947) Complete Works of Swami Vivekananda, Volume 1, 1st ed, India: Advaita Ashram

4,7 - Gibran, K., 2019. Prophet Wisehouse Classics Edition. Sweden. 1st ed. Wisehouse Classics (20 Sept. 2017)

5 - Sophocles, 2000. The Three Theban Plays: 'Antigone', 'Oedipus the King',

6 - Nietzsche, F., 2017. Thus Spoke Zarathustra. 1st ed. United Kingdom: Independently published (25 July 2017

Chapter 3 - No Philosophy
1 - B. Calne, D., 1999. Within Reason: Rationality and Human Behavior. 1st ed. United Kingdom: Pantheon Books; 1 edition (1 May 1999).
2 - Mohanty, D., 2015. The Curse of Damini. 1st ed. Partridge Publishing India (14 July 2015).

Chapter 4 - Patanjali
1 - Sadhguru (Jan 09, 2017) Recognizing the Adiyogi, Available at: https://isha.sadhguru.org/global/en/wisdom/sadhguru-spot/recognizing-the-adiyogi(Accessed: 1st March 2018).
2,8 - David Gordon White & Debra Diamond (2013) Yoga: The Art of Transformation , 1st edn., UK: Bravo Ltd.
3,4 - Iyengar, B., 2015. Light on Yoga: The Definitive Guide to Yoga Practice. 1st ed. .: Thorsons; Thorsons Classics edition edition (29 Jan. 2015).
5 - Rasamandala Das (2012) The Illustrated Encyclopedia of Hinduism, 3rd edn., UK: Lorenz Books.
6 - Light on Life: The Journey to Wholeness, Inner Peace and Ultimate Freedom. 2nd ed. U.K: Rodale; Reprints edition (2 May 2008) Google Play Online Version.
7 - Jagi Vasudev (Jun 26, 2014) Patanjali - The Father of Modern Yoga, Available at: https://isha.sadhguru.org/sg/en/wisdom/article/classical-yoga-the-influence-of-patanjali(Accessed: 22nd September 2018).

Chapter 5 - Introspection
1 - Light on Life: The Journey to Wholeness, Inner Peace and Ultimate Freedom. 2nd ed. U.K: Rodale; Reprints edition (2 May 2008) Google Play Online Version.
2 - Doctor, R., 2017. Ashtavakra GITA: Dialogues with King Janak. 1st ed. CreateSpace Independent Publishing Platform (25 Jan. 2017).
3 - Who Owns Yoga? | Al Jazeera Correspondent. 2019. Who Owns Yoga? | Al Jazeera Correspondent. [ONLINE] Available at: https://www.youtube.com/watch?v=LGvkki0tLoU&t=252s. [Accessed 12 March 2019].
4 - A. K. Ramanujan (translator),1973. Speaking of Siva (Penguin Classics). 1st ed. Penguin Classics; Reprint edition (August 30, 1973).

Chapter 6 - Mind
1 - Maitreya, A., 2001. The Dhammapada. 1st ed. Parallax Press; Reprint edition (August 9, 2001).
2, 3 - Olivia Goldhill. 2016. Scientists say your "mind" isn't confined to your brain, or even your body. [ONLINE] Available at: https://qz.com/866352/scientists-say-your-mind-isnt-confined-to-your-brain-or-even-your-body/. [Accessed 1 January 2019].
3 - Light on Life: The Journey to Wholeness, Inner Peace and Ultimate Freedom. 2nd ed. U.K: Rodale; Reprints edition (2 May 2008) Google Play Online Version.
4 - Vasudev, S., 2016. Inner Engineering: A Yogi's Guide to Joy. 1st ed. India: Random House Inc; 1 edition (20 Sept. 2016).
5 - Shah, I., 2018. The Sufis. 7th ed. .: ISF Publishing; 7th edition edition (6 Sept. 2018).

Chapter 7 - Yoga Gurus
1 - Richard Holloway (2017) A Little History of Religion (Little Histories), 2nd edn., US: Yale University Press.
2 - Yogananda, P., 2007. Yoga of the Bhagavad Gita: An Introduction to India's Universal Science of God-realization. 1st ed. U.S: Self-Realization Fellowship,U.S. (25 Oct. 2007).
3 - Adiga, A., 2012. The White Tiger. 1st ed. India: Atlantic Books; Main edition (1 Mar. 2012).
4 - Muralidharan, I., 2015. Reengineers, The. 1st ed. India: Element India (1 April 2015).
5,6 - Gibran, K., 2019. Prophet (Wisehouse Classics Edition. 1st ed. .: Wisehouse Classics (20 Sept. 2017).
7 - Varma, P., 2006. Being Indian. 1st ed. India: Penguin Books (30 Sept. 2006).
8 - Blaise Pascal, B., 1995. Pensees (Penguin Classics). 1st ed. Penguin Classics; Rev Ed edition (27 July 1995).
9 - Burrus, C. 1995. Frida Kahlo: 'I Paint my Reality' (New Horizons). 1st ed. Thames and Hudson Ltd; 01 edition (7 April 2008).

Chapter 8 - The Human Mind
1 - Swami Vivekananda (1947) Complete Works of Swami Vivekananda, Volume 1, 1st ed, India: Advaita Ashram
2 - Yogananda, P., 2007. Yoga of the Bhagavad Gita: An Introduction to India's Universal Science of God-realization. 1st ed. U.S: Self-Realization Fellowship,U.S. (25 Oct. 2007).
3 - By NANCY DILLON (OCT. 9, 2018) Ashtanga yoga guru Pattabhi Jois accused of sexual assault in new photos, Available at: https://www.sandiegouniontribune.com/news/ny-news-ashtanga-founder-photos-allege-sex-assault-20181009-story.html (Accessed: 3rd March 2019).
4 - Iyengar, B., 2015. Light on Yoga: The Definitive Guide to Yoga Practice. 1st ed. .: Thorsons; Thorsons Classics edition edition (29 Jan. 2015).

Understanding the Mind via Bhagavad Gita
1, 2, 3, - Swami Vivekananda (1947) Complete Works of Swami Vivekananda, Volume 1, 1st ed, India: Advaita Ashram.
4 - Light on Life: The Journey to Wholeness, Inner Peace and Ultimate Freedom. 2nd ed. U.K: Rodale; Reprints edition (2 May 2008) Google Play Online Version.
5 - Bertrand Russell (2004) History of Western Philosophy (Routledge Classics), 1st edn., UK: Routledge.
6 - Vasudev, S., 2017. Adiyogi: The Source of Yoga. 1st ed. India: Harper Collins India (1 Feb. 2017).
7 - Gibran, K., 2019. Prophet (Wisehouse Classics Edition. 1st ed. .: Wisehouse Classics (20 Sept. 2017).
8 - Friedrich Nietzsche (15 Mar 2015) Human, All Too Human & Beyond Good
9 - Allende, I., 2015. Ripper. 1st ed. Fourth Estate (29 Jan. 2015):

Understanding the Mind through The Gita of Ashtavakra
1,2,3,5,6&6a,7,8,9 - Doctor, R., 2017. Ashtavakra GITA: Dialogues with King Janak. 1st ed. CreateSpace Independent Publishing Platform (25 Jan. 2017).
4 - Swami Vivekananda (1947) Complete Works of Swami Vivekananda, Complete set in 8 volumes, 3rd edn., India: Advaita Ashram.
10 - Criss Jami (2015) Killosophy, 1st edn., UK: CreateSpace.
11 - C. G. Jung (1980) Psychology and Alchemy (Collected Works of C.G. Jung), 2nd edn., UK: Routledge.
12 - https://www.academia.edu. 2019. Wilkins, Kasinatha, Hastings, and the First English Bhagavad Gita. [ONLINE] Available at: https://www.academia.edu/15282813/Wilkins_Kasinatha_Hastings_and_the_First_English_Bhagavad_Gita. [Accessed 1 May 2019].

Chapter 9 - God
1 - Al-Biruni, Muhammad Ibn Ahmad Biruni (1993) Alberuni's India, 1st edn., UK: W. W. Norton & Company.
2 - Nietzsche, F., 2017. Thus Spoke Zarathustra. 1st ed. United Kingdom: Independently published.
3 - Alexander, E., 2017. My Experience In Coma. [ONLINE] Available at: http://ebenalexander.com/about/my-experience-in-coma/ [Accessed 4 March 2019].
4 - Sankaracharya (2012) The Crest-Jewel of Wisdom: and other writings of Sankaracharya, 1st edn., UK: THE FREEDOM RELIGION PRESS.
5 - Rumi, 2004. Selected Poems Penguin Classics. Penguin Classics; New Ed edition
6 - Gibran, K., 2019. Prophet Wisehouse Classics Edition. 1st ed. Wisehouse Classics
7 - Evelyn Einhaeuser. 2014. A YOGA THERAPIST'S PERSPECTIVE: MENAKA DESIKACHAR. [ONLINE] Available at: http://www.synergies-journal.com/healing/2014/12/19/a-yoga-therapists-perspective-menaka-desikachar. [Accessed 5 March 2019].
8 - David Gordon White & Debra Diamond (2013) Yoga: The Art of Transformation , 1st edn., UK: Bravo Ltd.
9, 9a - F. Yeats-Brown (1937) Yoga Explained, 1st edn., UK: Pilgrims Publishing.
10 - Alex Hern (Mon 17 Sep 2018 ) Instagram is supposed to be friendly. So why is it making people                              so                              miserable?, Available

at: https://www.theguardian.com/technology/2018/sep/17/instagram-is-supposed-to-be-friendly-so-why-is-it-making-people-so-miserable (Accessed: 2nd March 2019).
11 - Amit Ray (2012) Yoga and Vipassana : An Integrated Lifestyle, 1st edn., UK: Inner Light Publishers.

Chapter 10 - What is Yoga?
1 - Light on Life: The Journey to Wholeness, Inner Peace and Ultimate Freedom. 2nd ed. U.K: Rodale; Reprints edition (2 May 2008) Google Play Online Version

Chapter 11 - Modern Day Yoga

1 - James Mallinson (July 3rd 2016) The Amṛtasiddhi: Haṭhayoga's Tantric Buddhist Source Text, Available
at: https://www.academia.edu/26700528/The_Am%E1%B9%9Btasiddhi_Ha%E1%B9%AD hayogas_Tantric_Buddhist_Source_Text(Accessed: april 9 2019).
2 - Carl W Ernst (2016) Refractions of Islam in India (Sage Yoda), 1st edn., US: SAGE YODA Press.
3 - http://www.asianart.org (AY 25, 2014) Yoga and the Body, Available at: http://www.asianart.org/exhibitions_index/yoga-and-the-body (Accessed: april 9th 2019).
4,13 - David Gordon White & Debra Diamond (2013) Yoga: The Art of Transformation , 1st edn., UK: Bravo Ltd.
5 - Center of the Study of World Religions (October 14, 2015) Contesting Yoga's Past: A Brief History of Āsana in Pre-modern India, Available at: https://cswr.hds.harvard.edu/news/2015/10/14/contesting-yoga%E2%80%99s-past-brief-history-%C4%81sana-pre-modern-india (Accessed: April 9th 2019).
6,9 - Jan Schmidt-Garre, Breath of the Gods: A Journey to the Origins of Modern Yoga, Available at: https://www.amazon.co.uk/Breath-Gods-Journey-Origins-Modern/dp/B00FG1KAN0 (Accessed: April 9th 2019).
7,8,10 - A.G. Mohan (2010) Krishnamacharya: His Life and Teachings, 1st edn., US: Shambhala Publications Inc.
11 - Indra Devi (2015) Yoga for Americans, 4th edn., US: Martino Fine Books.
12 - Centre for Yoga Studies, What is the meaning and origin of the concept of the viniyoga of Yoga?, Available at: https://yogastudies.org/cys-journal/viniyoga/#viniyoga_style (Accessed: 1st March 2018).
14 - Swami Vivekananda (1947) Complete Works of Swami Vivekananda, Complete set in 8 volumes, 3rd edn., India: Advaita Ashram

Krishnamacharya Bibliography
• Kausthub Desikachar (2011) The Yoga of the Yogi: The Legacy of T. Krishnamacharya, 1st edn., US: North Point Press.
• Kausthub Desikachar (2011) Health, Healing, and Beyond, 1st edn., US: Farrar, Straus, and Giroux.
• A.G. Mohan (2010) Krishnamacharya: His Life and Teachings, 1st edn., US: Shambhala Publications Inc.

Chapter 11 - Asana
1 - Dr Mark Singleton (2010) Yoga Body: The Origins of Modern Posture Practice, First edn., USA: Oxford University Press. pages 60-63
2 - Dr Mark Singleton (2010) Yoga Body: The Origins of Modern Posture Practice, First edn., USA: Oxford University Press. pages 84-88
3 - Dr Mark Singleton (2010) Yoga Body: The Origins of Modern Posture Practice, First edn., USA: Oxford University Press. pages 95-97
4 - David Waller (2012) The Perfect Man: The Muscular Life and Times of Eugen Sandow, Victorian Strongman, 1st edn., UK: Victorian Secrets.
5 - Philip Rawson (1983) Erotic Art of India, First edn., London: Thames & Hudson Ltd.
6 - Phil Page & Clare Frank (2010) Assessment and Treatment of Muscle Imbalance, First edn., USA: Human Kinetics(ADVANTAGE).
7 - Light on Life: The Journey to Wholeness, Inner Peace and Ultimate Freedom. 2nd ed. U.K: Rodale; Reprints edition (2 May 2008) Google Play Online Version

8 - Sharon Begley (2009) The Plastic Mind, 1st edn., UK: Constable (26 Feb. 2009) pages 6-7
9 - Ramachandran, M., 2005. A Brief Tour of Human Consciousness: From Impostor Poodles to Purple Number. 2nd ed. US: Pi Press.
10 - Sharon Begley (2009) The Plastic Mind, 1st edn., UK: Constable (26 Feb. 2009) page 15
11, 12, 13,26 - Sharon Begley (2009) The Plastic Mind, 1st edn., UK: Constable (26 Feb. 2009)
14 - Annie Wright (Nov 26, 2016) Trust in God, but tie your camel., Available at: https://anniewrightpsychotherapy.com/trust-god-tie-camel/ (Accessed: 26 March 2019).
14 - Gibran, K., 2019. Prophet (Wisehouse Classics Edition. 1st ed. .: Wisehouse Classics (20 Sept. 2017).
16 - National Academy of Sports Medicine (NASM), B., 2016. NASM Essentials Of Personal Fitness Training (National Academy of Sports Medicine). 5th ed. Jones and Bartlett Publishers, Inc; 5th Revised edition edition (23 Jun. 2016): London.
17 - J. Alter, M., 2018. Science of Flexibility. 3rd ed. Human Kinetics (ADVANTAGE) (Consignment); 3rd Revised edition edition (15 May 2014): London.
18,23,24 - Jami, C., 2016. Healology. 1st ed. UK: CreateSpace Independent Publishing Platform.
19 - vivekananda.net. 2019. Swami Vivekananda - A biography. [ONLINE] Available at: https://www.vivekananda.net/PDFBooks/HTML/NikhilanandaBiography.html. [Accessed 1 May 2019].
20 - Iyengar, B., 2018. Light on Life: The Journey to Wholeness, Inner Peace and Ultimate Freedom. 2nd ed. U.K: Rodale; Reprints edition (2 May 2008) Google Play Online Version.
21 - Swami Vivekananda (1947) Complete Works of Swami Vivekananda, Complete set in 8 volumes, 3rd edn., India: Advaita Ashram.
22 - yoganatomy.com. 2019. Should the Knee Ever Go Past the Ankle or Toes in Warrior?. [ONLINE] Available at: https://www.yoganatomy.com/knee-past-ankle-in-warrior/. [Accessed 1 May 2019].
27 - Uddiyan, S., 2010. *Kalama Sutta: The Rediscovery of Conscience.* 1st ed. Nepal: Vajra Publications; 2010 edition.
28 - B. Pert, C., 2010. Molecules of Emotion: The Science Behind Mind-Body Medicine. 1st ed. New York: Scribne.
28a - Wei M.D., J.D.. 2015. Marlynn. [ONLINE] Available at: https://www.psychologytoday.com/gb/blog/urban-survival/201505/5-ways-stress-hurts-your-body-and-what-do-about-it. [Accessed 4 June 2019].
29 - rustydavisyogabreathwork.com. 2019. Rusty Davis - Yoga and Breathwork Awaken the seed of Transformation. [ONLINE] Available at: http://www.rustydavisyogabreathwork.com/blog/the-body-tells-a-story-and-never-lies-are-you-listening-where-do-you-store-emotions-and-how-to-let-go/. [Accessed 2 May 2019].
29 - suzanneheyn.com. 2019. http://suzanneheyn.com/the-body-stores-emotions/. [ONLINE] Available at: http://suzanneheyn.com/the-body-stores-emotions/. [Accessed 2 May 2019].
30 - Belluz. 2015. Julia. [ONLINE] Available at: <a href="https://www.vox.com/2015/7/22/9012075/yoga-health-benefits-exercise-science">https://www.vox.com/2015/7/22/9012075/yoga-health-benefits-exercise-science</a>. [Accessed 1 May 2019]

Meditation Chapter

1, 2 - Iyengar, B., 2018. Light on Life: The Journey to Wholeness, Inner Peace and Ultimate Freedom. 2nd ed. U.K: Rodale; Reprints edition (2 May 2008) Google Play Online Version.
3 - Aurelius, M., Hammond, M., & Clay, D. (2014). Meditations. London: Penguin Classics.
4 - Abhijit Naskar (2016) What is Mind?, 1st ed., CreateSpace Independent Publishing Platform; 1 edition (6 July 2016).
5 - Herbert Benson (2000) The Relaxation Response, 2nd edn. U.S: Avon Books; Revised edition edition (Feb. 2000).
6,12,13 - Sharon Begley (2009) The Plastic Mind, 1st edn., UK: Constable (26 Feb. 2009).
7 - Hippocrates,1983. Hippocratic Writings (Classics). 2nd ed UK, Penguin Classics; New Ed edition (24 Nov. 1983).
8 - David Mitchell (2014) Cloud Atlas, 1st edn., UK: Sceptre.

9 - Elizabeth Wurtzel (1996) Prozac Nation: Young and Depressed in America - A Memoir, 1st edn., US: Quartet Books.

10 - Russell C. Smith and Michael Foster (Aug 18, 2014) Why We've Got to Have Instant Gratification, Available at: https://www.psychologytoday.com/us/blog/reinvent-yourself/201408/why-we-ve-got-have-instant-gratification (Accessed: 2nd September 2018).

11 - Arthur Dobrin D.S.W. (Jan 25, 2013) Happiness is How You Are, Not How You Feel, Available at: https://www.psychologytoday.com/gb/blog/am-i-right/201301/happiness-is-how-you-are-not-how-you-feel (Accessed: 23 Jan 2019).

14 - Kurt Vonnegut (2008) Cat's Cradle, 1st edn., UK: Penguin Classics.

15 - Friedrich Nietzsche (1990) Twilight of the Idols and The Anti-Christ, 1st edn., UK: Penguin Classics.

16 - Swami Vivekananda (1947) Complete Works of Swami Vivekananda, Complete set in 8 volumes, 3rd edn., India: Advaita Ashram.

17 - Indu Muralidharan (2015) The Reengineers, 1st edn., India: HarperCollins.

18 - Harry Styles (2015) The Dhammapada (Penguin Little Black Classics), 1st edn., UK: Penguin Classics.

19 - Nyogen Senzaki; Paul Reps (1825) Zen Flesh, Zen Bones: A Collection of Zen and Pre-Zen Writings by Nyogen Senzaki , 1st edn., UK: Penguin.

20,21 - Gibran, K., 2019. Prophet Wisehouse Classics Edition. Sweden. 1st ed. Wisehouse Classics (20 Sept. 2017)

22 - Iyengar, B., 2018. Light on Life: The Journey to Wholeness, Inner Peace and Ultimate Freedom. 2nd ed. U.K: Rodale; Reprints edition (2 May 2008) Google Play Online Version.

23 - Vasudev, S., 2016. Inner Engineering: A Yogi's Guide to Joy. 1st ed. India:  -Random House Inc; 1 edition (20 Sept. 2016).

25 - Sadhguru (Unknown) How to Meditate, Available at: https://isha.sadhguru.org/yoga/meditations/how-to-meditate/ (Accessed: 24 Jan 2019).

26 - Jami, C., 2016. Healology. 1st ed. UK: CreateSpace Independent Publishing Platform.


Chapter - Kali

1 - C. G. Jung (1980) Psychology and Alchemy (Collected Works of C.G. Jung), 2nd edn., UK: Routledge.   2 - Theguardiancom. 2018. The Guardian. [Online]. [11 March 2019]. Available from:   https://www.theguardian.com/global-development/2018/jun/28/poll-ranks-india-most-dangerous-country-for-women

3 - By Joe Coscarelli (June 8, 2015) Art of the Rolling Stones: Behind That Zipper and That Tongue, Available at: https://www.nytimes.com
/2015/06/08/arts/music/art-of-the-rolling-stones-behind-that-zipper-and-that-tongue.html?_r=0 (Accessed: 3 March 2018).


Chapter - Reflection

1 - M. Sapolsky, R., 2004. Why Zebras Don't Get Ulcers -Revised Edition. 2nd ed. New York: St Martin's Press.

2 - Burns, D., 2005. Feeling Good: The New Mood Therapy. 2nd ed. London: Harper.

3 - Chuang Tzu, Martin Palmer, Elizabeth Breuilly, 2017. The Book of Chuang Tzu. 1st ed. United Kingdom: Penguin Classics; 1 edition (30 Nov. 2006) pages 309-310

Printed in Great Britain
by Amazon